INTESTINAL ISCHEMIA

edited by

MARC COOPERMAN, M.D.
Associate Professor of Surgery
The Ohio State University College of Medicine
Columbus, Ohio

FUTURA PUBLISHING COMPANY
Mount Kisco, New York
1983

Published by
Futura Publishing Company, Inc.
295 Main Street
Mount Kisco, New York 10549

LCCN: 83-80584
ISBN: 0-87993-197-3

Dedication

To my wife, Jo.

Acknowledgment

The editor wishes to thank Mrs. Helene Ayres without whose assistance the completion of this book would not have been possible.

Contributors

From
The Ohio State University College of Medicine
Columbus, Ohio

Wynn Wygal Adam, M.D.
Assistant Professor of Radiology

Eric D. Anderson, M.D.
Clinical Instructor in Surgery

Mary Pat Borgess, M.D.
Assistant Professor of Radiology

James H. Caldwell, M.D.
Professor of Medicine

Kathryn P. Clausen, M.D.
Associate Professor of Pathology

Marc Cooperman, M.D.
Associate Professor of Surgery

E. Christopher Ellison, M.D.
Clinical Instructor in Surgery

William E. Evans, M.D.
Clinical Professor of Surgery

Peter J. Fabri, M.D.
Assistant Professor of Surgery

John J. Ferrara, M.D.
Clinical Instructor in Surgery

Warren L. Garner, M.D.
Clinical Instructor in Surgery

Denis R. King, M.D.
Assistant Professor of Pediatric Surgery

Joel G. Lucas, M.D.
Assistant Professor of Pathology

Michael J. Luzar, M.D.
Assistant Professor of Medicine

Hagop S. Mekhjian, M.D.
Professor of Medicine

William L. Smead, M.D.
Assistant Professor of Surgery

John M. Stang, M.D.
Assistant Professor of Medicine

Patrick S. Vaccaro, M.D.
Assistant Professor of Surgery

Foreword

In an aging population, circulatory disorders clearly can be expected to become increasingly common. No disorders of inadequate blood flow have eluded detection and treatment as subtly as ischemic conditions of the digestive tract. To the average physician, acute intestinal ischemia portends a uniformly fatal outcome. The diagnosis is obscure and often made long after effective treatment might have been possible. No single laboratory test or combination of diagnostic maneuvers has proved to be sufficiently accurate to be wholly reliable. Greater uncertainty confounds the recognition of chronic intestinal ischemia. Even at the operating table where direct inspection is possible, recognition of impaired bowel may be equivocal.

Spurred by an early interest in intraoperative recognition of ischemic bowel, Dr. Cooperman has assembled a "state of the art" series of essays on the multifaceted problem of ischemia of the intestinal tract. In twenty carefully written chapters, subjects include the anatomy, pathophysiology, and pathology of ischemic bowel disease; laboratory diagnosis and radiographic manifestations; and the preparation and surgical management of patients. These form the keystone for informative chapters on specific, even esoteric manifestations of intestinal ischemia. Various current modes of evaluating the viability of the bowel are discussed and evaluated, with special attention paid to proposed techniques that may yet prove to be useful improvements. Frustration with the specificity of current techniques may provide the stimulus for continued efforts to improve diagnostic precision.

This book is, at present, a benchmark in the understanding of ischemic disease of the bowel, and will serve as a useful reference for those faced with treating the problem.

—Larry C. Carey, M.D.
Robert M. Zollinger Professor and Chairman
The Ohio State University College of Medicine
Columbus, Ohio

Preface

Despite advances in diagnostic techniques, operative management, and postoperative care, ischemic disease of the intestine continues to be associated with high morbidity and mortality. The care of the patient with intestinal ischemia remains one of the most formidable challenges facing the internist or surgeon caring for patients with gastrointestinal disease. The purpose of this book is to present the current state of knowledge concerning ischemic disease of the intestine. It is hoped that it will be a useful reference text for practicing physicians as well as for students and those in training.

Prompt diagnosis and effective care of patients with ischemic bowel disease require a knowledge of the relevant anatomy, pathophysiology, and pathology. These topics have been covered in early chapters and are intended to serve as a useful review for the clinician. Diagnosis often depends on keen clinical suspicion, with the laboratory and the radiologist providing suggestive or confirmatory evidence of ischemic bowel disease. The uses as well as the limitations of current laboratory and radiologic procedures are reviewed in chapters on these subjects. A separate chapter on the preoperative preparation is also included, as these patients must be rapidly and adequately resuscitated prior to operation.

The accurate intraoperative assessment of intestinal viability has been a major problem for the surgeon, as clinical judgment must be subjective. Now, the use of Doppler ultrasound or fluorescein dye provides objective evidence of bowel viability, and both are superior to clinical assessment alone. The research background as well as the clinical uses of these techniques are described in a chapter devoted to this problem.

The remainder of the book is devoted to the various clinical entities that comprise the spectrum of ischemic bowel disease. Ischemia may involve any part of the gastrointestinal system and may arise from a variety of causes ranging from emboli to autoimmune disorders. Some forms of intestinal ischemia, such as strangulated hernia, are common, while others are quite rare. It is the purpose of this book to be comprehensive, yet to describe the scope of ischemic bowel disease in sufficient depth to be of help to both the student and the practicing clinician.

As more people grow older, ischemic disease of the intestinal tract will become more common. It will become increasingly important to be aware of this group of diseases, to recognize them early, and to treat them effectively. It is hoped that this volume will help to meet those needs.

—**Marc Cooperman,** M.D.
Associate Professor of Surgery
The Ohio State University College of Medicine
Columbus, Ohio

Contents

1

Vascular Anatomy of the Intestinal Tract

Warren L. Garner, M.D.

The vascular supply to the intestinal tract consists of three main vessels, the celiac axis, and the superior and inferior mesenteric arteries. There are widespread interconnections between their branches as well as important connections to the vessels of the thorax and the iliac systems. The venous drainage tends to follow the organization of the arterial system, except that the major veins join to form the portal vein which enters the liver, rather than emptying directly into the inferior vena cava.

Celiac Axis

The celiac axis (Figure 1) is the arterial supply to the abdominal structures derived from the foregut. It arises as a short, thick trunk just distal to the aortic hiatus of the diaphragm, where it is embedded in the celiac ganglion and plexus. After 1–3 cm, it divides into its three branches, the left gastric, the common hepatic, and the splenic. These three arise as independent vessels about 90% of the time.

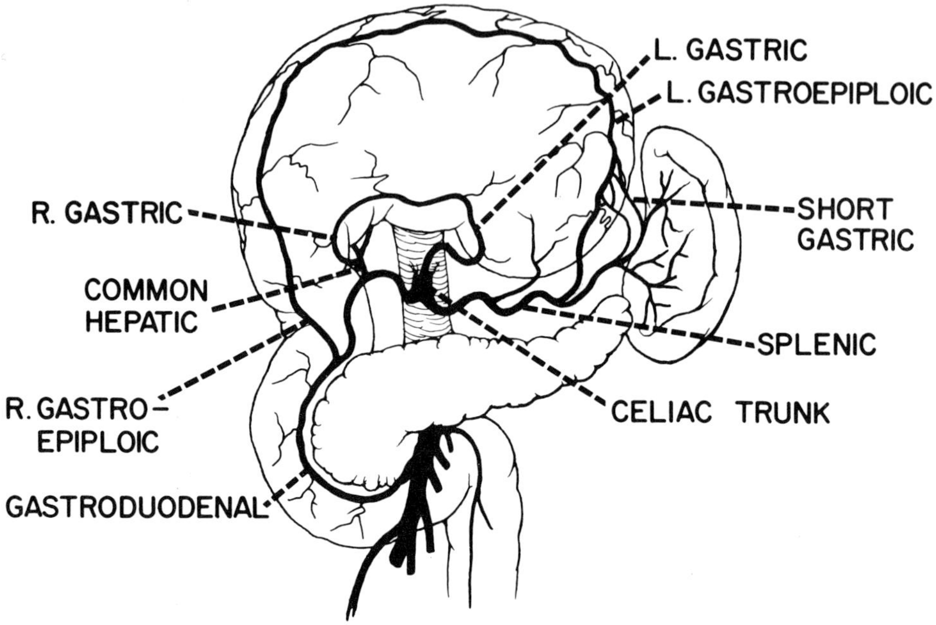

Figure 1. Celiac axis with major arterial tributaries.

A gastrosplenic trunk occurs in approximately 5% of individuals, with the hepatic artery derived directly from the aorta or from the superior mesenteric artery. A hepatosplenic trunk is found in 3–4%, with the left gastric arising from the aorta, hepatic, or splenic arteries. In 1–2% of people, a hepatogastric trunk exists, with the splenic artery derived from the aorta or the superior mesenteric artery. Rare anomalies exist, including a combined celiac trunk and superior mesenteric artery.

The left gastric is most commonly the first branch of the celiac trunk, arising from its midportion. In other cases (25%) it is a terminal branch with the splenic and hepatic arteries. Its course is upward and to the left in the gastropancreatic fold. It bifurcates into two main branches, a ventral branch distributed to the anterior surface of the stomach, and a dorsal branch which gives branches to the posterior stomach, where it usually anastomoses with the right gastric artery. An esophageal branch arises before this bifurcation and is distributed to the cardia and esophagus.

An aberrant left hepatic artery is frequent (23%), arising from the left gastric artery just proximal to its bifurcation. About half the time, this vessel replaces completely the left hepatic branch of the common hepatic. When present, it runs cephalad about 5–6 cm and then crosses the caudate lobe to enter the liver substance at the fissure for the ligamentum venosum.

The common hepatic arises from the celiac trunk with the splenic artery but is usually slightly smaller. It runs along the upper border of the pancreas to the pylorus or first part of the duodenum. At this point, halfway between the origin and bifurcation of the hepatic artery, the gastroduodenal artery branches downward, and the main hepatic artery turns upward and continues in the edge of the lesser omentum to the liver, where it divides into left and right branches. The right gastric arises at varied locations along the hepatic artery.

The gastroduodenal descends behind the duodenum, giving off several duodenal branches. After reaching the pancreas, it divides into right gastroepiploic and anterior-superior pancreaticoduodenal arteries. The right gastroepiploic is usually larger and passes from right to left along the greater curvature of the stomach. It gives off branches to the pylorus, stomach, and greater omentum. It terminates by anastomosing with the left gastroepiploic artery. The superior pancreaticoduodenal passes between the pancreas and the descending portion of the duodenum. At varying locations, it anastomoses with the inferior pancreaticoduodenal arteries to form the anterior pancreatic arcade.

The common hepatic branches into its subdivisions at varying distances from the liver hilum. The cystic artery arises from the right hepatic in most cases.

The splenic artery, the largest branch of the celiac,

passes to the left along the upper edge of the pancreas. It is usually tortuous and varies in length by as much as 400%. There are numerous pancreatic branches supplying the body and tail of the gland. The left gastroepiploic artery arises from either the distal splenic artery or one of its terminal branches. It passes through the greater omentum and then passes from left to right along the greater curvature of the stomach. There are branches to both the stomach and the greater omentum. Several (5–7) small short gastric arteries arise from the terminal splenic artery and its end branches. These pass to the greater curvature of the stomach and anastomose with branches of the left gastric and left gastroepiploic. The splenic artery terminates by dividing into terminal branches 3–4 cm from the splenic hilum. These end vessels are variable in exact origin and distribution; superior and inferior hilar vessels occur and may be derived from the left gastroepiploic. These extensive interconnections make ischemic disease infrequent in the distribution of the celiac axis.

Superior Mesenteric Artery

The superior mesenteric artery (Figure 2) is the artery of the midgut. It supplies the distal duodenum, jejunum, ileum, cecum, ascending colon, and about half of the transverse colon. It arises from the anterior aorta about 1¼ cm distal to the celiac artery. Passing just beneath the splenic vein and the body of the pancreas, it descends in front of the uncinate process and the third part of the duodenum into the base of the mesentery. Its first branch, the inferior pancreaticoduodenal artery, courses to the right between the duodenum and the head of the pancreas, then ascends to anastomose with the superior pancreaticoduodenal artery. It supplies the head of the pancreas and the descending and inferior duodenum.

The blood supply to the small bowel is derived from a

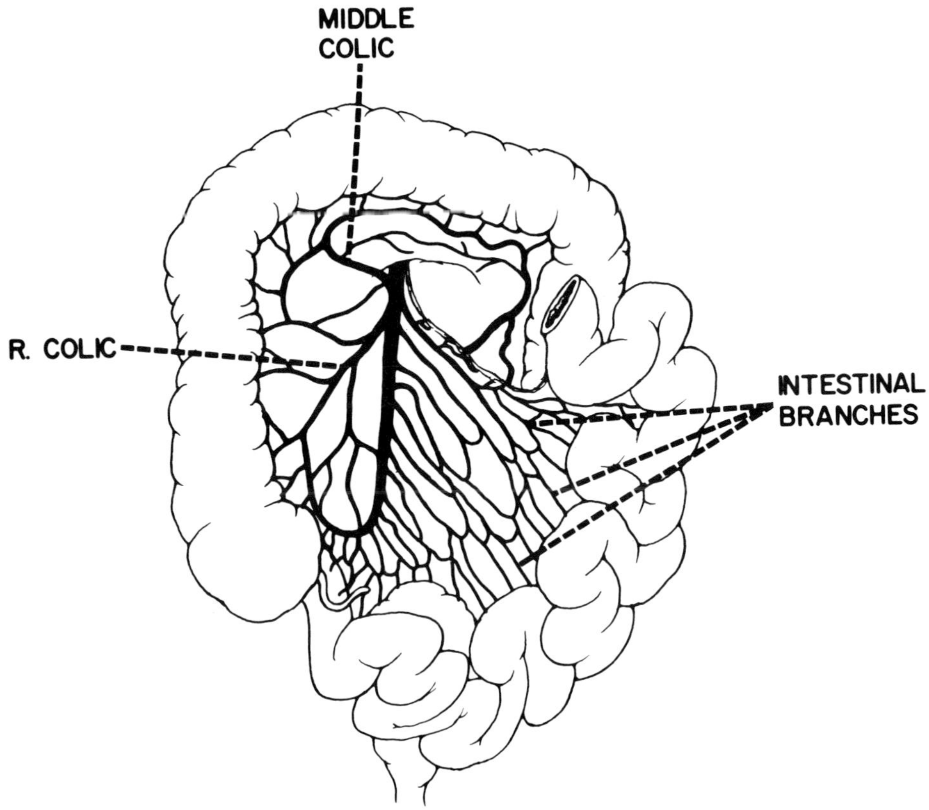

Figure 2. Superior mesenteric artery with its major branches.

variable number of arteries, usually 12–15, which arise from the left side of the superior mesenteric artery as it proceeds downward. These intestinal arteries branch into a series of arcades, connecting to the branch above and below. The branching and arch formation continue through four or five series of arches, becoming continually smaller as the vessels approach the intestine. Small vessels arise from the terminal arches that encircle the small bowel and provide branches to the lymph nodes and mesentery.

The right colic arises at the midpoint of the superior mesenteric artery. It passes right, ventral to the ureter and gonadal vessels, toward the middle of the ascending colon. It then divides, sending branches down to anastomose with the ileocolic and up to anastomose with the middle colic. The branches form arcades which supply the ascending colon.

The middle colic artery arises proximal to the previous vessels just distal to the pancreas. It proceeds upwards between the layers of the transverse mesocolon and divides into right and left branches. A series of arches is again formed, which are about 2 cm below the transverse colon. Those branches anastomose with the right colic on the right and the left colic on the left.

Inferior Mesenteric Artery

The inferior mesenteric artery (Figure 3) supplies structures derived from the embryonic hindgut. It arises from the aorta 3–4 cm above the bifurcation, passes ventrally and slightly to the left, then crosses back across the left common iliac artery. After crossing the inlet of the pelvis, it becomes the superior rectal artery. The left colic artery arises to the left 2–3 cm below the origin of the inferior mesenteric. After a varying length, it branches into superior and inferior branches. The superior branch anastomoses with the middle colic at the left transverse colon; this part of the arterial system is referred to as the "marginal artery of Drummond." The inferior branch supplies the lower descending colon and anastomoses to the sigmoid arcades. The sigmoid arteries, two or three in number, run downward and to the left to supply the descending colon and sigmoid colon by a series of interconnected arcades. The superior rectal artery is the continuation of the inferior mesenteric. It descends into the pelvis between layers of the sigmoid mesocolon. It divides into anterior and posterior branches, which descend on either side of the rectum.

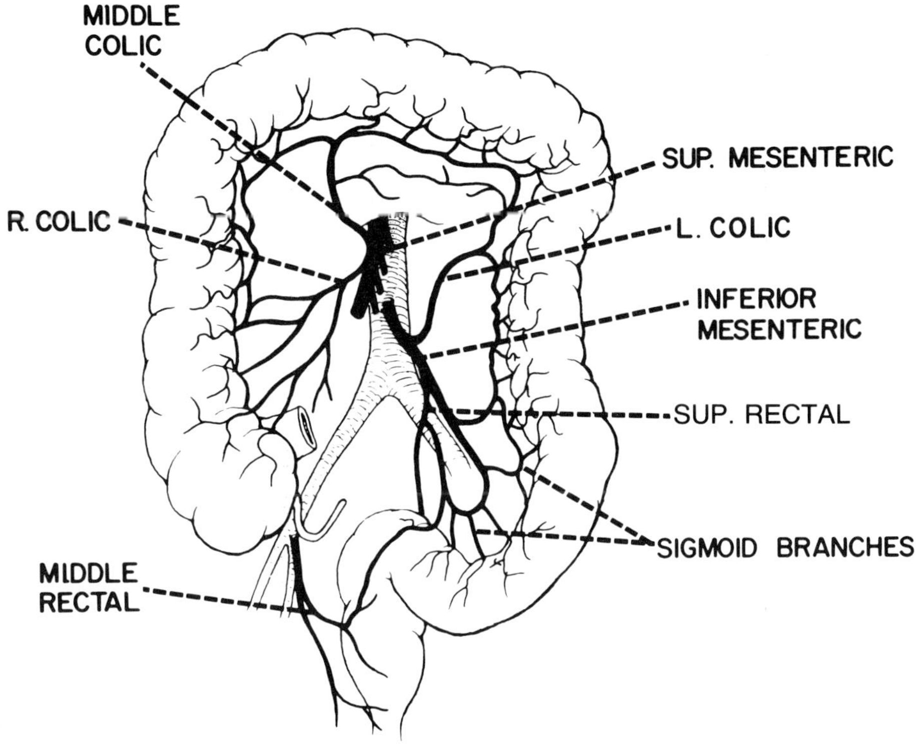

Figure 3. Inferior mesenteric artery with its major branches.

These form a series of loops around the lower rectum and anastomose with the middle rectal branch of the internal iliac and with the inferior rectal branch of the inferior pudendal.

Collateral Circulation

The preceding anatomic descriptions show the extensive collateralization between the major intestinal arteries and their branches. The connection between the superior and inferior mesenteries, the marginal artery, is sufficient to supply either system, should one of these vessels become occluded. It must be noted, however, that this collateral is not constant, with flow that is minimal or absent in some individuals. This makes the splenic flexure an area with intrinsically tenuous blood supply, a fact that correlates with the frequency of ischemic colitis at this location. This is sometimes called Griffin's point. The extensive collaterals around the pancreas via the superior and inferior pancreatic duodenals connect the celiac and superior mesenteric arteries.

Collateral circulation from above is carried on by anastomoses between descending branches of the esophageal arteries and ascending branches of the left gastric and inferior phrenic arteries. Collateralization from below is maintained by connection between the inferior mesenteric by the superior rectal artery and either the internal iliac via the middle rectal artery or the internal pudendal via the inferior rectal. This region, Sudeck's point, is important in patients who have had interruption of the inferior mesenteric artery as in aortic aneurysm surgery as an alternative site of ischemia.

Venous Drainage

The venous drainage of the intestinal tract is via the portal system. The majority of veins in the abdominal cavity follow closely the anatomic pattern of corresponding arteries. Tributaries from the spleen, pancreas, and the greater curvature of the stomach join to form the splenic vein, which is also joined by the inferior mesenteric vein, which drains the left, transverse, descending, and sigmoid colon. The superior mesenteric vein drains the right transverse and ascending colon, cecum, small bowel, pancreas and duodenum. The confluence of the splenic and superior mesenteric veins forms the portal vein. Small branches from the pylorus, gallbladder, and lesser curvature via the coronary vein join the portal vein. The portal blood enters the liver where it is filtered through hepatic sinusoids and then drains into the inferior vena cava by way of the hepatic veins.

There are several important anastomoses between the portal and systemic venous systems. The inferior mesenteric drains directly into the inferior vena cava by way of the superior rectal vein. The gastric veins anastomose to the esophageal veins which drain into the azygous system connecting to the superior vena cava. There are small veins in the falciform and round ligaments which drain into the superior and inferior epigastric via subcutaneous vessels around the umbilicus. Retroperitoneal veins drain the posterior surface of nonperitonealized organs such as the duodenum, pancreas, and ascending and descending colon.

References

1. Gardner E, Gray DJ, O'Rahilly R: Anatomy. *A Regional Study of Human Structure.* 4th ed, WB Saunders Co, Philadelphia, 1975.
2. Gray H, Goss CM: *Anatomy of the Human Body.* 2nd ed, Lea & Febiger, Philadelphia, 1973.

2

Pathophysiology of Ischemic Bowel Disease

Hagop S. Mekhjian, M.D.

One of the least understood areas in medicine is the pathophysiology of ischemic bowel disease. The reasons for this are the difficulty of doing studies in humans and the significant differences that exist among various species in response to ischemia. Occlusion of a major mesenteric vessel or its branches has been used as an experimental animal model for the study of the pathophysiology of intestinal ischemia in the laboratory. Although the relevance of the observations made in these experiments remains in doubt, a knowledge of the pathophysiologic phenomena associated with intestinal ischemia is useful for the rational approach to the treatment of patients. A basic understanding of the mesenteric circulation and the mechanisms controlling intestinal blood flow is essential for the understanding of the pathophysiology of ischemic bowel disease.

The Mesenteric Circulation[1–2]

The blood supply of the gastrointestinal tract is provided by three major vessels. The celiac axis originates at the level of the first lumbar vertebra at almost a 90° angle from the aorta. Its branches supply blood primarily to the liver, the stomach, and the duodenum, where collateral communications with branches of the superior mesenteric artery occur. The superior mesenteric artery originates just distal to the celiac axis at a relatively acute angle, and because of its large size and angle of origin is in direct line of blood flow from the aorta. The superior mesenteric artery is the most important source of blood supply to the gastrointestinal tract. The colic and ileocolic branches supply blood to the right and transverse colon respectively. The smaller intestinal branches supply blood to the jejunum and ileum. Prior to entering the intestinal wall, the small intestinal branches form a series of arcades, thus creating a rich network of collaterals in the mesentery of the small intestine. The arteriae rectae penetrating the bowel wall, however, are end arteries that enter the intestinal wall tangentially. Thus, a selective occlusion of one of these end arteries results in focal ischemia and necrosis. The network of arcades is much less developed in the colonic vessels. Instead, the marginal artery runs parallel the length of the colon and provides branches to the colon as well as collaterals to the branches of the inferior mesenteric artery in the region of the splenic flexure. Occasionally, the marginal artery may be absent, however, making the splenic flexure more vulnerable to ischemic diseases of the colon.

The inferior mesenteric artery originates at the level of the third lumbar vertebra and supplies blood to the rest of the colon. Collaterals exist between the branches of the marginal artery of the meandering artery which communicates directly with the middle colic artery. A rich network of collaterals also exists at the rectosigmoid junction between the branches of the mesenteric and iliac arteries.

In the event of slow and progressive occlusion of the mesenteric vessels, it is possible for the entire gastrointestinal tract to be supplied by one artery without causing ischemia. The most vulnerable areas for segmental ischemia and necrosis are the splenic flexure, the rectosigmoid junction, and in the case of small vessel disease, the arteriae rectae. Reduced blood flow in these areas more readily produces segmental necrosis or infarction.

Intestinal Microcirculation

The arteriae rectae penetrate the muscular layer of the intestine and form a rich network of collaterals in the submucosa. A parallel venous plexus also exists in the submucosa, but there is no convincing evidence in man that functionally significant arteriovenous communications are present in the small intestine.[3] Straight arterioles originate from this submucosal plexus and enter the individual villi. In the villus, the main arteriole takes a hairpin turn, forming the distributing arteriole. The branches of the distributing arterioles arborize along the villus to a rich capillary network which eventually communicates with the venous system.

The hairpin arrangement of the central arteriole creates a situation whereby it is in close proximity to the venules in which blood is flowing in the opposite direction.[4,5] There is ample evidence for the presence of a countercurrent exchange mechanism between the arteriole and the vein, similar to the absorptive mechanism in the nephron.[0,7] This mechanism also contributes to the intestinal absorption of sodium and water. Thus, alterations of blood flow in the villus alters the efficiency of absorption.[8] Perhaps more important to the pathophysiology of intestinal ischemia is the fact that oxygen can diffuse from the arteriole to the vein by the countercurrent exchange mechanism at the base of the villus. During slow or reduced blood flow this mechanism becomes even more efficient, resulting in the "shunting" of oxygen from the villous tip and producing ischemic injury.[9,10]

Regulation of Intestinal Blood Flow

The blood flow through the gastrointestinal tract is approximately 1500–1800 ml/min, or 25 ml/kg/min. The earliest experimental technique for the measurement of intestinal blood flow was the simple transection of the portal vein and measurement of the drained blood.[11] Newer and more sophisticated techniques using electromagnetic flow meters, microsphere distribution, indicator dilution curves, and washout or absorption of highly diffusible gases have given remarkably similar results for total intestinal blood flow in the experimental animal.[8] Studies using the distribution and disappearance of the lipophilic gases such as ^{85}Kr have provided valuable information about the distribution of blood in the intestinal wall.[12,13] From these studies, it has become apparent that there are marked differences in the vascularity of the different layers of the intestinal wall.[14–16] For example, the mucosa receives about three times more blood than the muscularis. The region of the submucosa and the crypts is also two times more vascular than the full intestinal wall.

The determinants of blood flow to the intestine comprise the cardiac output, arterial blood pressure, patency of the major blood vessels, and the local regulatory mechanisms in the intestinal wall.[17] The intestinal blood flow remains remarkably constant despite wide fluctuations in arterial and venous pressure, but dramatic decreases in blood flow occur during physical exercise, and increases in blood flow occur after a meal.[14,18,19]

The autoregulation of intestinal blood flow is controlled by two functionally and anatomically distinct areas. The first and the more important of these is the intestinal arteriole.[20] Although the mechanisms involved in the autoregulation of blood flow by the arteriole are controversial, it is clear that the arteriole is capable of responding to a variety of hormonal, chemical, and neural stimuli (Table I) producing dramatic alterations or redistribution of blood

Table I
Agents Affecting Splanchnic Circulation

Vasodilators	*Vasoconstrictors*
Urotensin I	Digitalis Glycosides
Urokinase	Propranolol
Phenoxybenzamine	Vasopressin
Methyl Prednisolone	PGF 2α
Dopamine	VIP
PGE1	Adrenaline
Perhexiline	Noradrenaline
Papaverine	Angiotensin II
Acetylcholine	Calcium
Histamine	Hyperkalemia
Isoprenaline	
GI hormones—CCK Gastrin, Glucagon, Secretin	
5HT	
Magnesium	
Acetate, Pyruvate	

flow in the intestine. Some of these factors are operative during physiological phenomena as well as during intestinal ischemia. The second switching mechanism is the precapillary sphincter.[21] It controls the number and distribution of open capillaries. The capillaries themselves play little or no role in the regulation of blood flow. The tissue need for oxygen seems to be the primary factor controlling the precapillary sphincters. It should be pointed out that the autoregulatory mechanism fails following a severe fall in blood pressure or with distention of the bowel.[22,23] The intestinal vascular bed escapes autoregulation after continuous stimulation with vasopressors or catecholamines.[24] In summary, it can be said that the adequacy of the intestinal circulation is determined by the critical interaction of the anatomic state of the intestinal blood vessels, temporal events that alter flow in the major vessels, and the adequacy of the physiological phenomena that regulate the distribution of intestinal blood flow.

Causes of Intestinal Ischemia

The two major causes for intestinal ischemia are occlusive disease of the mesenteric vessels and nonocclusive causes resulting in reduced intestinal blood flow and ischemia.[8,25] The incidence of occlusive vessel disease as a cause of ischemic bowel disease has varied in different series. It has become increasingly clear that nonocclusive causes account for the majority of cases of ischemic bowel disease. In one series of extensive ischemic bowel disease, less than one-third of the patients had occlusive vessel disease.[26,28] Furthermore, occlusive vessel disease is not an uncommon postmortem finding in asymptomatic patients dying from unrelated causes. Progressive and slow atherosclerotic obstruction and thrombosis of one or two major mesenteric vessels rarely results in ischemia because of the rich collateral circulation between the branches of the major mesenteric vessels.

Ligation of a mesenteric artery or one of its branches has been used as the experimental model for the study of intestinal ischemia. In clinical practice, acute occlusion of a major mesenteric artery is an infrequent but important cause of intestinal ischemia because it is a potentially curable condition.[29,30] Acute obstruction of a mesenteric artery can be the result of embolic disease, dissection from an aortic aneurysm, or vascular trauma.[31–33] The superior mesenteric artery is the most frequently involved vessel in embolic disease because of its large size and the acute angle of origin from the aorta, putting it in the direct line of blood flow from the aorta.

Occlusive disease of the intestines can also be a manifestation of other systemic collagen vascular diseases.

Small or medium sized vessels can be involved in periarteritis nodosa, systemic lupus erythematosus, Henoch-Schönlein purpura, and rheumatoid arteritis. In these diseases the vasa recta or the arterioles are most frequently involved, causing segmental infarction or focal necrosis and ulceration. Intestinal ischemia in these diseases is usually suspected on the basis of the clinical findings and the known association of vasculitis with the underlying collagen vascular diseases. A more detailed discussion of the association of collagen vascular diseases and intestinal ischemia can be found in Chapters 19 and 20.

Venous occlusive disease is the least common cause of intestinal ischemia. It is usually associated with hyperviscosity and hypercoagulation syndromes. It has also been reported in association with liver cirrhosis, abdominal neoplasms, sepsis, and as a complication of the intake of oral contraceptives.

The nonocclusive causes account for the majority of cases of intestinal ischemia or infarction. The common denominator in all of these causes is a fall in cardiac output and vasoconstriction of the mesenteric vessels.[34–37] Undoubtedly, a patient with otherwise clinically insignificant mesenteric arterial obstruction is more likely to develop intestinal ischemia following a hypotensive episode. In spite of this, the fact that intestinal ischemia and infarction can occur in the absence of obstructive lesions of the mesenteric vessels has been established beyond doubt. The factors incriminated in nonocclusive intestinal ischemia are listed in Tables I and II. Digitalis glycosides have vasoconstrictive effects on the mesenteric circulation;[38–44] used in a patient with congestive heart failure, they have a beneficial effect on intestinal circulation by improving cardiac output. The injudicious use of digitalis glycosides, however, in patients with atherosclerosis can precipitate intestinal ischemia. The role of vasoactive peptides in the pathophysiologic events associated with ischemia remains controversial.[45–48] It is difficult to determine with certainty whether com-

Table II

Etiology of Intestinal Ischemia

Occlusive Mesenteric Arterial Disease
Atherosclerosis
Embolic disease
Atrial fibrillation
Prosthetic heart valves
Rheumatic heart disease
Angiographic procedures
Mural thrombi
Dissecting aneurysms
Peripheral small vessel disease
Arteritis
Atherosclerosis
Clostridial infection
Intestinal obstruction
Vascular trauma
Venous Thrombosis
Hypercoagulation states
Oral contraceptives
Nonocclusive Ischemia
Heart failure
Shock
Vasoconstrictor drugs
Digitalis
Propanolol
Vasopressin

pounds such as vasoactive intestinal polypeptide (VIP) or prostaglandins have a causative role in ischemia or are simply released from the intestinal wall as a result of ischemic necrosis. Regardless of their exact role in ischemia, it is likely that vasoactive compounds are important in mediating some of the systemic effects of intestinal ischemia.

Effects of Intestinal Ischemia

Very rapid structural changes are observed following intestinal ischemia.[49–52] The earliest changes are the formation of subepithelial blebs followed by loss of surface epithelium. These are most severe at the tip of the villi, so that in mild or early ischemia the crypt cells are relatively spared. With more severe or prolonged ischemia, complete denudation of the villi and lamina propria occurs, followed by hemorrhage and ulceration. In this respect, the changes become indistinguishable from the sequelae of an infarct in other organs.

Important alterations in intestinal function accompany the structural changes of ischemia. Generally, these functional changes correlate well with the histologic changes. The earliest change is the loss of the active absorption of sugars, amino acids, and sodium.[53,54] The latter is accompanied by a lowering of the activity of sodium potassium-activated ATPase in the basolateral membrane of the enterocyte.[55] In addition to the loss of absorptive function, there is net secretion of water and electrolytes.[53–56] The degree and extent of this secretion depends on the degree of damage and can be modified by the intraluminal infusion of glucose and oxygen.[57,58] The explanation for the net intestinal secretion is a matter of debate, but recent studies seem to provide the best answer.[59] It is postulated that following ischemia and loss of the mature enterocytes located at the tip of the villi, the absorptive function of the intestine is lost, but the secretory function of the crypt cells is maintained. This is analogous to the conditions that exist in nontropical sprue, where because of the villous atrophy, absorptive function is abolished and a secretory state is present in the intestine. The secretory theory is supported by recent studies in which undirectional fluxes were measured in the ischemic ileum of the dog.[60] In these studies, the lumen-to-blood movement of sodium was markedly diminished, whereas the blood-to-lumen flux of sodium was unchanged. The latter results in net secretion of fluid into the intestinal lumen. The accumulation of fluid in the intestinal lumen creates a vicious cycle by producing intestinal distension which further aggravates the ischemia. In addition to distention, the loss of fluid into the intestinal lumen aggravates also the hemodynamic disturbances accompanying the intestinal ischemia. While the exact mechanism for this secretion is not known, it is tempting to speculate that it might be mediated by potent secretagogues such as prostaglandins and vasoactive intestinal peptide, both of which are associated with intestinal ischemia.[46–48]

The intestine possesses tremendous regenerative activity so that after a brief attack of ischemia, histologic and functional recovery is fairly rapid. In the dog, after a brief and reversible ischemia of one hour, histological recovery occurs in 24 hours. Similar results are obtained in other experimental animals. On the basis of experiments performed in several other animal models, it can be concluded that full intestinal functional recovery occurs in seven days,[55] provided surgical revascularization of the intestine has been performed promptly. It may take longer for the secretory process to return to normal.

The factors involved in the progression of reversible ischemic changes to irreversible intestinal ischemia are poorly understood. Undoubtedly, the duration of the ischemic episode is of utmost importance. Local factors such as the production of lactates, release of lysosomal hydrolases, presence of proteolytic enzymes, as well as body temperature and hemoglobin concentration, all play a role in determining the severity of the ischemic injury.[60–62] Once ischemia is established, three major pathophysiological events follow. (See Table III.) These are the massive losses of fluid, the release of vasoactive substances, and the bacterial invasion of the bowel wall, with the resultant endotoxemia and septicemia.[63,64]

Table III

Sequelae of Intestinal Ischemia

- Exudation of Plasma
  - Contraction of blood volume
  - Hypoxia
  - Acidosis
- Release of Vasoactive Substances
  - Myocardial depressant factor—low cardiac output
  - Histamine
  - VIP
- Bacterial Invasion
  - Endotoxin release
  - Septicemia

One major factor in the fluid loss is the intestinal secretion of fluids which has already been mentioned. Additional factors include the exudation of fluid into the bowel wall and the peritoneal cavity, resulting in further compromise of the intestinal circulation.

Several compounds have been implicated in the pathogenesis of the circulatory collapse associated with intestinal ischemia. (See Table I.) Of these, histamine seems to be one of the more important. Following a brief episode of ischemia, there is a decrease in intestinal activity of diamine oxidase, an enzyme important in the breakdown of histamine.[65,66] This results in high levels of histamine in portal blood and plasma with resultant hypotension. The survival of experimental animals with ischemia can be improved by the administration of H_2 receptor antagonists,[67] and mortality is increased by the administration of agents that inhibit diamine oxidase activity.[67,68] These observations lend further support to the theory that histamine is important in the pathogenesis of hypotension associated with intestinal ischemia.

Another peptide, vasoactive intestinal peptide (VIP), is elevated in the venous blood following the occlusion of the mesenteric artery.[45–47] Since VIP has potent vasodilator, hypotensive, and secretory properties, it would only tend to aggravate the circulatory disturbances associated with ischemic bowel disease. The myocardial depressor factor is another peptide that is presumably absorbed from the ischemic intestine leading to a decrease in cardiac output and a fall in coronary artery blood flow.[60,69]

Summary and Conclusions

The pathophysiology of intestinal ischemia is poorly understood because of the inadequacy of animal models and the difficulties associated in extrapolating animal data to human beings. It is clear that the intestinal tract is a very vascular organ with a rich network of collaterals between the major vessels. The intestinal blood flow remains relatively constant by a process of autoregulation under a wide range of variations in blood pressure and flow. The main components of the autoregulatory mechanism are the intestinal arteriole and, to a lesser extent, the precapillary sphincter. The central arteriole forms a hairpin arrangement in the villus, creating a mechanism for countercurrent exchange of oxygen and solutes. This arrangement also makes the villous tip most vulnerable to the effects of ischemia.

Intestinal ischemia can result from occlusive and nonocclusive causes for the reduction of intestinal blood flow. The nonocclusive causes account for the majority of cases of intestinal ischemia.

Acute intestinal ischemia results in distinct alterations in the histology and function of the intestine. The final outcome is determined by the severity and duration of ischemia. The major pathophysiological changes that account for the clinical picture include the massive losses of fluid, the absorption of vasoactive compounds, and the endotoxemia and septicemia with resultant fall in cardiac output and ultimate circulatory collapse.

References

1. Tepperman BL, Jacobson ED: Mesenteric circulation. In *Physiology of the Gastrointestinal Tract.* Johnson LR (Ed), Raven Press, New York 1981.
2. Baum S: Normal anatomy and collateral pathways of the mesenteric circulation. In *Vascular Disorders of the Intestine.* Boley SJ (Ed), Appleton Century Crofts, New York 1971.
3. Boulter PS, Parks AG: Submucosal vascular patterns of the alimentary tract and their significance. *Br J Surg* 47:546, 1960.
4. Lundgren O: Studies on blood flow distribution and countercurrent exchange in the small intestine. *Acta Physiol Scand (Suppl)* 303:1, 1967.
5. Lundgren O: The circulation of the small bowel mucosa. *Gut* 15:1005, 1974.
6. Hallback DA, Hulten L, Jodal M, et al: Evidence for the existence of a countercurrent exchanger in the small intestine in man. *Gastroenterology* 74:683, 1978.
7. Bond JH, Levitt DG and Levitt MD: Quantitation of countercurrent exchange during passive absorption from the dog small intestine. *J Clin Invest* 59:308, 1977.
8. Lanciault G, Jacobson ED: The gastrointestinal circulation. *Gastroenterology* 71:851, 1976.
9. Bynum TE, Jacobson ED: Gastrointestinal mechanisms. In *Pathophysiology: Altered Regulatory Mechanisms in Disease.* Frohlich ED (Ed), JB Lippincott Co, Philadelphia 1972.
10. Kamp M, Lundgren O, Nilsson NJ: Extravascular shunting of oxygen in the small intestine of the cat. *Acta Physiol Scan* 72:396, 1968.
11. Burns GP, Schenk WG: Intestinal blood-flow in the conscious dog. *Surg Forum* 18:313, 1967.
12. Hulten L, Jodl M, Lldhagen J, et al: Blood flow in the small intestine of cat and man as analyzed by an inert gas washout technique. *Gastroenterology* 70:45, 1976.

13. Zierler KH: Equations for measuring blood flow by external monitoring of radioisotopes. *Circ Res* 16:309, 1965.
14. Bond JH, Prentiss RA, Levitt MD: The effects of feeding on blood flow to the stomach, small bowel and colon of the conscious dog. *J Lab Clin Med* 93:594, 1979.
15. Nyhof R, Sit SP, Gallavan R, et al: A mechanism for postprandial intestinal hyperemia in the dog. *The Physiologist* 21:85, 1978.
16. Norris HT, Sumner DS: Distribution of blood flow to the layers of the small bowel in experimental cholera. *Gastroenterology* 66:973, 1974.
17. Lundgren O, Svanik J: Mucosal hemodynamics in the small intestine of the cat during reduced perfusion pressure. *Acta Physiol Scand* 88:551, 1973.
18. Burns GP, Schenk WG: Effect of digestion and exercise on intestinal blood flow and cardiac output. *Arch Surg* 98:790, 1969.
19. Brandt JL, Castleman L, Ruskin HD, et al: The effect of oral protein and glucose feeding on splanchnic blood flow and oxygen utilization in normal and cirrhotic subjects. *J Clin Invest* 34:1017, 1955.
20. Johnson PC, Intaglietta M: Contributions of pressure and flow sensitivity to autoregulation in mesenteric arterioles. *Am J Physiol* 231:1686, 1976.
21. Johnson PC, Wayland H: Regulation of blood flow in single capillaries. *Am J Physiol* 212:1405, 1976.
22. Brobmann GF, Underwood LD, McCoy J, et al: Early regional vascular responses to hemorrhage and reinfusion in dogs. *Surg Gynecol Obstet* 131:409, 1970.
23. Ohman U: Blood flow and oxygen consumption in the feline small intestine and responses to artificial distension and intestinal obstruction. *Acta Chir Scand* 142:329, 1976.
24. Lautt WW, Graham SC: Effect of nerve stimulation of precapillary sphincters, oxygen extraction and hemodynamics in the intestine of cat. *Circ Res* 41:32, 1977.
25. Lanciault G, Fang WF, Jacobson ED, et al: Evaluation of potential agents for treatment of nonocclusive mesenteric ischemia in the dog. *Circ Shock* 3:239, 1976.
26. Williams CF, Anastasia LF, Hasiotis CA, et al: Experimental nonocclusive mesenteric ischemia. *Am J Surg* 115:82, 1968.

27. Ottinger LW: Nonocclusive mesenteric infarction. *Surg Clin North Am* 54:689–698, 1974.
28. Williams LF, Wittenberg J: Vascular insufficiency of the intestine. Separating fact from fad and fiction. *Viewprints Dig Dis* 5:1, 1973.
29. Wangenstein SL, Golden GL, Stapleton SL: Successful superior mesenteric artery embolectomy. *Am J Surg* 123:601, 1972.
30. MacKenzie RL, Provan JL: Recognition and management of embolism to the superior mesenteric artery. *Can Med Assoc J* 7:1207, 1970.
31. Singh RP, Shah RC, Lee ST: Acute mesenteric vascular occlusion: A review of thirty-two patients. *Surgery* 78:613, 1975.
32. Skinner DB, Zarius CK, Moossa AR: Mesenteric vascular disease. *Am J Surg* 128:835, 1974.
33. Boley SJ, Brandt SJ, Veith FJ: Ischemic disorders of the intestines. *Current Problems in Surgery* 15:1, 1978.
34. Ottinger LW: Nonocclusive mesenteric infarction. *Surg Clin North Am* 54:689, 1974.
35. Bynum TE, Jacobson ED: Nonocclusive intestinal ischemia. *Arch Int Med* 139:281, 1979.
36. Jordan PH, Boulafendis D, Guinn GA: Factors other than major vascular occlusion that contribute to intestinal infarction. *Ann Surg* 171:189, 1970.
37. Aldrete JS, Han SY, Laws HL, et al: Intestinal infarction complicating low cardiac output states. *Surg Gyncol Obstet* 144:371, 1977.
38. Levinsky RA, Lewis RM, Bynum TE, et al: Digoxin induced intestinal vasoconstriction. The effects of proximal arterial stenosis and glucagon administration. *Circulation* 52:130, 1975.
39. Pawlik W, Jacobson ED: Effects of digoxin on the mesenteric circulation. *Cardiovascular Res Center Bull* 12:80, 1974.
40. Vlano HB, Treat E, Chang ACK, et al: Splanchnic circulatory responses to ouabain in shock. *Surgery* 70:678, 1971.
41. Treat E, Vlano B, Jacobson ED: Effects of intraarterial ouabain on mesenteric and carotid hemodynamics. *J Pharmacol Exp Ther* 179:144, 1971.
42. Bynum TE, Jacobson ED: Shock intestinal, ischemia and digitalis. *Circ Shock* 2:235, 1975.

43. Shanbour LL, Jacobson ED, Brobmann GF, et al: Effects of ouabain on splanchnic hemodynamics in the rhesus monkey. *Am Heart J* 81:511, 1971.
44. Bynum TE, Hanley H, Cole JS: Effect of digitalis glycosides on splanchnic blood flow in man. *Clin Res* 21:509, 1973.
45. Bateson PG, Buchanan KD, Stewart DM, et al: The release of vasoactive intestinal peptide during altered mid-gut blood flow. *Br J Surg* 67:131, 1980.
46. Modlin IM, Bloom SR, Mitchell SC: Vasoactive intestinal plasma polypeptide (VIP) levels and intestinal ischemia. *Experientia* 34:535, 1978.
47. Mailman D: Effects of vasoactive intestinal polypeptide on intestinal absorption and blood flow. *J Physiol (London)* 279:121, 1978.
48. Kobold EE, Thal AP: Quantitation and identification of vasoactive substances liberated during various types of experimental intestinal ischemia. *Surg Gyncol Obstet* 117:315, 1963.
49. Chin CJ, Scott HJ, Guzd FN: Volume deficit versus toxic absorption—A study of canine shock after mesenteric arterial occlusion. *Ann Surg* 175:476, 1972.
50. Chin CJ, McArdle AH, Brown R, et al: Intestinal mucosal lesion in low flow states. (I.) A morphological, hemodynamic and metabolic reappraisal. *Arch Surg* 101:478, 1970.
51. Wagner R, Gabbert H, Höhn P: The mechanism of epithelial shedding after ischemic damage to the small intestinal mucosa. A light and electron microscopic investigation. *Virchows Arch (cell Pathol)* 30:25, 1979.
52. Marston A: Causes of death in Mesenteric arterial occlusion. (I.) Local and general effects of devascularisation of the bowel. (II.) Observations on devascularisation of the ischaemic bowel. *Ann Surg* 158:952, 1963.
53. Robinson JWL, Menge H, Sepulveda, et al: The functional response of the dog ileum to one hour's ischemia. *Clin Sci Molec Med* 50:115, 1976.
54. Menge H, Robinson JWL: Early phase of jejunal regeneration after short-term ischemia in the rat. *Lab Invest* 40:25, 1979.
55. Robinson JWL, Haroud M, Winistörfer B, et al: Recovery of function and structure of dog ileum and colon following two hour's acute ischemia. *Europ J Clin Invest* 4:443, 1974.

56. Cook BH, Wilson ER, Taylor AE: Intestinal fluid loss in hemorrhagic shock. *Am J Physiol* 221:1494, 1971.
57. Mirkovitch V, Menge H, Robinson JWL: Protection of the intestinal mucosa during ischemia by intraluminal perfusion. *Res Exp Med* 166:183, 1975.
58. Hueckel HJ, Chiu CJ, Hinchey EJ: The effect of intraluminally administered glucose in reducing fluid and electrolyte loss from the ischemic intestine. *Surg Gynecol Obstet* 136:780, 1973.
59. Robinson JWL, Winistörfer B, Mirkovitch V: Source of net water and electrolyte loss following intestinal ischemia. *Res Exp Med* 176:263, 1980.
60. Haglund U, Lundholm K, Lundgren O, et al: The relationship between the intestinal release of lysosomal enzymes and cardiotoxic material during regional simulated shock: An experimental study in the cat. *Circ Shock* 2:49, 1975.
61. Bounous G, Menard D, de Medicis E: Role of pancreatic proteases in the pathogenesis of ischemic enteropathy. *Gastroenterology* 73:102, 1977.
63. Manohar M, Tyagi RPS: Experimental intestinal ischemic shock in dogs. *Am J Physiol* 225:887, 1975.
63. Tjiong B, Bella E, Weiner M, et al: Fluid shifts and metabolic changes during and after the occlusion of the superior mesenteric artery. *Surg Gynecol Obstet* 139:217, 1974.
64. Gaus H, Matsumoto K: The escape of endotoxin from the intestine. *Surg Gynecol Obstet* 139:395, 1974.
65. Wollin A, Navert H, Bounous G: Effect of intestinal ischemia on diamine oxidase activity in rat intestinal tissue and blood. *Gastroenterology* 80:349, 1981.
66. Kusche J, Lorenz W, Stahlknecht C-T, et al: Intestinal diamine oxidase activity and histamine release in rabbit mesenteric ischemia. *Gastroenterology* 80:980, 1981.
67. Altura BM, Halevy S: Beneficial and detrimental actions of histamine H1 and H2 receptor antagonists in circulatory shock. *Proc Nat'l Acad Sci USA* 75:2941, 1978.
68. Bieganski T, Kusche J, Freussner KD, et al: Human intestinal diamine oxidase: Substrate specificity and comparative inhibitory study. *Agents Actions* 10:108, 1980.
69. Lefer AM: Role of myocardial depressant factor in the pathogenesis of circulatory shock. *Fed Proc* 29:1836, 1970.

3

Pathology of Ischemic Bowel Disease

Kathryn P. Clausen, M.D.
Joel G. Lucas, M.D.

Ischemic lesions of the bowel can result from a variety of primary lesions of blood vessels as well as from low flow states not directly related to regional vascular disease. The distribution and severity of the lesions in the bowel depend upon the size and degree of occlusion of a vessel and the extent of collateral circulation.

The vascular lesions and hemodynamic events leading to ischemic damage are essentially the same for small and large bowel, as are the intestinal lesions that result.[11] However, the small bowel seems somewhat more likely to develop acute ischemic necrosis with infarction. The colon is more frequently involved with chronic ischemic colitis or ulceration with stricture.[1]

Consideration of the pathology of the vasculature is followed by a description of the resulting lesions of the bowel.

Vascular Lesions

Arterial

The most common occlusive lesions of mesenteric arteries are atheromata, thrombi, or emboli.[10,11]

Atherosclerosis of the mesenteric arteries is usually most severe in the proximal 2 cm and has a strong association with aortic atherosclerosis (Figure 1). Distal vessels are

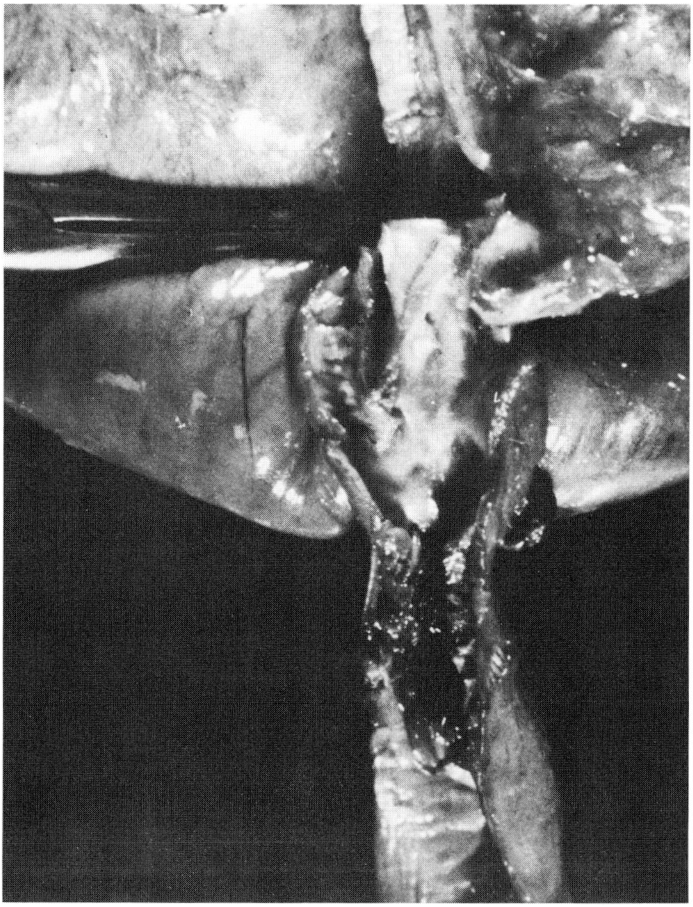

Figure 1. Opened superior mesenteric artery with atherosclerotic plaque and associated thrombosis in proximal portion.

uncommonly affected. Atheromata are rarely totally occlusive but can cause severe luminal narrowing and predispose to occlusive thrombosis (Figure 2). Occlusion can also result from hemorrhage into an atheromatous plaque. Ischemic symptoms from atherosclerosis usually do not occur until the luminal diameter is reduced by at least 50%.[13]

Occlusive Embolism does not require underlying vascular disease. Thus, surgical cure can result from prompt embolectomy.[14] The sources are usually cardiac; emboli result from mural thrombi associated with atrial fibrillation or myocardial infarction. Atheroembolism can also result from surgical manipulation of the aorta in aneurysmectomy (Figure 3).

Occlusion by extrinsic compression can result from dis-

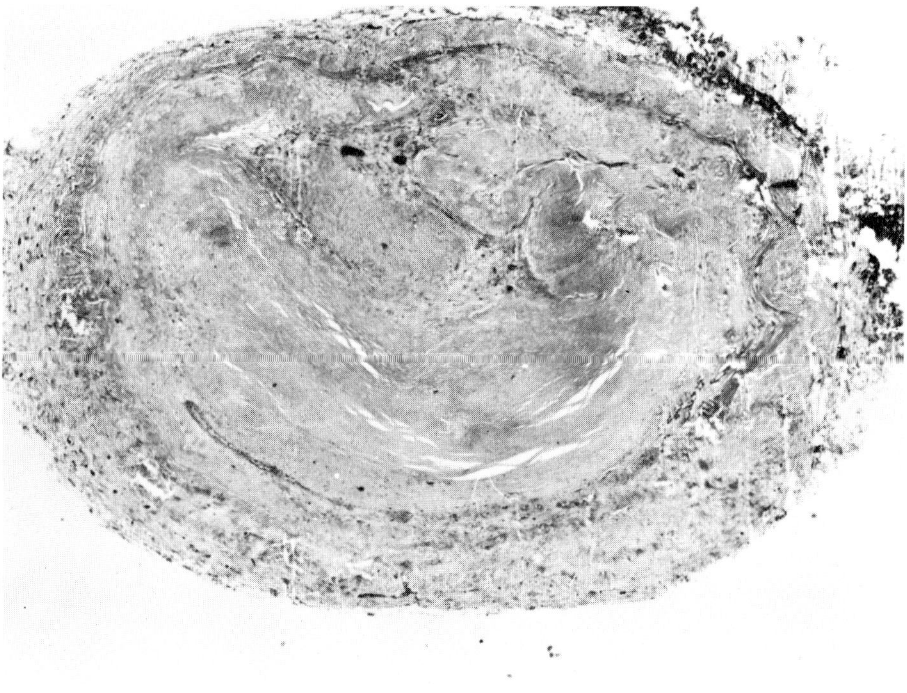

Figure 2. Artery with marked narrowing of lumen due to atherosclerotic plaque. Hematoxylin and eosin. Magnification 23×.

secting aortic aneurysm, tumor, or previous operations. There is a syndrome of abdominal pain attributed to congenital bands or anomaly of the celiac axis, but whether such an entity really exists remains controversial.[10] No histopathologic lesions of the bowel can be attributed to "celiac axis syndrome."

Vasculitis of several types can affect the mesenteric vasculature.[5,16] Periarteritis nodosa typically involves the small and medium sized muscular arteries of intestinal mesentery as well as nervous system, skin, genitourinary tract, and kidneys. It is frequently associated with hypertension. The lesions are segmental and have a propensity to develop near bifurcations and branches. Acute lesions

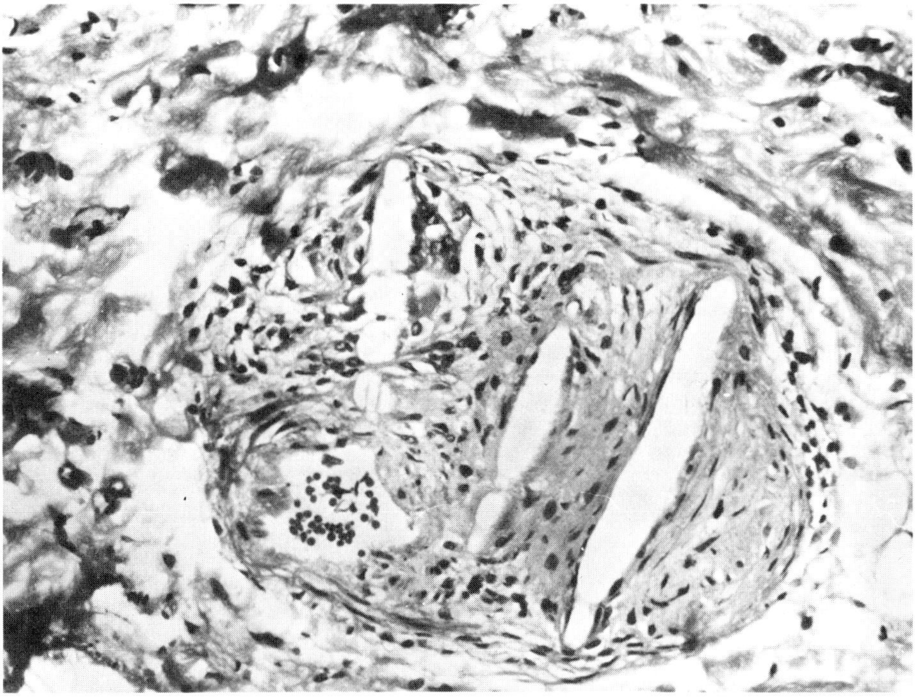

Figure 3. Small bowel. A submucosal artery is occluded by an atherosclerotic embolus. There is a small recanalized lumen. The large slits represent cholesterol clefts. Hematoxylin and eosin. Magnification 255×.

are characterized by fibrinoid necrosis of arterial wall with acute transmural inflammation and thrombosis[5] (Figure 4). Healed lesions can result in small aneurysms. A morphologically identical form of vasculitis has been associated with hepatitis B antigen.[5]

A more diffuse, acute, and uniform type of vasculitis involving arterioles and capillaries has been described as hypersensitivity angiitis. This can affect any organ, including the gut. Vasculitis is often associated with systemic autoimmune disease such as lupus erythematosus, and intestinal ischemia can be a resulting complication. Henoch-Schönlein purpura is usually associated with abdominal pain and ischemic lesions of bowel. The vascular lesion is a necrotizing vasculitis of small arteries and arterioles.

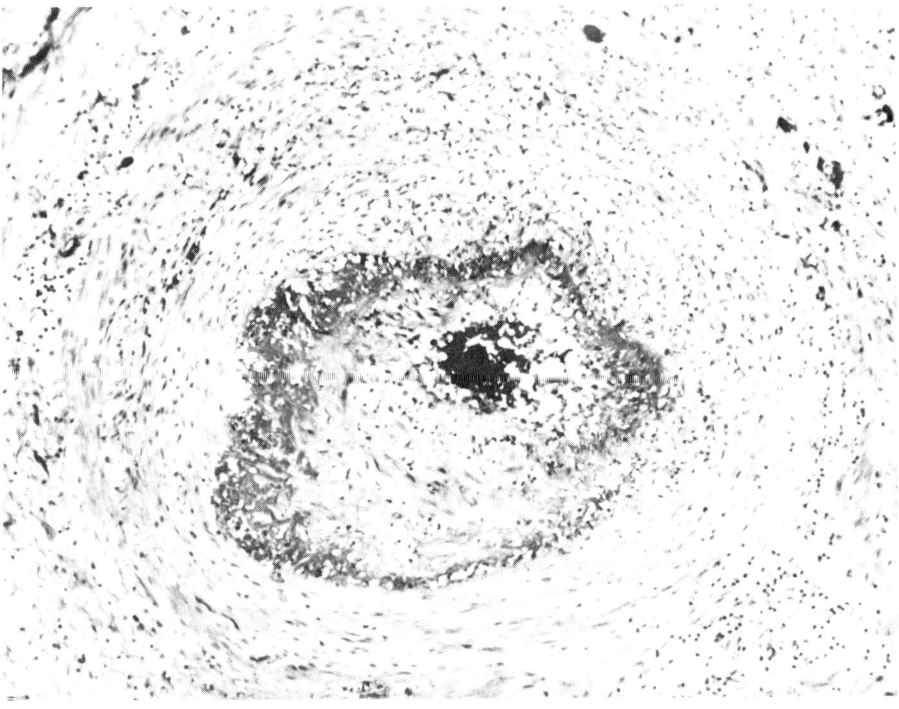

Figure 4. Mesentery. Polyarteritis nodosa in a medium sized artery with fibrinoid necrosis and infiltration of wall by inflammatory cells. Hematoxylin and eosin. Magnification 97×.

There is associated vasculitis of skin and glomerulonephritis.

Buerger's disease (thromboangiitis obliterans) is distinctive in that it involves both arteries and veins of small to medium caliber.[8] It involves the extremities in particular; but lesions can also be found in brain, heart, and abdominal viscera. It usually affects young men between 20 and 45 years of age. There is segmental inflammation of the full thickness of artery or vein with thrombosis. No fibrinoid necrosis is present. Thrombi can organize in later stages.

Intravascular coagulation can affect the bowel just as it can affect any other organ in the body.[1]

Venous

Mesenteric vein thrombosis can result from a variety of causes. Retrograde congestion leading to thrombosis can result from cirrhosis or extrinsic compression. It is seen in hyperviscosity and hypercoagulability states such as sickle cell disease, polycythemia rubra vera, and antithrombin III deficiency. Parasites can invade and occlude veins. Abdominal sepsis can result in pyelophlebitis.[1] Volvulus produces a venous occlusive lesion.

Mesenteric venous thrombosis has been reported in young women taking oral contraceptives[2] (Figures 5 and 6). Strictures of the bowel attributed to the use of enteric-coated potassium tablets are now thought to be the result of healed localized venous infarcts.[1]

Nonocclusive Mesenteric Ischemia

It has been estimated that at least 20% of patients with ischemic necrosis of the bowel have no totally occluding mesenteric vascular lesions.[11] Preexisting narrowing due to atherosclerosis is common. The underlying mechanism seems to be splanchnic vasoconstriction secondary to low

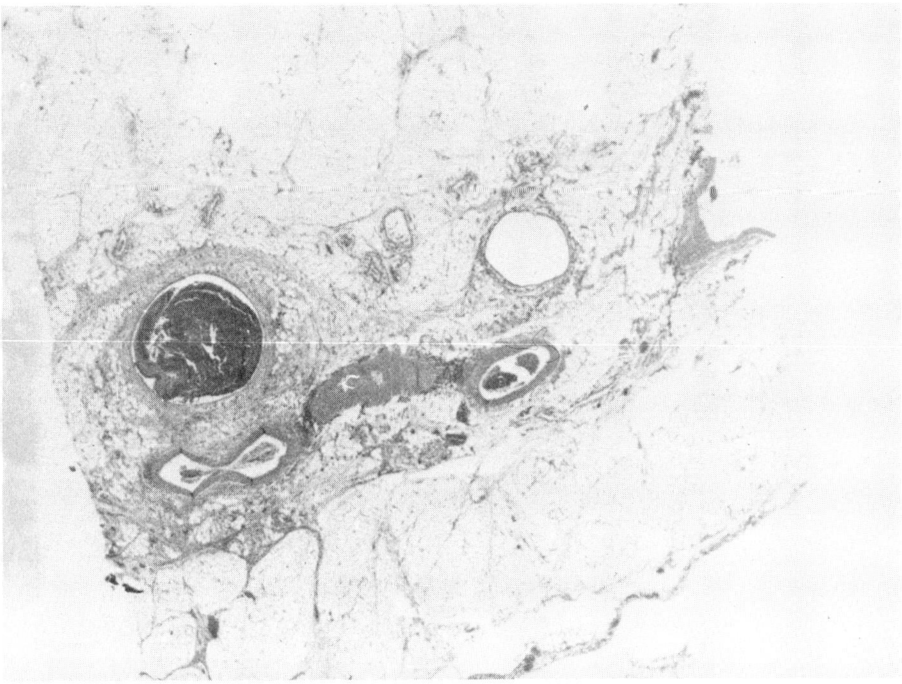

Figure 5. Mesentery. Veins with recent thrombus associated with oral contraceptive use. Hematoxylin and eosin. Magnification 8.7×.

flow states.[1,6,7,12] These include heart failure, cardiac arrhythmia, dehydration, sepsis, hypovolemic shock, and the use of pressor drugs.[1]

The lesions resulting from nonocclusive ischemia are similar to those produced by vascular occlusion; but they tend to be patchy, very widespread, and may vary in severity.

Ischemic Lesions of Bowel

The basic pathologic process of ischemic injury to bowel is the same for both small and large intestine, although the

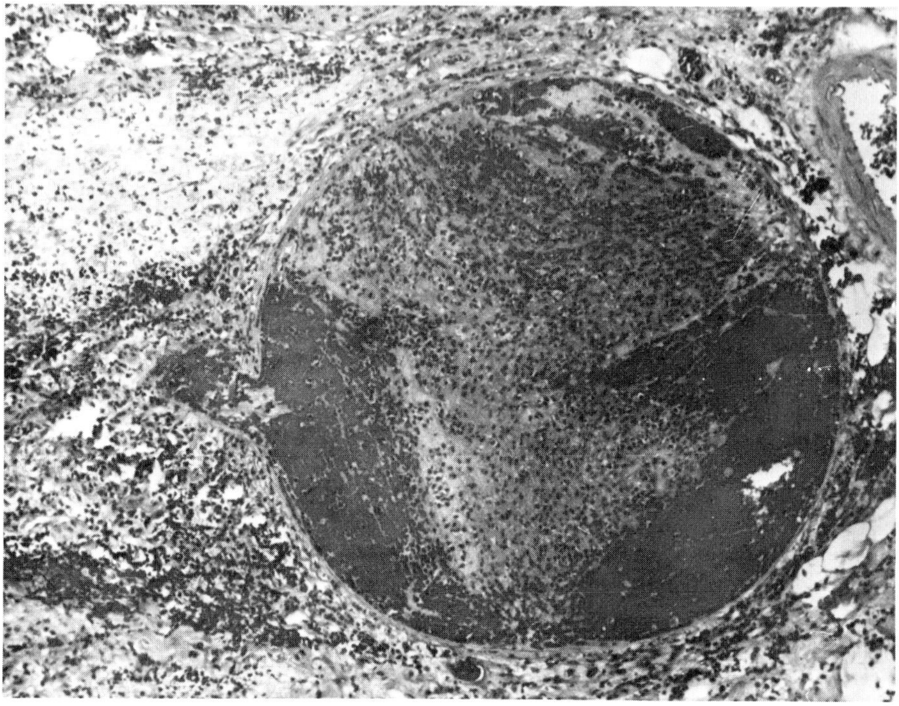

Figure 6. Small bowel. Markedly distended submucosal vein with thrombosis and surrounding hemorrhage. Hematoxylin and eosin. Magnification 100×.

frequency and clinical manifestations may vary, depending on location.[11]

As with ischemic injury to any other organ, intestinal ischemia can range from minimal hypoxia to massive infarction with gangrene. Its onset can be acute or gradual; it can be reversible up to a certain point. Healing may occur by complete resolution or by scarring with stricture. There is no need to coin a new descriptive term for each variation in pattern. The lesions to be described all fall generally within the following categories:

- acute ischemic necrosis (infarction)
- acute and subacute ischemic enterocolitis
- ischemic stricture and ulcer (healed infarct)
- transient ischemic colitis (reversible)

Infarction

Both arterial and venous obstruction can produce intestinal infarction. Venous infarcts progress somewhat more slowly and are always hemorrhagic.[11]

The early gross appearance of infarcted bowel is characterized by edema and violaceous color. The mucosa appears necrotic and nodular. Totally necrotic bowel may be purple or nearly black in color, foul-smelling, and thin-walled. It may be extremely friable. There may be gas bubbles in the wall or veins.

The mucosa is most vulnerable to hypoxic injury and manifests the first visible changes.[13] It undergoes necrosis and ulceration with hemorrhage into the lumen. A surface membrane composed of fibrin, blood, or necrotic tissue may develop (Figure 7). Intravascular thrombi may be present in the mucosa and submucosa.[1,11] There is marked submucosal edema and hemorrhage (Figures 8 and 9). Later, the cells will lose their nuclei, lyse, and be widely separated by edema.

The inflammatory reaction tends to be poor[13] in the early phases (Figure 10). Gangrene represents total necrosis of the bowel wall with superinfection by intestinal organisms (Figure 11). At this stage, the mesentery and its vessels may be heavily inflamed, but this does not imply primary vasculitis.

Acute and Subacute Ischemia

This lesion is somewhat less severe than total infarction and does not progress to total necrosis of all layers of the bowel wall. The mucosal lesion is the same as that in the early stages of infarction, i.e., superficial hemorrhage, effacement or "bursting" of glands, mild acute inflammation, and sometimes a necrotic surface membrane. Crypt abscesses may occasionally be seen. Inflammation can increase and be followed by sloughing and ulceration. This

(Text continued on page 42)

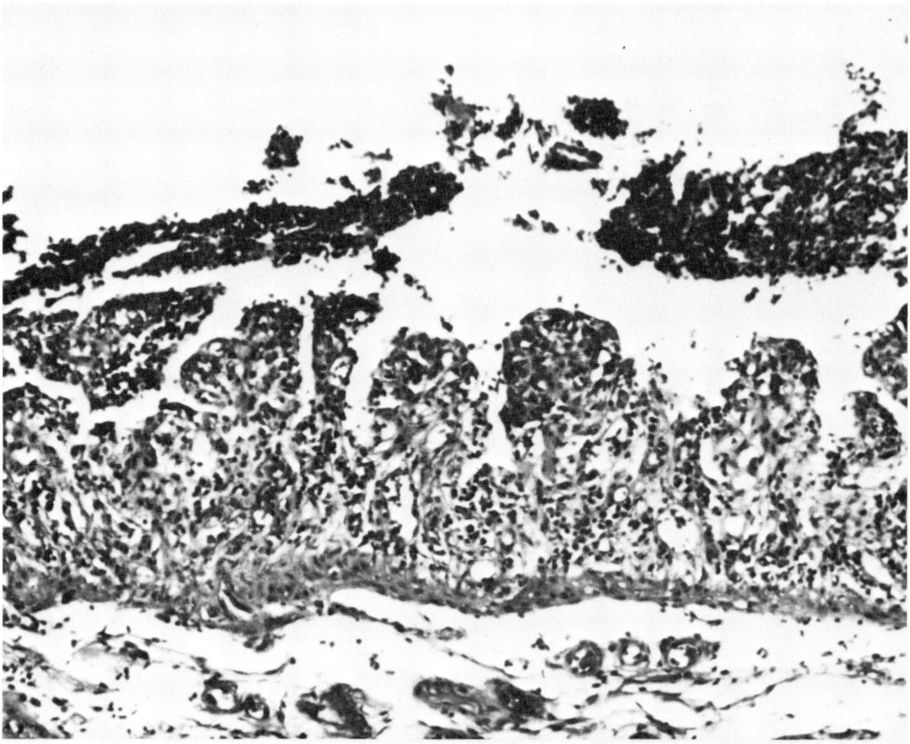

Figure 7. Small bowel. Surface membrane composed of exuded protein with many polymorphonuclear leukocytes. The mucosal epithelium is denuded, and the lamina propria is infiltrated by polymorphonuclear leukocytes. The submucosa is edematous. Hematoxylin and eosin. Magnification 150×.

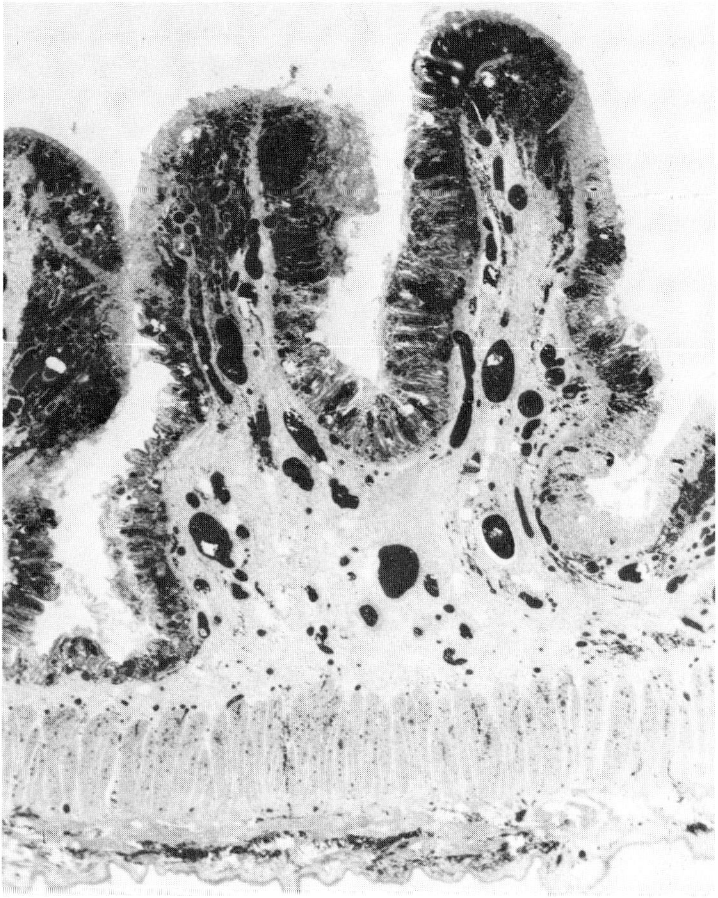

Figure 8. Small bowel. Early ischemic injury with hemorrhagic necrosis of mucosa and congestion of submucosal vessels. Hematoxylin and eosin. Magnification 16×.

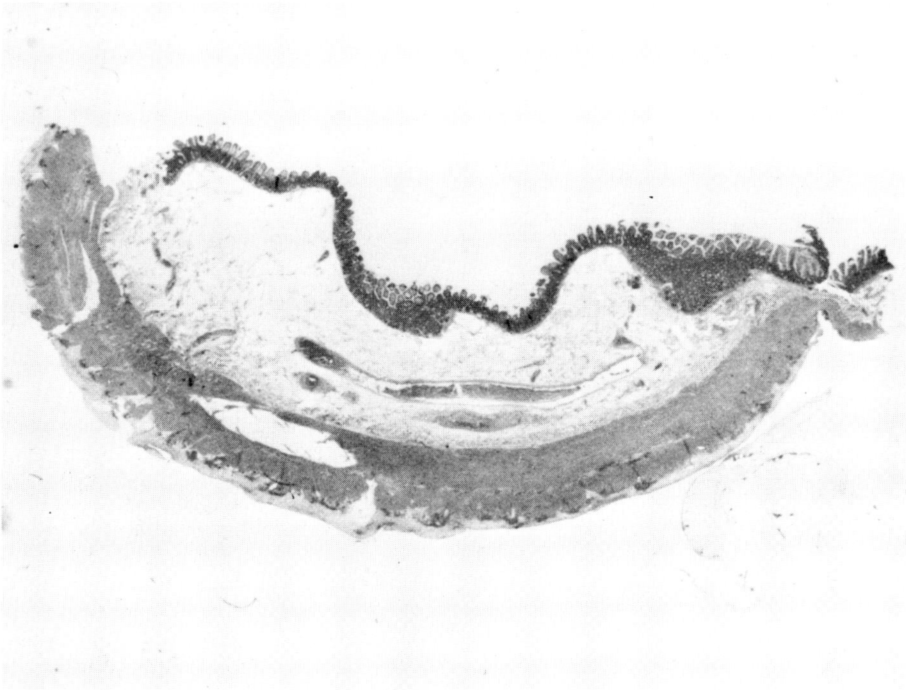

Figure 9. Small bowel. Marked submucosal edema. Hematoxylin and eosin. Magnification 5.2×.

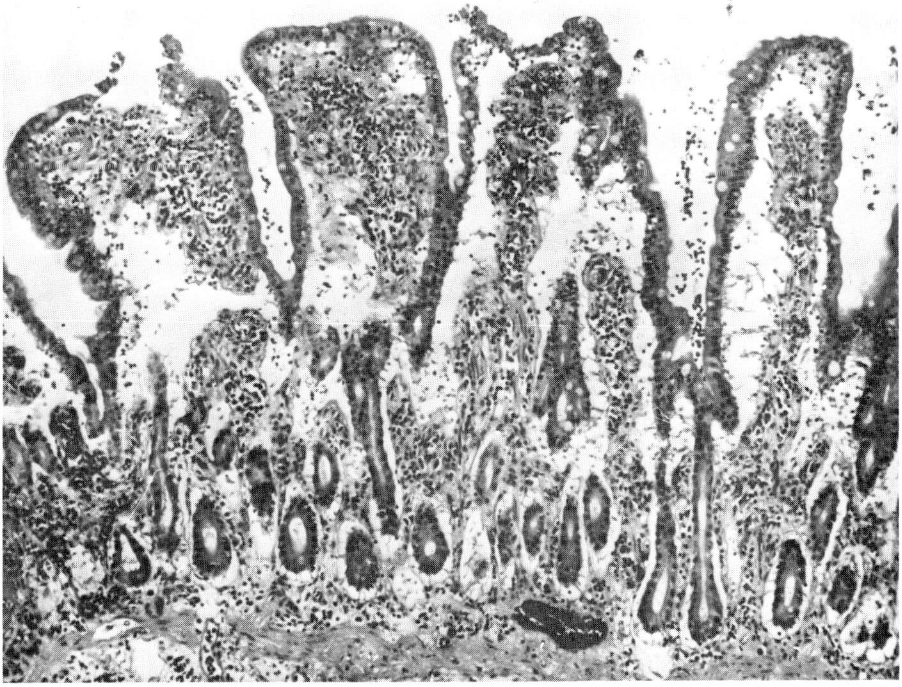

Figure 10. Small bowel. Early ischemic mucosal injury with edema and polymorphonuclear leukocyte infiltration of lamina propria. Note focal mucosal disruption. Hematoxylin and eosin. Magnification 90×.

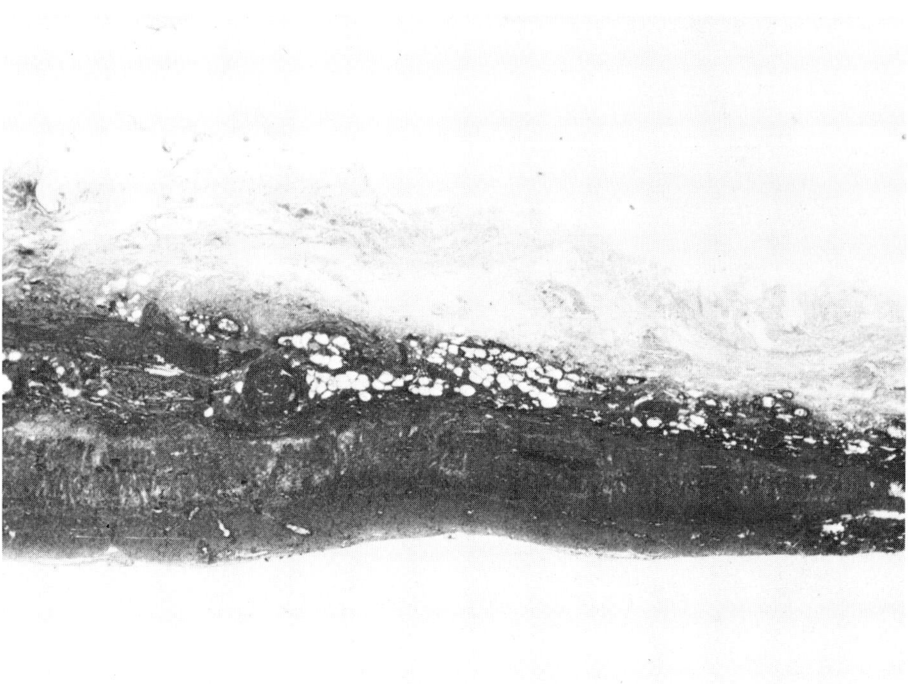

Figure 11. Small bowel. Infarction of entire bowel wall. Hematoxylin and eosin. Magnification 17×.

is particularly true in the colon and can produce a picture superficially resembling ulcerative colitis.[3,9] The distinguishing feature of the acute lesion, however, is the presence of mucosal hemorrhage and intravascular thrombi (Figure 12).

The more chronic or reparative phase of this lesion is characterized by granulation tissue, chronic inflammation, and repair. The bases of the ulcerated areas fill in with proliferating capillaries, fibroblasts, and macrophages (Figures 13A, 13B and 14). Inflammation is predominantly lymphocytic and plasmacytic. There may be hemosiderin pigment and an occasional foreign body giant cell. Persistent normal mucosa may give the appearance of pseudo-

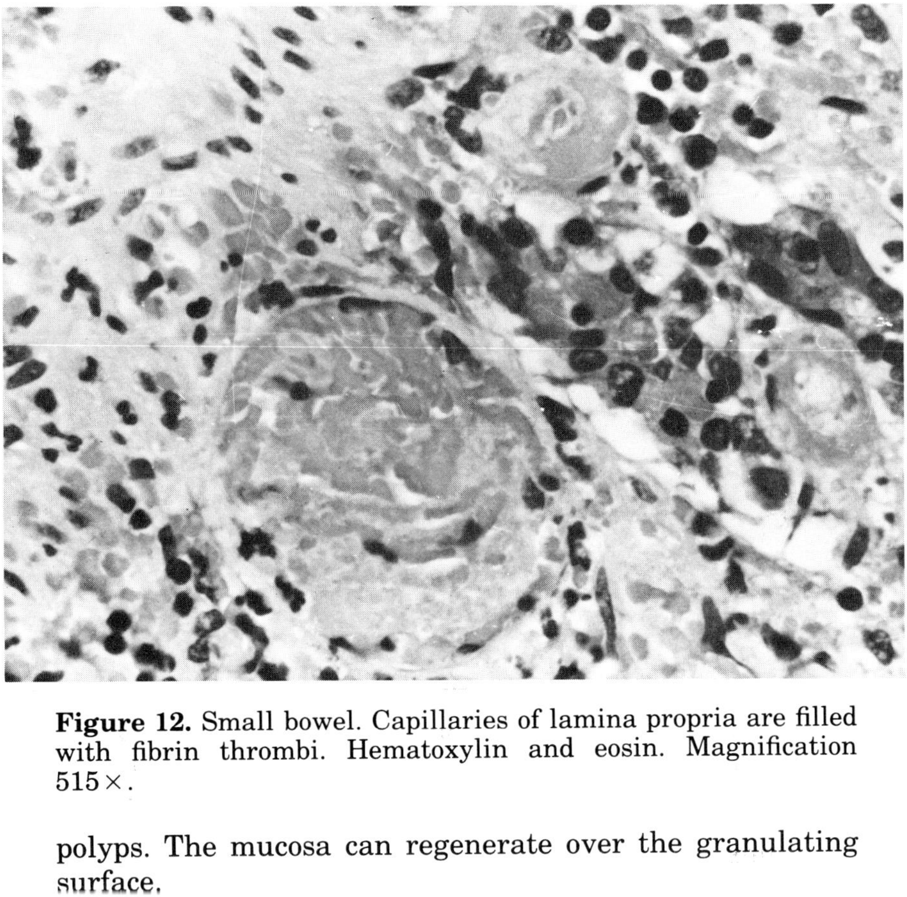

Figure 12. Small bowel. Capillaries of lamina propria are filled with fibrin thrombi. Hematoxylin and eosin. Magnification 515×.

polyps. The mucosa can regenerate over the granulating surface.

Ischemic Stricture and Ulcer

This can occur in small bowel or colon as the acute ischemic process resolves and can be solitary or multiple. There can be a resulting bowel obstruction. In the colon, the splenic flexure is the most common site. Any focal ischemic injury can cause this lesion, but it is particularly distinctive in the small bowel in association with the use of enteric-coated potassium tablets.[1]

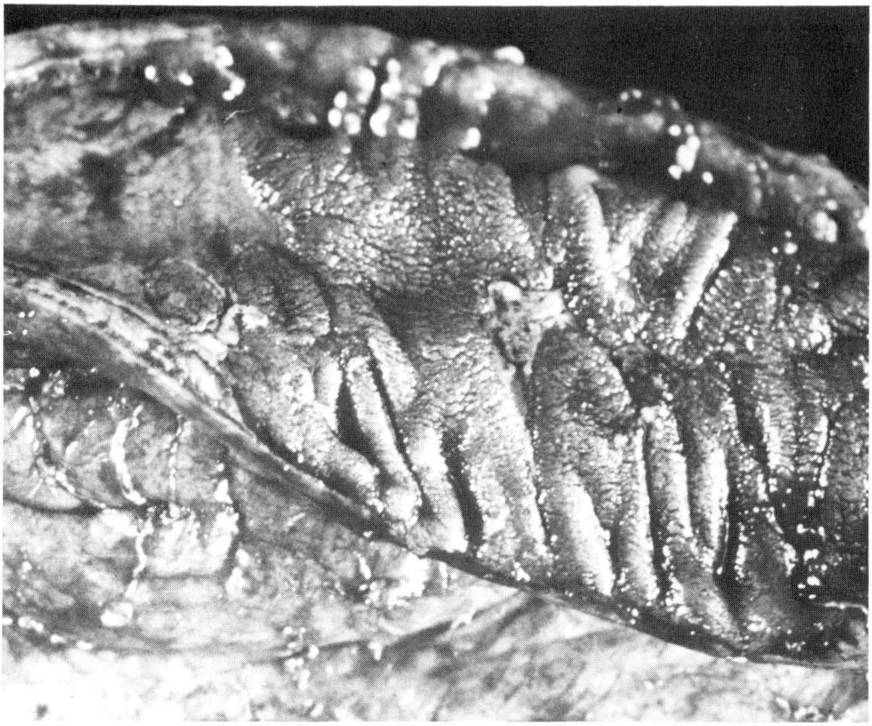

Figure 13A. Small bowel. Chronic ischemic changes with flattened granular mucosa.

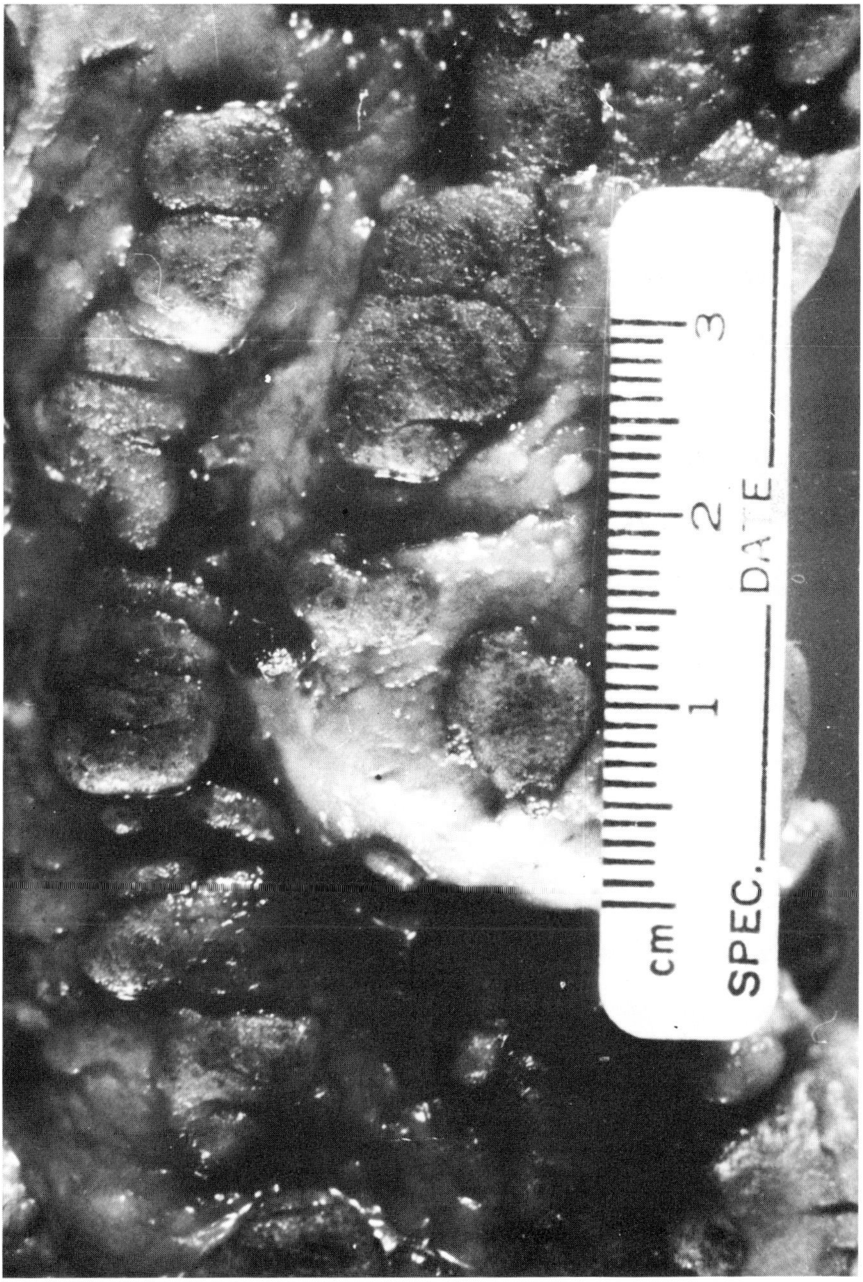

Figure 13B. Colon. Chronic ischemia with ulceration and granulation tissue.

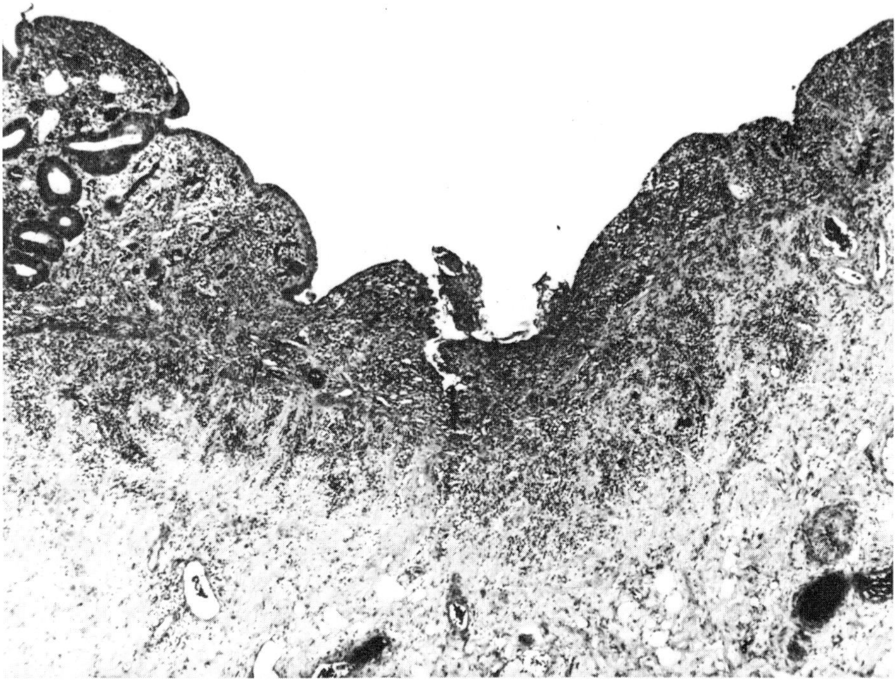

Figure 14. Small bowel. Chronic ischemic ulcer with inflammation and fibrosis in the base. Portions of the ulcer, as well as mucosa at the edge, are covered by regenerating epithelium. Hematoxylin and eosin. Magnification 65×.

Ischemic strictures are concentric.[11] The mucosa is frequently ulcerated. The submucosa is filled with granulation or scar tissue which extends beyond the ulcer and can penetrate the entire thickness of the muscle wall to serosa (Figure 15). There may be hemosiderin remaining from previous hemorrhages. The segmental pattern can strongly simulate Crohn's disease, but inflammatory fistulae and granulomata are absent.

Miscellaneous

It has been suggested that an angiomatous lesion of the bowel in older patients may have an ischemic basis. "An-

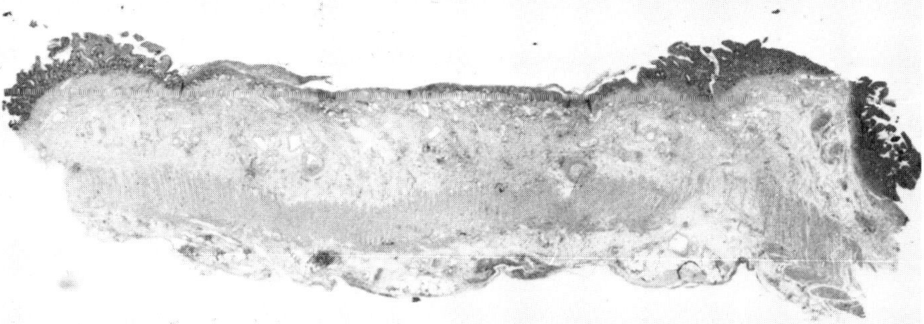

Figure 15. Ischemic stricture of small bowel. Chronic ulcer with submucosal fibrosis. Hematoxylin and eosin. Magnification 5.4×.

giodysplasia" is characterized by telangiectasis of veins, venules, and capillaries in the submucosa and lamina propria of the colon. It may be age-related change due to obstruction of submucosal veins.[11,13]

References

1. Boley SJ, Brandt LJ, Veith FJ: Ischemic disorders of the intestines. *Curr Probl Surg 25,* Year Book Medical Publishers, Chicago 1978.
2. Civetta JM, Kolodny M: Mesenteric venous thrombosis associated with oral contraceptives. *Gastroenterology* 58:713, 1970.
3. Dawson MA, Schaeffer MW: The clinical course of reversible ischemic colitis. *Gastroenterology* 60:577, 1971.
4. Drucker WR, Davis JH, Holden WD, Reagan JR: Hemorrhagic necrosis of the intestine. *Arch Surg* 89:42, 1964.
5. Fauci AS, Haynes BF, Katz P: The spectrum of vasculitis: Clinical, pathologic, immunologic and therapeutic considerations. *Ann Intern Med* 89 (Part 1):660, 1978.
6. Freiman DC: Hemorrhagic necrosis of the gastrointestinal tract. *Circulation* 32:329, 1965.

7. Grosh JL, Mann RH, O'Donnell WM: Nonthrombotic intestinal infarction in heart disease. *Am J Med Sci* 250:613, 1975.
8. Herrington JL, Grossman MD: Surgical lesions of the small and large intestines resulting from Buerger's disease. *Ann Surg* 168:1079, 1968.
9. McGovern VJ, Goulston SJM: Ischaemic enterocolitis. *Gut* 6:213, 1965.
10. Marston DM, Keiny R, Szilagyi DE, Taylor EW: Intestinal ischemia. *Arch Surg* 111:107, 1976.
11. Morson BC, Dawson JM: *Gastrointestinal Pathology*. Blackwell Scientific Publications, Oxford 1979.
12. Ming S: Hemorrhagic necrosis of the gastrointestinal tract and its relation to cardiovascular status. *Circulation* 32:322, 1965.
13. Price WE, Rohrer GV, Jacobson ED: Mesenteric vascular diseases. *Gastroenterology* 57:599, 1969.
14. Skinner DB, Zarius CK, Moossa AR: Mesenteric vascular disease. *Am J Surg* 128:835, 1974.
15. Wolff WI, Grossman MB, Shinya H: Angiodysplasia of the colon: Diagnosis and treatment. *Gastroenterology* 72:329, 1977.
16. Zeek PM: Periarteritis nodosa: A critical review. *Am J Clin Path* 22:777, 1952.

4

Laboratory Diagnosis of Mesenteric Infarction

James H. Caldwell, M.D.

Articles on the clinical problem of acute intestinal ischemia usually emphasize the need for early diagnosis but only occasionally deplore the unavailability of specific laboratory tests that might help to achieve this. Many studies in animals suggest a variety of laboratory abnormalities that might be relevant. In every case, information extending these data to the clinical situation is absent, incomplete, or lacks information regarding specificity and sensitivity. The clinician, faced with the frustrating combination of nonspecific physical signs and laboratory tests of unknown value, is aided little in his efforts to confirm a tentative diagnosis of intestinal ischemia. The urgency of early diagnosis has been confirmed by Barnett et al. who found mortality twice as high in patients operated upon 36 or more hours after the onset of symptoms than in patients operated upon earlier.[1] A screening test that could be ordered by nonsurgical clinicians would probably hasten surgical referral and lead to earlier and more appropriate supporting investigations. Radiologic studies of this problem are reviewed in Chapter 5 of this book, and Boley et al. have summarized the difficulties encountered in employing an angiography-based protocol for detection and management of acute mesenteric ischemia.[2] This chapter critically reviews the laboratory tests currently employed and surveys the experimental literature for studies that have not yet been applied clinically (Table I).

Leukocytosis and Hemoconcentration

Elevations of white blood count and hematocrit are widely cited as aids to diagnosis of mesenteric infarction, even though their nonspecificity is recognized.[2,3] Although early experience suggested that 100% of patients had se-

Table I

Laboratory Tests in Diagnosis of Mesenteric Ischemia

Currently Used Hematological Tests
Leukocyte count (leukocytosis)
Hematocrit (hemoconcentration)
Biochemical Tests of Proposed Diagnostic Value
Blood gases (metabolic acidosis)
Serum phosphate (hyperphosphatemia)
Serum Enzymes
No established role
Amylase
Lactic dehydrogenase
Alanine aminotransferase (SGOT)
Proposed for clinical application
Serum intestinal alkaline phosphatase
Creatine kinase isoenzymes
Diamine oxidase

vere leukocytosis,[4] the more recent literature shows that mesenteric infarction with a normal leukocyte count is not uncommon. In seven recent series reporting a total of 389 patients, only 74% had white cell counts greater than 10,000.[5–11] Of the elevated counts reported, about half were greater than 20,000, and values of 50,000 to 90,000 have been reported infrequently.[12] The percent of patients with leukocytosis appears to be the same regardless of the etiology of ischemia,[5] and the presence of leukocytosis has no impact on the outcome.[6] Thus, the determination of blood leukocyte count lacks sensitivity as well as specificity in the early diagnosis of bowel infarction.

Increases in hematocrit reflecting hemoconcentration are regularly seen in the early phases of experimental intestinal ischemia. Like the white cell count, the frequency of an elevated hematocrit is less than universal in spontaneous human disease, probably due to variables such as early fluid therapy, coexisting chronic illness, and gastrointestinal blood loss. In recent series where the data were recorded, only about half of the patients showed laboratory evidence of hemoconcentration or dehydration.[7,9]

Acidosis and Hyperphosphatemia

It is widely recognized that metabolic acidosis complicates the natural course of intestinal necrosis as part of the cycle of tissue hypoxia, release of systemic vasoactive materials, and refractory hypotension.[13] Brooks and Carey reported experience with mesenteric infarction in seven patients in whom base deficits developed before hypotension. The mean base deficit was significantly greater than that of a group of patients with other acute abdominal diseases, and it was proposed that early recognition of metabolic acidosis should have diagnostic value.[14] This conclusion was supported by experiments in which dogs with superior mesenteric artery ligation developed acidosis prior to hypotension, while dogs with pancreatitis, perforation, and other conditions became acidotic only when shock supervened. Other investigators have not confirmed the discriminating value of pH studies in experimental models, finding base deficits in bowel perforation, common bile duct obstruction, intestinal obstruction, and pancreatitis, as well as in mesenteric infarction.[15] Perhaps more important is the fact that no report of clinical experience since the report of Brooks and Carey has provided data on the specificity and sensitivity of base deficit as an aid to early diagnosis. Accordingly, it is not yet clear whether metabolic acidosis represents an aid to early diagnosis or a complication of established bowel necrosis.

Following the retrospective observation that seven patients with massive intestinal infarction had impressive elevations of serum phosphate, Jamieson, Durand, and coworkers studied this phenomenon in a canine model. They found significantly elevated serum phosphate associated with metabolic acidosis 4 hours after superior mesenteric artery ligation, and proposed that hyperphosphatemia might be a useful diagnostic sign.[16] In additional animal studies they found increased peritoneal fluid phosphate parallel with the serum elevation[17] and related this to loss of phosphate from necrotic intestinal muscle.[18] They have estimated the sensitivity of the serum phosphate elevation to be 70% in patients with three or more feet of ischemic intestine and believe the test to be highly specific, except in patients with renal failure and bone disease.[17,19] Details on numbers of patients, time of appearance or duration of hyperphosphatemia, or impact on outcome have not been reported. Although it is implied that hyperphosphatemia is more specific than metabolic acidosis for mesenteric infarction,[18] the association of similar elevations of serum phosphate with lactic acidosis from other causes[20] suggests that serum phosphate may not be a highly specific test for intestinal ischemia. While it is likely to be useful in the proper clinical context, it might be difficult to interpret in patients with severe cardiac or pulmonary disease, or in other circumstances where widespread tissue hypoxia precedes intestinal infarction. As with metabolic acidosis, other investigators have not yet reported their experience with serum phosphate as a diagnostic aid. Further clinical study of both serum pH and phosphate is urgently needed. Both assays are readily available and data supporting their use for diagnosis in gut ischemia could be obtained in a relatively short time.

Serum Enzymes

Amylase

There is a general awareness that the serum amylase may be elevated in intestinal infarction as well as in several other nonpancreatic abdominal emergencies. Although serum amylase is the only enzyme assay rapidly and widely performed in the assessment of acute abdominal disease, there is relatively little information on the frequency of amylase elevation in acute mesenteric vascular insufficiency. In an early survey of serum amylase in patients with an acute abdomen, elevations due to mesenteric thrombosis or necrosis complicating intestinal obstruction were less frequent than in patients with cholecystitis or visceral perforation.[21] Abruzzo et al. reported serum amylase elevations in two of six cases of mesenteric thrombosis in a series of 494 patients with elevated amylase, most of whom had pancreatic disease.[22] A more recent series reported hyperamylasemia in 21% of patients with mesenteric infarction.[7] Elevations are usually in the range of no more than two to three times the upper limit of normal. It is clear that the serum amylase is neither specific nor sensitive in the detection of ischemic bowel. The major importance of these observations is to alert the reader to the nonspecificity of elevations of the serum amylase.

Lactic Dehydrogenase and Transaminase

Early in the era of diagnostic enzymology, abnormalities of LDH and SGOT were described in some patients with intestinal infarction.[23, 24] It is now generally accepted that these tests are too nonspecific to be of value and are probably insensitive as well.[3] There appears to be no contemporary enthusiasm for using these tests in an effort to improve early diagnosis.

Intestinal Alkaline Phosphatase (SIAP)

This isoenzyme has been widely studied in animal models and provides an assay specific for intestinal injury. Bounous and Hugon, studying three different levels of hemorrhagic shock in dogs, showed reduced intestinal tissue alkaline phosphase and elevation of serum isoenzyme that correlated with the degree of intestinal necrosis at 4 and 48 hours.[25] The relationship among rate of rise, height of elevation, and severity of the intestinal lesion has been confirmed in a canine model using selective ligation of branches of the superior mesenteric artery.[26]

In another study, *de novo* intestinal alkaline phosphatase appeared in the serum of 6 of 7 dogs six hours after mesenteric artery occlusion, but did not appear in dogs with intestinal perforation, intestinal obstruction, pancreatitis, or ligation of the common bile duct.[15] This apparent specificity of SIAP for intestinal ischemia contrasts with peritoneal fluid alkaline phosphatase, which is increased with ischemia,[27] intestinal trauma,[28] and experimental perforation.[29] In spite of a decade of interest and encouraging animal experiments, serum intestinal alkaline phosphatase assay has not been studied in the clinical setting and no conclusion is available regarding potential usefulness in man at this time. Investigators have been deterred by the fact that the presence of intestinal alkaline phosphatase in man is normal in blood groups B and O individuals and rises in the serum normally after a meal.[30] In spite of this, the isoenzyme is rarely found in fasted or ill hospitalized patients,[31] so it remains a test that could be interpreted in the appropriate clinical context. Prospective studies and additional clinical experience with this assay should be carried out and reported.

Creatine Kinase

This enzyme is widely used in clinical diagnosis of myocardial infarction and skeletal muscle disease. Three isoenzymes are readily separated by electrophoresis. CPK-MM is the form normally present in human serum, and CPK-MB appears with myocardial infarction. CPK-BB is found in smooth muscle and brain and is not found in normal adult human serum, usually appearing only after significant brain injury. Since 1976 there has been increasing evidence that CPK-BB may appear after intestinal injury. Itano reported 16 cases associated with the detection of this isoenzyme, all but one having proved or probable cerebral sources for the appearance of CPK-BB. One case of fatal membranous enterocolitis and bowel necrosis had the isoenzyme.[32] In a brief report of 41 patients with diverse illnesses associated with the appearance of CPK-BB, five patients with bowel necrosis were included, and some had elevated total CPK as well.[33] Doran has reported in detail a case of colon infarction associated with renal failure and diffuse skeletal muscle necrosis following probable drug overdose. As total CPK was very high, serial electrophoretic studies were done, and both MB and MM were elevated. CPK-BB appeared 24 hours before emergency laparotomy for acute abdominal signs revealed necrosis of the descending colon, and was absent after resection of this segment of bowel.[34] Because of this suggestive human evidence, Graeber et al. studied total and isoenzyme CPK following superior mesenteric artery ligation in dogs. Compared with sham-operated or peritonitis controls, animals with bowel infarction had significant elevations in total CPK from 3 to 30 hours after onset, with the predominant elevation in CPK-MM. However, CPK-BB rose between 3 and 12 hours with a peak around 6 hours, while CPK-MB peaked in the second 12 hours after occlusion.[35] These results suggest that determination of CPK and all three of its isoenzymes might be of great value in clinical assessment of mesenteric vascular events in man. Although prospective human studies have not yet been carried out, the reported clinical experience and the similarity of canine and human intestinal CPK content suggest promise for clinical application.

Diamine Oxidase (DAO)

This is a histamine-catabolizing enzyme found in intestinal epithelium, studied because of the evidence that histamine released during intestinal ischemia contributes to the "intestinal factor" in the pathogenesis of shock. A recent study of DAO in experimental ischemia suggested that the enzyme assay may have a role in diagnosis as well as in studies of pathophysiology.

Previous studies established that DAO in intestinal mucosa plays a role in modulating the response to several conditions including intestinal ischemia.[36] Wollin et al. studied DAO content in intestinal tissue, lumen, lymph, and peripheral blood following superior mesenteric artery occlusion of varying duration in rats. DAO content of tissue fell with increasing duration of ischemia, while luminal, lymphatic, and serum concentrations of the enzyme rose significantly after 30, 60, or 90 minutes of ischemia.[37] The duration of the elevation in serum depended in part on the duration of clamping and probably on the severity of initial mucosal injury, suggesting that in some circumstances the serum enzyme may be elevated for only a brief time. Human studies of the enzyme have been reported to show decreased plasma levels in patients with chronic small intestinal mucosal disease,[38] but have not at this time been extended to clinical ischemic disease. The assessment of this assay as a clinically applicable diagnostic aid in acute intestinal vascular disease is of obvious promise.

Vasoactive Intestinal Polypeptide (VIP)

This gut peptide was examined in experimental ischemia in pigs in order to determine whether it may play a role in the hemodynamic sequelae of intestinal infarction. Modlin et al. showed increased levels of VIP in portal but not peripheral blood during clamping of the mesenteric vessels, and proposed that it may have pathophysiological significance.[39] More recently, elevations in peripheral blood VIP have been reported during graded reductions in mesenteric artery flow in dogs, and the assay has been proposed to have potential diagnostic value.[40] Although VIP assay is presently available on a limited basis in the evaluation of secretory diarrhea due to functioning pancreatic neoplasm, there is insufficient information about VIP in other clinical conditions at this time. Future human studies of VIP should address its potential as a diagnostic marker for intestinal ischemia.

Summary

This review of the status of laboratory studies in the early stages of acute intestinal vascular disease must conclude that there is at present no specific, sensitive, reproducible and readily available test to improve early diagnosis. The hematologic aberrations often seen are nonspecific and insensitive. There is not yet wide experience or agreement among authorities on the value of blood gas and serum phosphate determinations, but further study of acidosis and hyperphosphatemia appears to have the greatest promise. The new appreciation that certain serum enzymes may be specific for gut injury in the proper clinical context suggests obvious directions for further clinical investigation. Of the gut enzymes available, CPK-BB appears most promising, since human experience has been reported and the methodology is already in place. If the retrospective clinical experience is confirmed by prospective study, additional study of the comparative value of different enzymes will be in order. Finally, since the clinical conditions under study are relatively infrequent, one may hope that systematic data gathering will establish the utility of the several possible laboratory approaches in the near future. It is unlikely that evolving therapy will have a noticeable impact on the mortality of gut ischemia until major advances in earlier diagnosis are made.

References

1. Barnett WO, Petro AB, Williamson JW: A current appraisal of problems with gangrenous bowel. *Ann Surg* 183:653, 1976.
2. Boley SJ, Brandt LJ, Veith FJ: Ischemic disorders of the intestines. *Curr Probl Surg* 15:1, 1978.
3. Vyden JK: The systemic effects of acute superior mesenteric vascular insufficiency. In *Vascular Disorders of the Intestines*. Ch 14, p 279, Boley SJ, Schwartz SS, Williams LF (Eds), Appleton-Century-Crofts, New York 1971.
4. Uricchio JF, Calenda DG, Freedman D: Mesenteric vascular occlusion. *Ann Surg* 139:206, 1954.
5. Ottinger LW, Austen WG: A study of 136 patients with mesenteric infarction. *Surg Gynecol Obstet* 124:251, 1967.
6. Delany HM: Prognostic factors in infarction of the intestine. *Surg Gynecol Obstet* 135:253, 1972.
7. Mattox KL, Guinn GA: Mesenteric infarction. Diagnostic and therapeutic enigmas. *Am J Surg* 126:332, 1973.

8. Singh RP, Shah RC, Lee ST: Acute mesenteric vascular occlusion. A review of 32 patients. *Surgery* 78:613, 1975.
9. Kairaluoma MI, Karkola P, Heikkinen E, et al: Mesenteric infarction. *Am J Surg* 133:188, 1977.
10. Ver Stegg KR, Broders CW: Gangrene of the bowel. *Surg Clin North Am* 59:869, 1979.
11. Hildebrand HD, Zierler RE: Mesenteric vascular disease. *Am J Surg* 139:188, 1980.
12. Saris DS, Uricchio JF: Superior mesenteric arterial embolectomy. *Arch Surg* 81:90, 1960.
13. Mavor GE: Acute occlusion of the superior mesenteric artery. *Clinics in Gastroenterology* 1:639, 1972.
14. Brooks DH, Carey LC: Base deficit in superior mesenteric artery occlusion, an aid to early diagnosis. *Ann Surg* 177:352, 1973.
15. Barnett SM, Davidson ED, Bradley EL: Intestinal alkaline phosphatase and base deficit in mesenteric occlusion. *J Surg Res* 20:243, 1976.
16. Jamieson WG, Wall WJ, Durand D: Changes in serum phosphate levels associated with intestinal infarction and necrosis. *Surg Gynecol Obstet* 140:19, 1975.
17. Sawer BA, Jamieson WG, Durand D: The significance of elevated peritoneal fluid phosphate level in intestinal infarction. *Surg Gynecol Obstet* 146:43, 1978.
18. Taylor BM, Jamieson WG, Durand D: Preinfarction diagnosis of acute mesenteric ischemia by simple measurement of inorganic phosphate in body fluids. *Can J Surg* 22:40, 1979.
19. Jamieson WG, Taylor BN, Troster M, et al: The significance of urine phosphate measurements in the early diagnosis of intestinal infarction. *Surg Gynecol Obstet* 148:334, 1979.
20. O'Connor LR, Klein KL, Bethune JE: Hyperphosphatemia in lactic acidosis. *N Engl J Med* 297:707, 1977.
21. Burnett W, Ness TD: Serum amylase and acute abdominal disease. *Br Med J* 2:770, 1955.
22. Abruzzo JL, Homa M, Houch JC, et al.: Significance of the serum amylase determination. *Ann Surg* 147:921, 1958.
23. Claman C, Hershberg TB, Sleaggs JO, et al: Serum lactic dehydrogenase in diagnosis of acute surgical abdomen. *Surgery* 44:43, 1958.

24. Zimmerman HJ, West M: Serum enzymes in gastrointestinal diseases. *Med Clin North Am* 48:189, 1964.
25. Bounous G, Hugon J: Serum levels of intestinal alkaline phosphatase in relation to shock. *Surgery* 69:238, 1971.
26. Bonakdarpour A, Ming SC, Esterhai JA, et al: Serum alkaline phosphatase and glutamic oxalacetic transaminase in experimental intestinal ischemia. *J Surg Res* 21:409, 1976.
27. Rush BF, Host WR, Fewel J, et al.: Intestinal ischemia and some organic substances in serum and abdominal fluid. *Arch Surg* 105:151, 1972.
28. Delany HM, Moss CM, Carnevale N: The use of enzyme analysis of peritoneal blood in the clinical assessment of abdominal organ injury. *Surg Gynecol Obstet* 142:161, 1976.
29. Moss CM, Baron N, Bernstein L, et al: The origin of the elevated peritoneal fluid alkaline phosphatase activity in small intestinal injury. *J Surg Res* 23:172, 1977.
30. Langman MSJ, Leuthold E, Rakou EB, et al: Influence of diet on the "intestinal" component of serum alkaline phosphatase in people of different ABO blood groups and secretor status. *Nature* 212:41, 1966.
31. Beckman L, Beckman G, Dahlgren S: Isoenzyme variations of serum alkaline phosphatase and naphthyl amidase in biliary and gastrointestinal disease. *Scand J Gastroenterol* 3:241, 1968.
32. Itano M: The detection of CPK_1 (BB) in serum. *Am J Clin Pathol* 65:351, 1976.
33. Lamar W, Woodard L, Statland BE: Clinical implications of creatine kinase-BB isoenzyme. *N Engl J Med* 299:834, 1978.
34. Doran GR: Appearance of creatine kinase BB isoenzyme in the serum of a patient suffering from infarction of the colon. *Clin Chim Acta* 92:415, 1979.
35. Graeber GM, Cafferty PJ, Reardon MJ, et al: Changes in serum total creatine phosphokinase (CPK) and its isoenzymes caused by experimental ligation of the superior mesenteric artery. *Ann Surg* 193:499, 1981.
36. Kusche J, Stahlknecht CD, Lorenz W, et al: Diamine oxidase activity and histamine release in dogs following acute mesenteric artery occlusion. *Agents Actions* 7:81, 1977.
37. Wollin A, Navert H, Bounous G: Effect of intestinal ischemia

on diamine oxidase activity in rat intestinal tissue and blood. *Gastroenterology* 80:349, 1981.
38. Bayless TM, Luk GD, Baylin SB, et al: Decreased plasma diamine oxidase levels with Crohn's disease and celiac disease. *Gastroenterology* 80:1106, 1981.
39. Modlin IM, Bloom SR, Mitchell S: Vasoactive intestinal plasma polypeptide (VIP) levels and intestinal ischemia. *Experientia* 34:535, 1978.
40. Bateson PG, Buchanan KD, Stewart DM, et al: The release of vasoactive intestinal peptide during altered mid-gut blood flow. *Br J Surg* 67:131, 1980.

5

Radiographic Manifestations of Ischemic Bowel Disease

Mary Pat Borgess, M.D.
Wynn Wygal Adam, M.D.

Impairment of arterial or venous blood flow to the gastrointestinal tract results in a variety of radiographic findings. These range from subtle thickening of the mucosal folds of the bowel to gas in the portal veins, suggestive of intestinal gangrene. The consequences of vascular occlusion depend upon the duration of the ischemia, length of the intestine involved, the rapidity of onset, and collateral channels available.

The role of the radiologist in the diagnosis and management of patients with ischemic bowel disease has changed considerably over the past ten years with the advent of specific angiographic criteria for the diagnosis of intestinal ischemia. If the angiogram shows the changes of vasospasm, the radiologist may play a role in treatment with an intraarterial vasodilator infusion shown to decrease the mortality of mesenteric ischemia.

Radiologic Management

Plain abdominal radiographs should be made immediately. These will suggest intestinal ischemia in a significant number of cases, and alternatively, they may give a clue to previously unsuspected other causes of the patient's symptoms, such as a perforated viscus.

If the plain radiographs suggest ischemia in the distribution of the superior mesenteric artery, an angiogram should be performed. Even if the plain films are unremarkable and there is a strong clinical suspicion of intestinal ischemia, angiography is indicated. If the angiogram shows emboli, thrombosis, or changes of nonocclusive mesenteric ischemia, specific therapy can be started.

If the radiographs or clinical presentation are compatible with inferior mesenteric ischemia, a barium enema should be performed, ideally within 48 hours of the onset of symptoms.

If these procedures are not diagnostic and the clinical presentation is confusing, an upper gastrointestinal and small bowel barium study may be helpful.

Plain Film Findings

The plain films should include an upright chest film, and supine, erect, and decubitus films of the abdomen. Chest films are important because patients with an apparent abdominal process may, in fact, have chest disease. Lung parenchymal or pleural disease may stimulate sensory nerves in the diaphragm and lower chest wall, causing referred pain to the abdomen that may closely mimic acute abdominal disease. Pneumonia, esophageal perforation, and diaphragmatic hernias commonly present with epigastric symptoms. Furthermore, chest film findings may point to a specific underlying cause of the intraabdominal problem, such as congestive heart failure or cardiomegaly in nonocclusive mesenteric ischemia. In cases of subphrenic or subhepatic abscesses, the chest film findings may precede the abdominal film changes. As little as one or two cubic centimeters of free intraperitoneal air from a perforated viscus can frequently be detected on erect chest and abdominal films or decubitus abdominal films.

The supine abdominal film gives the best overall view of the abdomen in terms of gas pattern, calcifications, bony structures, and soft tissue masses. The erect film is helpful in the evaluation of free intraperitoneal air, air-fluid levels, pseudotumors,[1,2] and the presence of fixed or rigid bowel loops.[3] The decubitus film may also demonstrate free air, fixed and rigid loops, and is very helpful in differentiating large from small bowel. Generally, the left side down decubitus film (left lateral decubitus) is the most useful, since air trapped in the lesser sac from posterior duodenal perforation can escape into the right flank through the foramen of Winslow.[4] The hepatic contour and iliac crest are the most superior portions of the peritoneum in the left lateral decubitus position, so attention is focused on these areas in an inspection for free air. The right side down (right lateral decubitus) usually is not obtained unless the patient is unable to lie on his left side.

The simplest way to classify ischemic bowel is to distinguish between mild and severe forms. Mild cases result from transient ischemia and may resolve with complete healing, or may result in strictures. Severe cases are the result of transmural infarction with gangrene. Some authors feel that radiology contributes little to the diagnosis in these patients, whereas others have found that plain films and barium studies may be important in detecting the presence of gangrene, leading to earlier surgical intervention.[5]

Positive plain radiographic findings have been reported in 20 to 60% of cases.[6,7] In one series, 21% of the plain abdominal radiographs were specific and an additional 18% were suggestive of ischemia.[8] Early in the course of the disease the findings are nonspecific. In the presence of colonic ischemia, there is a mild increase in the amount of gastrointestinal gas in both the large and small bowel. The appearance is one of paralytic ileus (Figure 1). When superior mesenteric ischemia is present, a moderate to marked amount of gas is located primarily in the small bowel. In 50% of patients the pattern suggests a bowel obstruction (Figure 2).[8,9] Occasionally, the abdomen may show no abdominal gas, or have intraperitoneal fluid.[6]

The most reliable finding is "thumbprinting". Allen et al. believe the submucosa is the layer most sensitive to vascular insult and first manifests changes.[10] Edema and congestion develop in the submucosa and localized hemorrhage can occur. If the mucosa is intact, the intestinal lumen has a scalloped contour on the radiographs termed thumbprinting (Figure 3).[2,6,8,11–14] Such a pattern can also occur in hemophilia, allergic reactions, Henoch-Schönlein purpura, anticoagulant therapy, or trauma due to submucosal hemorrhage (Figure 4).[15] As the edema and hemorrhage become more diffuse, discrete thumbprinting will be lost and replaced by blunting and thickening of the mucosal folds. This is termed transverse ridging and gives a corrugated pattern to the bowel contour (Figure 5).[8,13]

Still later in the course of the disease, all the mucosal pattern will be lost and the bowel will have a narrowed tubular appearance. At this stage the gas filled loops frequently appear separated, mostly due to edema of the bowel wall and mesentery, but also due to overfilling of the lumen with fluid. These loops commonly appear rigid at fluoroscopy and fixed in the abdomen, showing no positional change between the supine and erect abdominal films (Figure 6).[3] As ischemia progresses, the bowel becomes flaccid, dilated, and noncontractile. A loop with this appearance should raise the suspicion of transmural infarction. (See Figure 3.)[9–11,13,19] If the transmural infarction occurs in the colon, the pattern resembles that of toxic megacolon; the transverse colon is greatly dilated and has an ulcerated,

(Text continued on page 78)

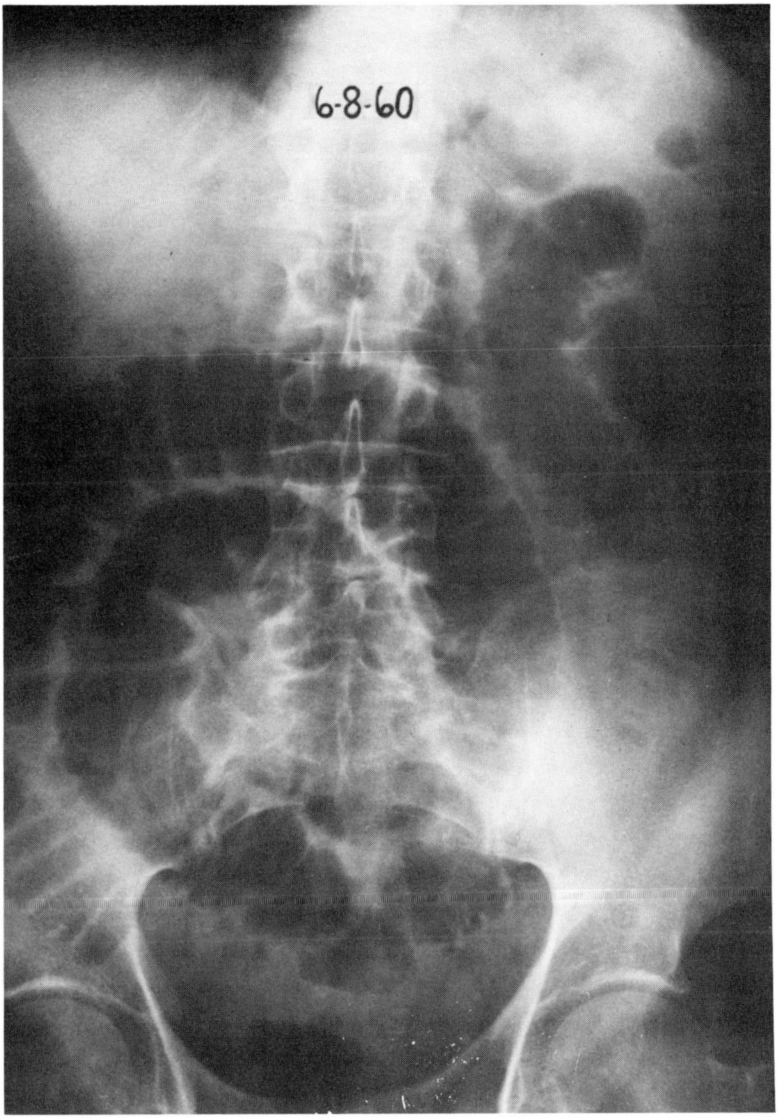

Figure 1A. A supine abdominal film shows several dilated loops of small bowel.

(Illustration continued on the following page)

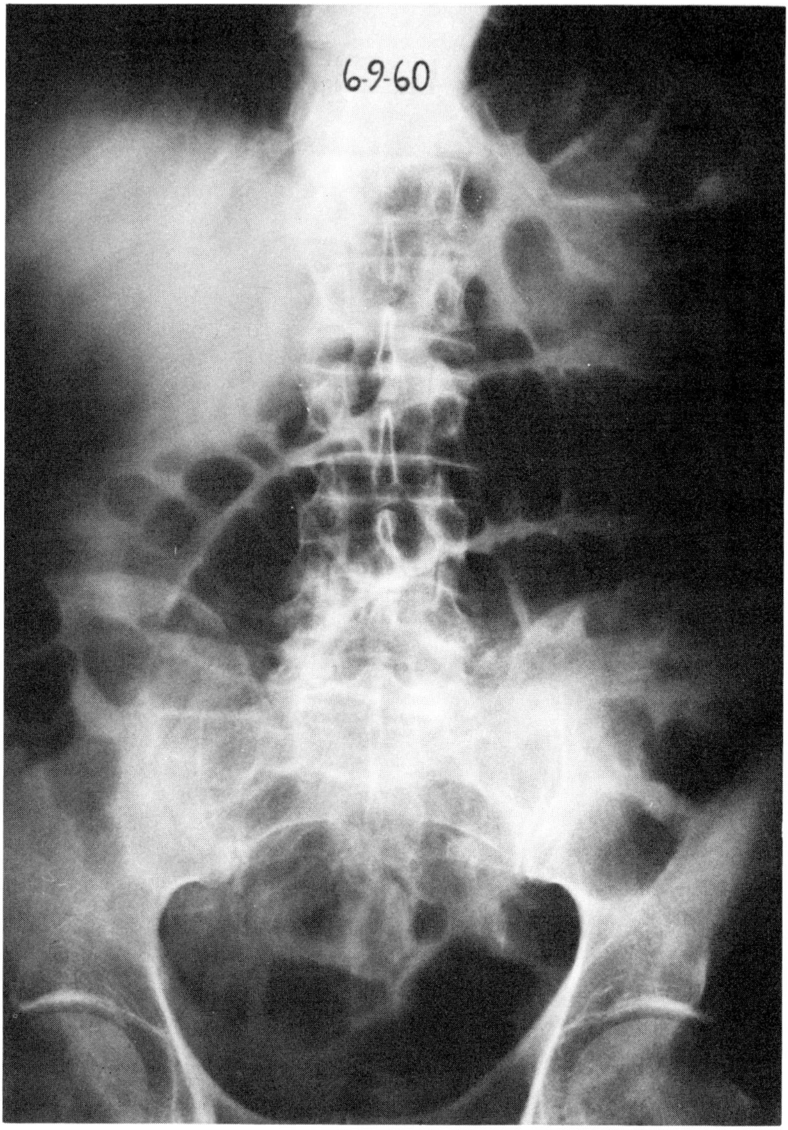

Figure 1B. Another film made one day later shows gas in a distended colon. The progression of gas makes obstruction unlikely. This was proved mesenteric ischemia.

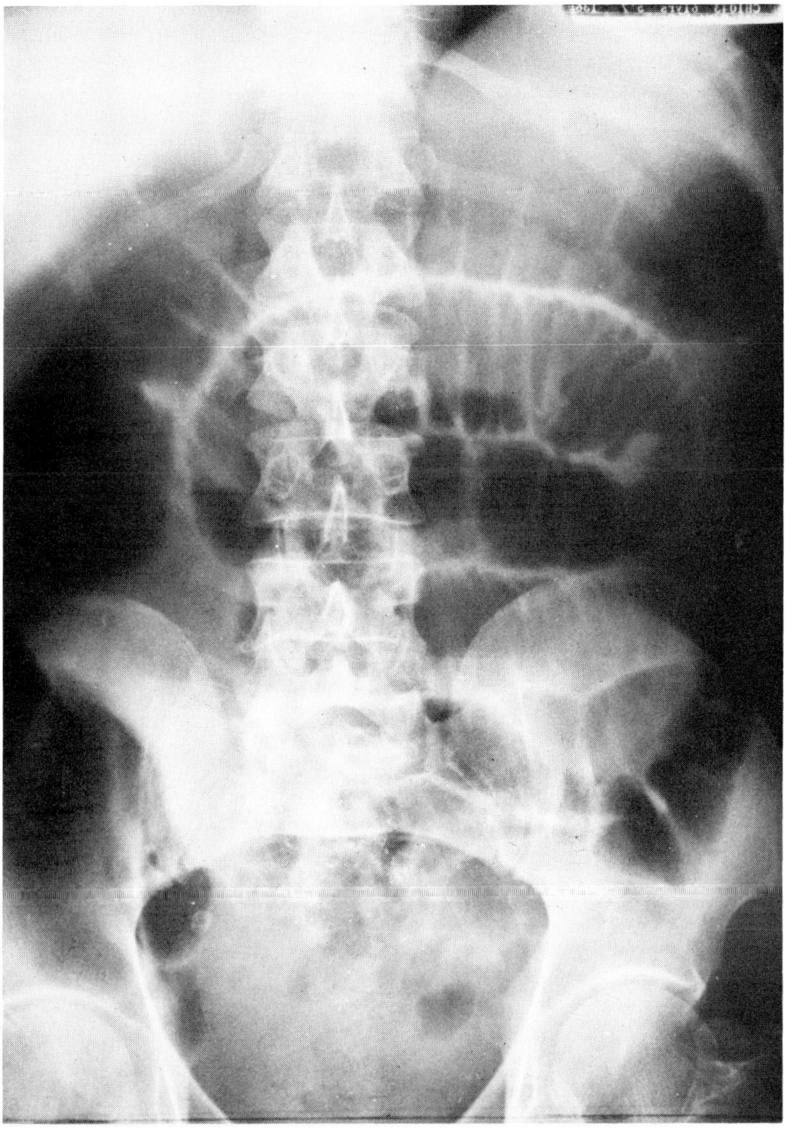

Figure 2. Patient was an elderly man with an acute abdomen. Supine (A) and erect (B) abdominal films show marked small bowel dilatation and colonic dilatation proximal to splenic flexure. The radiologic picture cannot be distinguished from an obstructing lesion at the splenic flexure. He had an acute superior mesenteric artery embolus.

(Illustration continued on the following page)

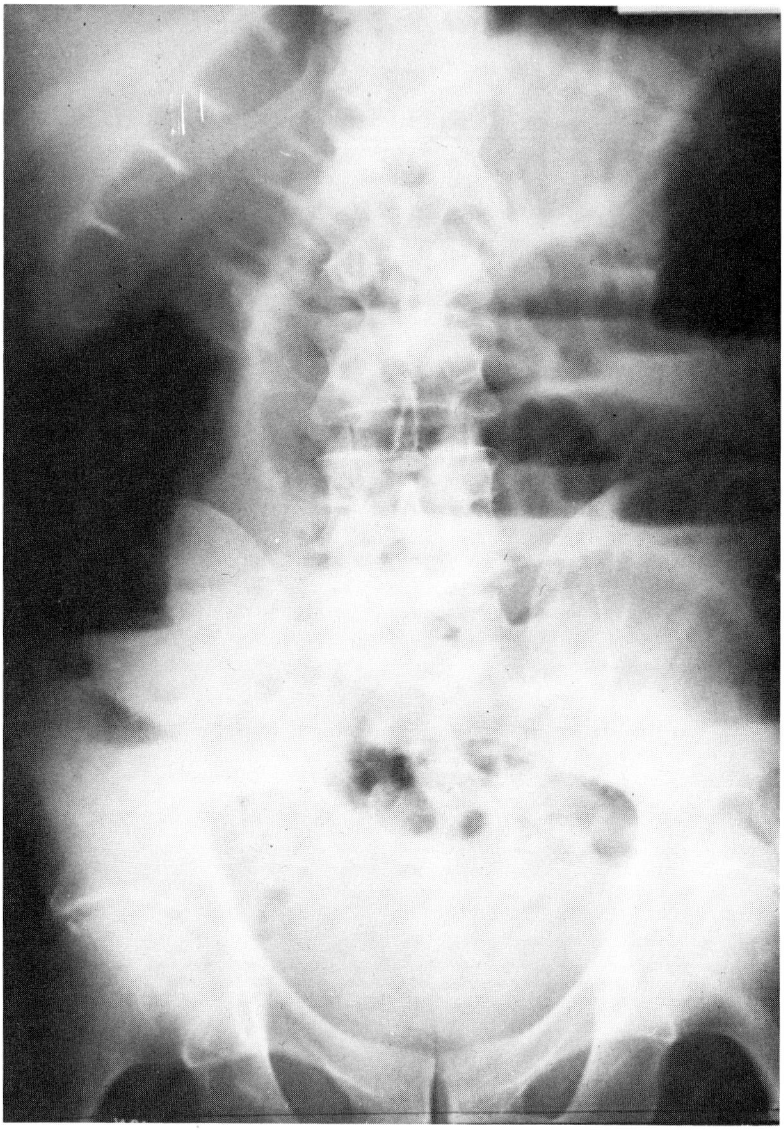

Figure 2B.

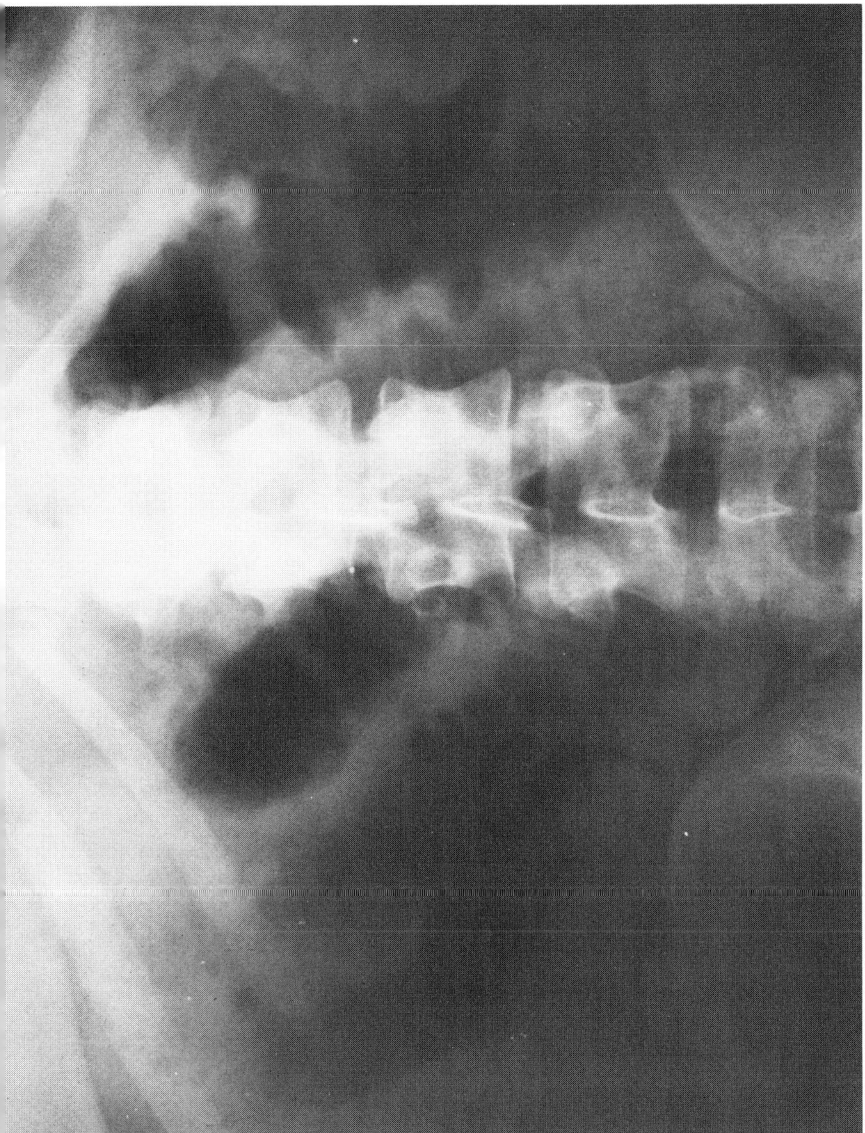

Figure 3A. Supine abdominal film of a 23-year-old woman 2-3 weeks after Caesarean section. Separation of mildly dilated proximal small bowel with some areas of thumbprinting are present.

(Illustration continued on the following page)

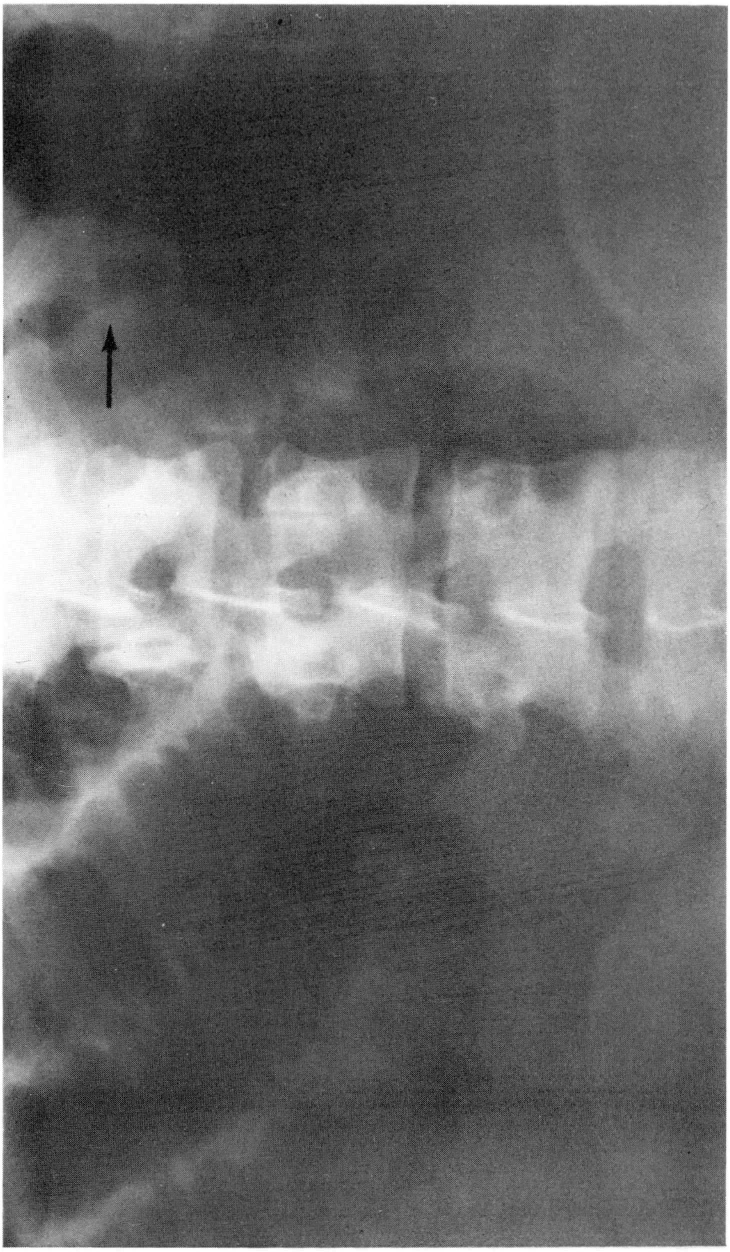

Figure 3B. Preliminary and (C) 2-hour films from a small bowel examination 3 days after (A) show a flaccid aperistaltic loop of bowel (arrow) which is seen in transmural infarction. This was confirmed at operation; however, the etiology was not established. This could have been secondary to a postpartum hypercoagulable state.

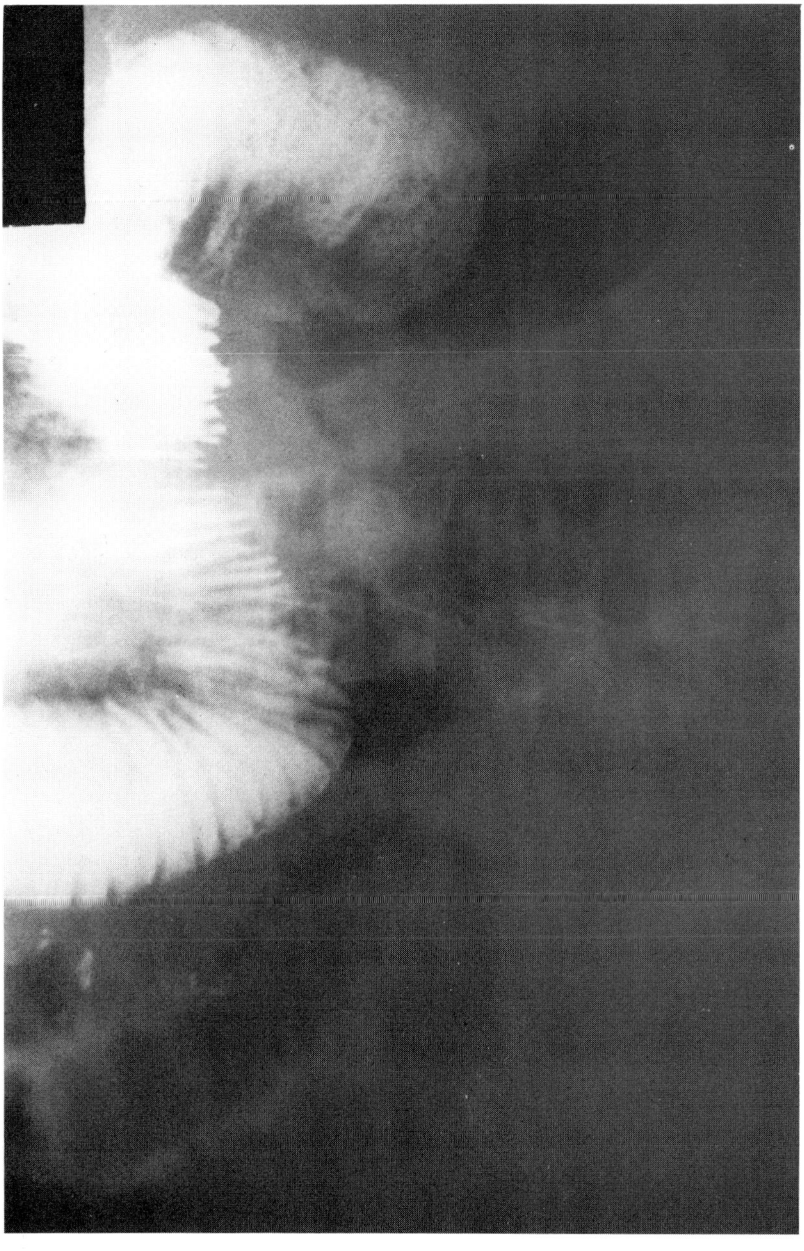

Figure 3C.

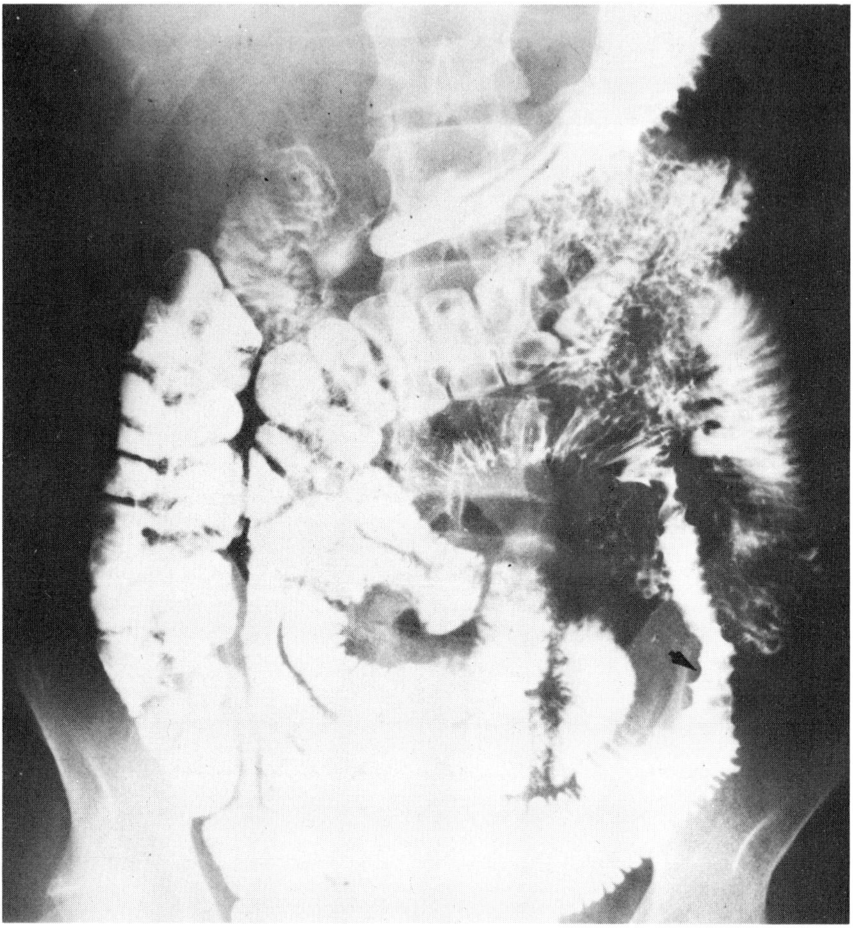

Figure 4. Patient was a young man with hemophilia who had crampy abdominal pain. Small bowel series shows a long loop of jejunum with thumbprinting (→) and separation of bowel loops consistent with intramural and mesenteric hemorrhage.

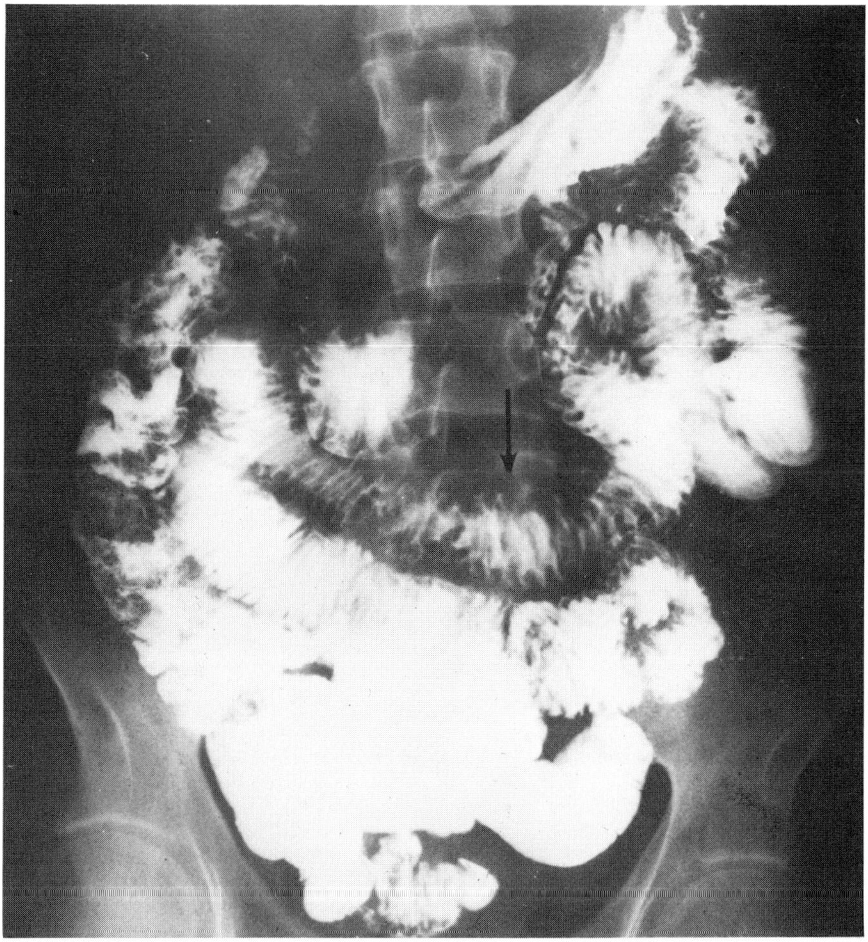

Figure 5. Small bowel study shows straight, regularly aligned, thickened folds in a loop of jejunum (arrow). This is called transverse ridging.

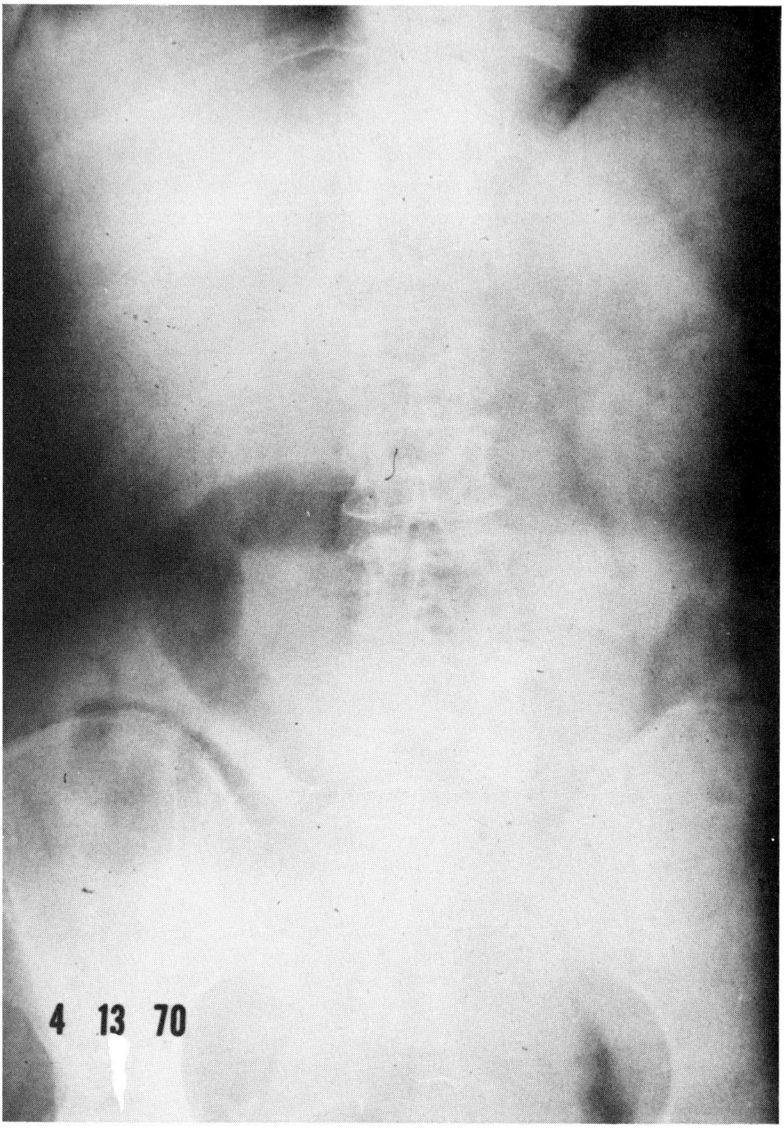

Figure 6. Patient was a middle-aged woman with an acute abdomen. Initial abdominal film (A) and those obtained 8 days later (B) demonstrate a long, smoothly contoured, slightly narrowed loop of small bowel that appears fixed in the abdomen without change. Haziness suggests free peritoneal fluid. Findings are highly suggestive of small bowel infarction, which was confirmed at operation.

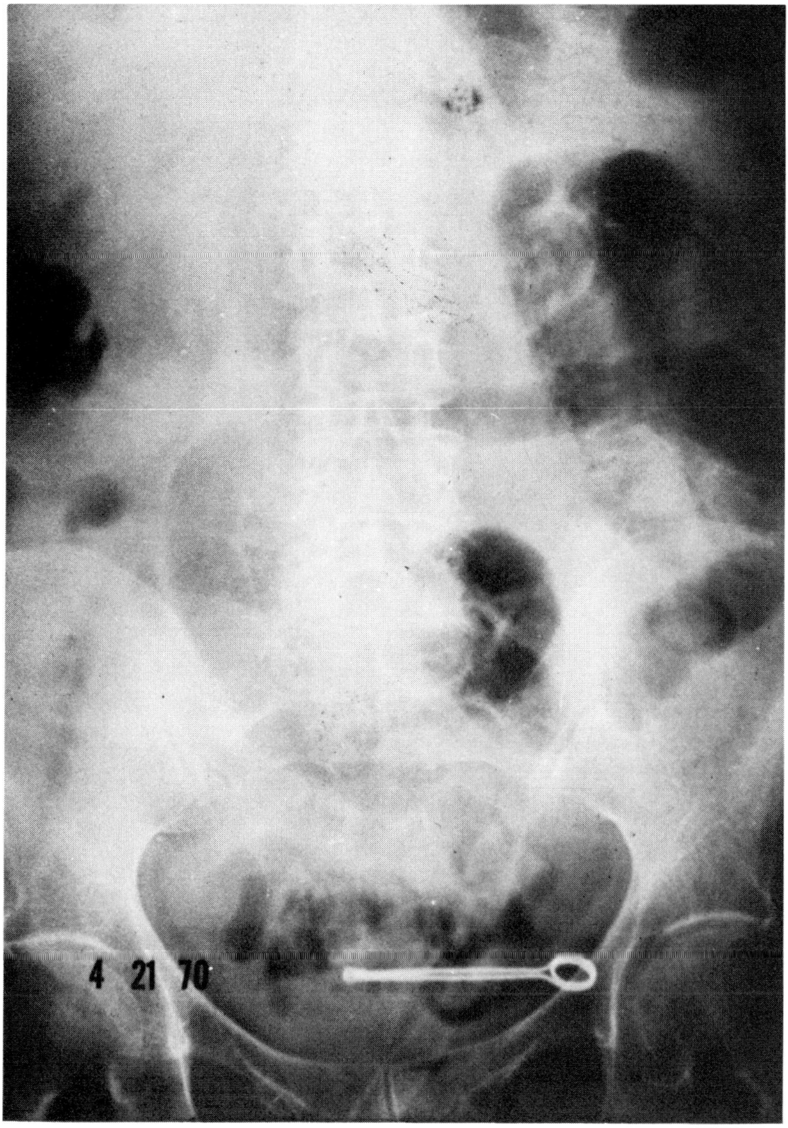

Figure 6B.

pseudopolypoid mucosa.[17] Air-fluid levels may be seen in this segment.[5] The appearance may be radiographically indistinguishable from that of ulcerative or granulomatous colitis.[11]

Uncommonly, free intraperitoneal gas, intramural gas, or portal venous gas can be seen (Figure 7). Gas in the portal vein may be seen either in association with gas in the bowel wall or as an isolated finding. Although 72% are secondary to necrotic bowel, this finding has been associated with intraabdominal abscesses, bowel obstructions,

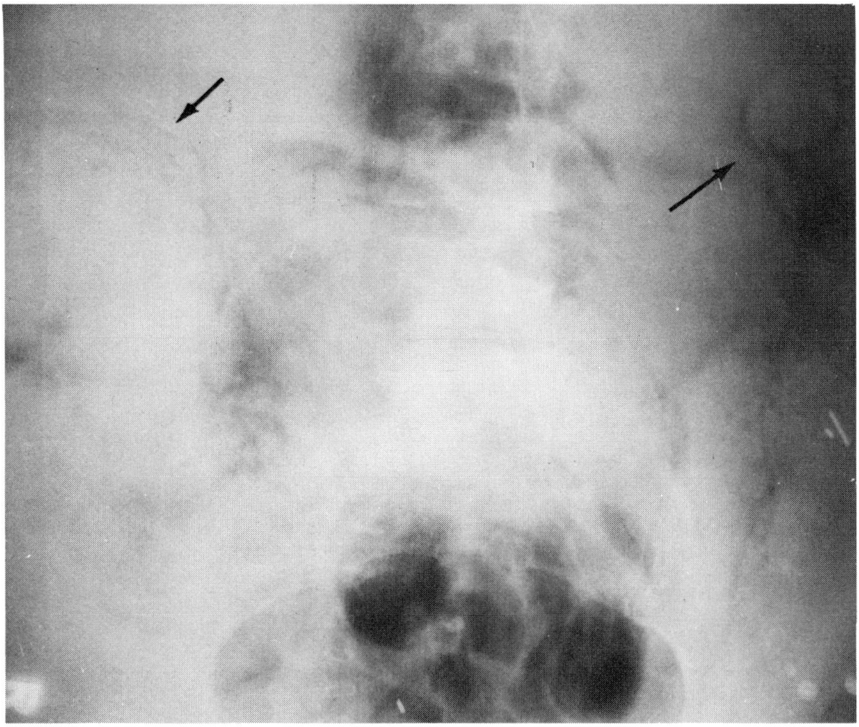

Figure 7. Supine abdominal film shows crescent-shaped and linear gas collections paralleling the bowel lumen. This appearance is characteristic of intramural gas. At autopsy, patient was found to have occlusion of the celiac axis, superior mesenteric and inferior mesenteric arteries with gangrenous bowel.

and peptic ulcer disease.[20] The presence of gas in the portal vein or bowel wall does not correlate with the extent of intestinal necrosis. Intramural air may occasionally be seen after sigmoidoscopy in patients with ulcerative or granulomatous colitis.[20]

Intramural gas is caused by dissection of the bowel wall by air, but in all probability, gas-producing bacteria also play a major role. Intramural gas may occur alone or in association with gas in the branches of the portal vein. This appears as a branching, radiolucent pattern that extends peripherally nearly to the liver capsule (Figure 8). The peripheral location is helpful in distinguishing this from air in the biliary tree, which tends to have a more central position. The difference in location is due to the centripetal flow of bile in contrast to the centrifugal flow of portal blood.[12,20,21] Hepatic gangrene, liver abscesses, and necrotic tumors may also be associated with liver gas, but these entities do not have a branching pattern. Intramural or portal venous gas implies a poor prognosis, and mortality is about 81%.[12]

Barium Studies

A barium enema study should be done as soon as possible if ischemic colitis is suspected. The findings on an initial barium study may not be diagnostic of ischemia, and therefore sequential studies are recommended.[13]

Early in the course of the disease, the barium studies reflect the plain abdominal radiographic findings, but provide better visualization. Thumbprinting or thickened, blunted folds are seen with submucosal edema or hemorrhage (Figures 9–13). More severe ischemia results in mucosal damage. The blood and fluid are then discharged through a break in the mucosa into the lumen, forming ulcers (Figures 14 and 16).[10–22] The presence of ulcerations may denote a worse prognosis than simple exudate.

(*Text continued on page 88*)

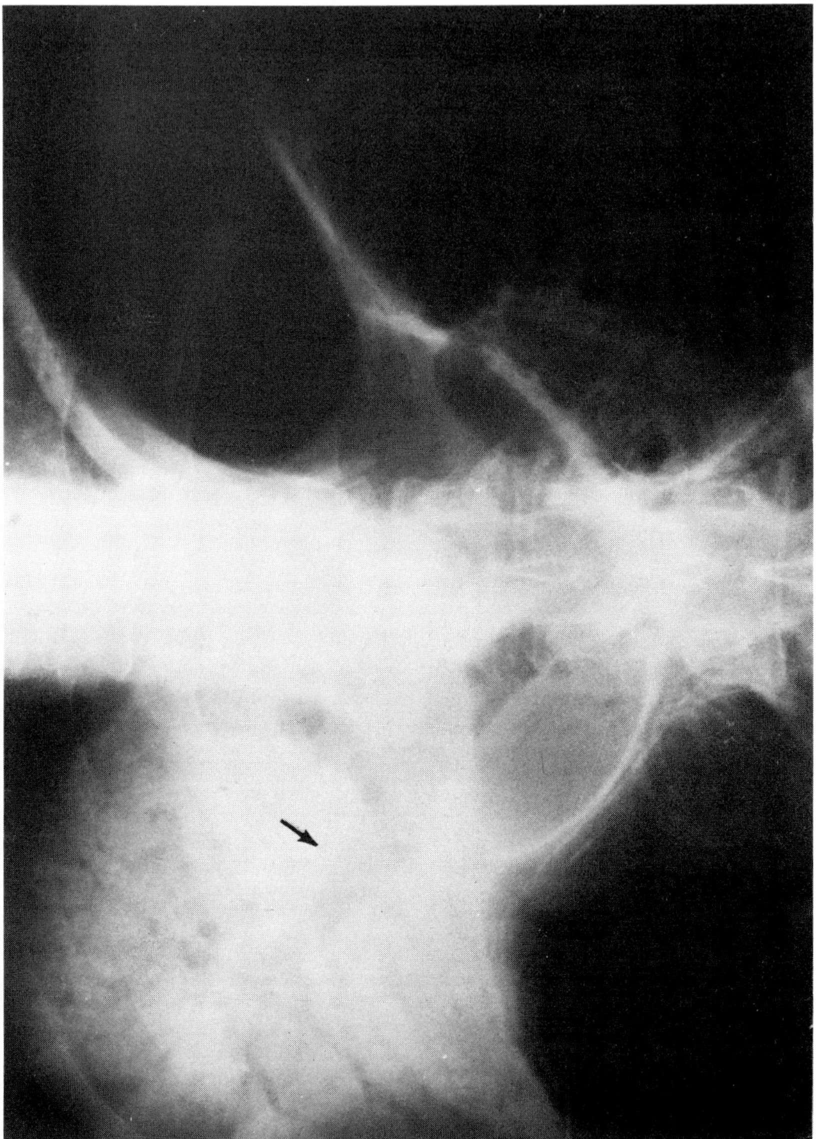

Figure 8. Supine abdominal film nicely demonstrates the classic pattern of hepatic portal venous gas in association with linear streaks of gas in the wall of dilated loops of bowel. Autopsy revealed extensive gangrenous bowel secondary to multiple thrombosis of the superior mesenteric, inferior mesenteric, and gastric arteries.

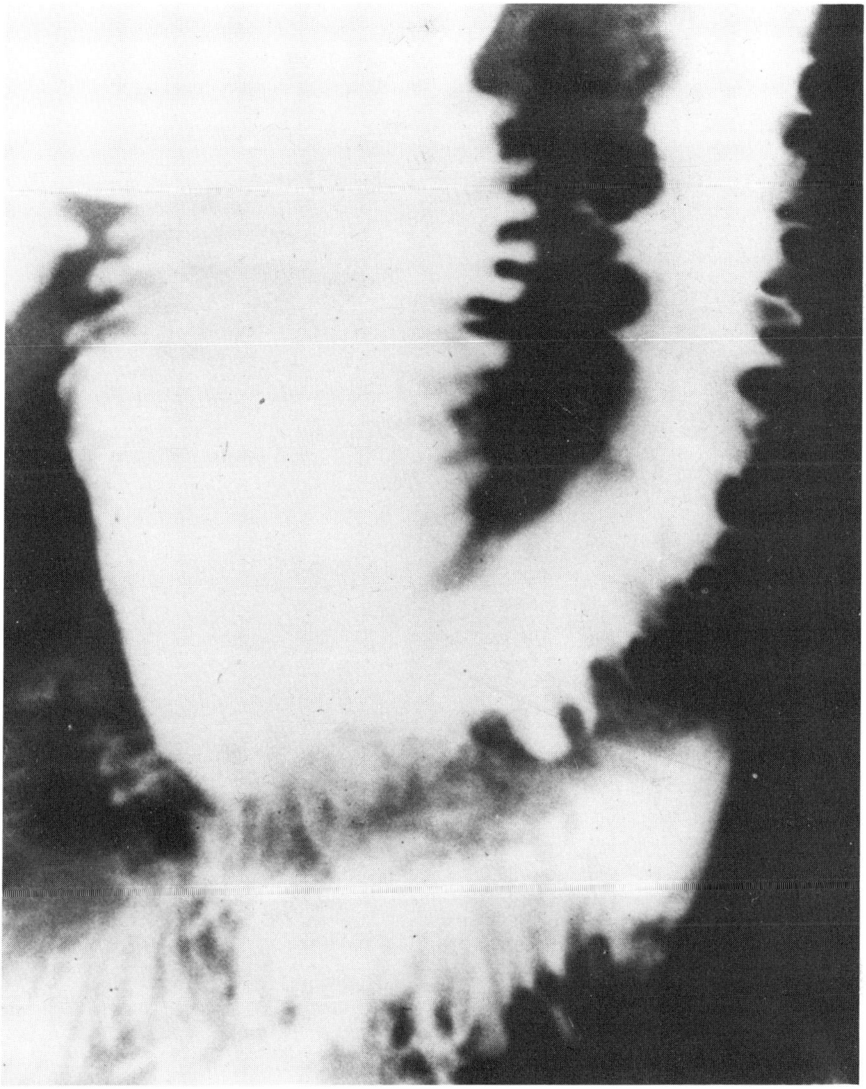

Figure 9. Spot film of small bowel demonstrates marked thumbprinting. (Published with permission of Dunbar JD, Nelson SW: *Am J. Radiol. Ther.* 99:127–135, 1967.)

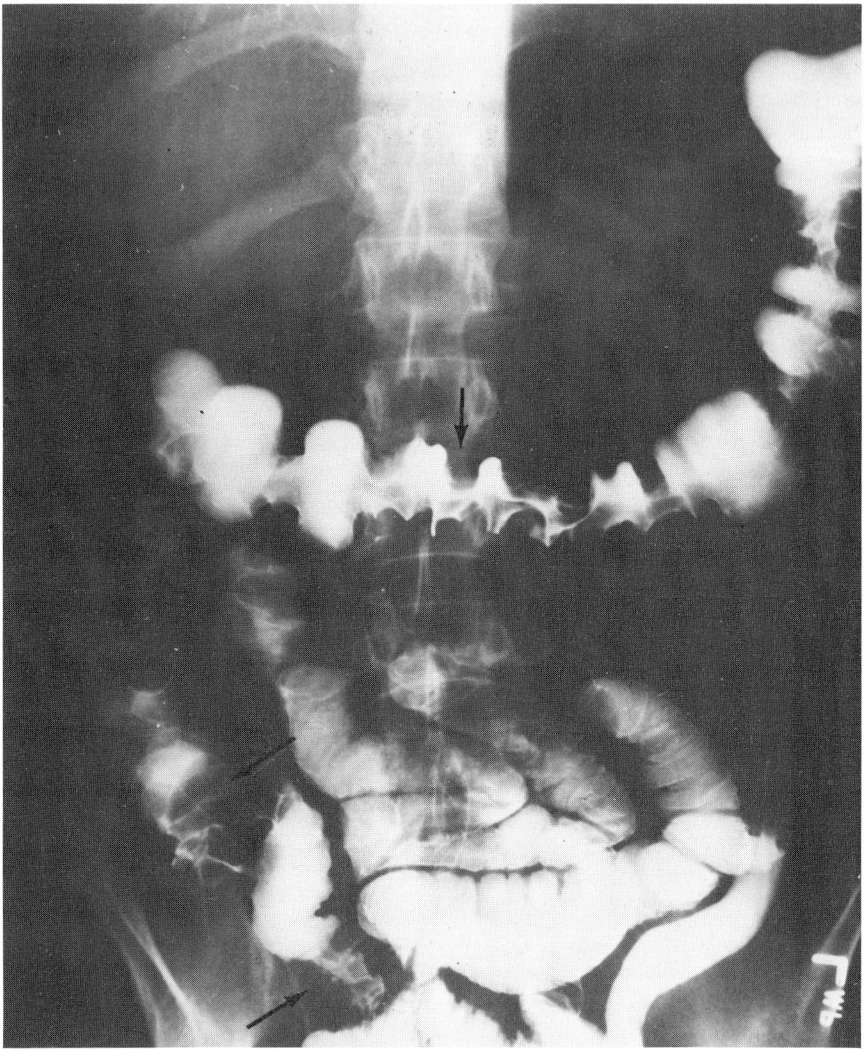

Figure 10. Patient was middle-aged woman with abdominal pain localizing to right lower quadrant. Barium enema film demonstrates striking thumbprinting of the terminal ileum, the right and transverse colons, presumed to be superior mesenteric ischemia. She did well with expectant therapy.

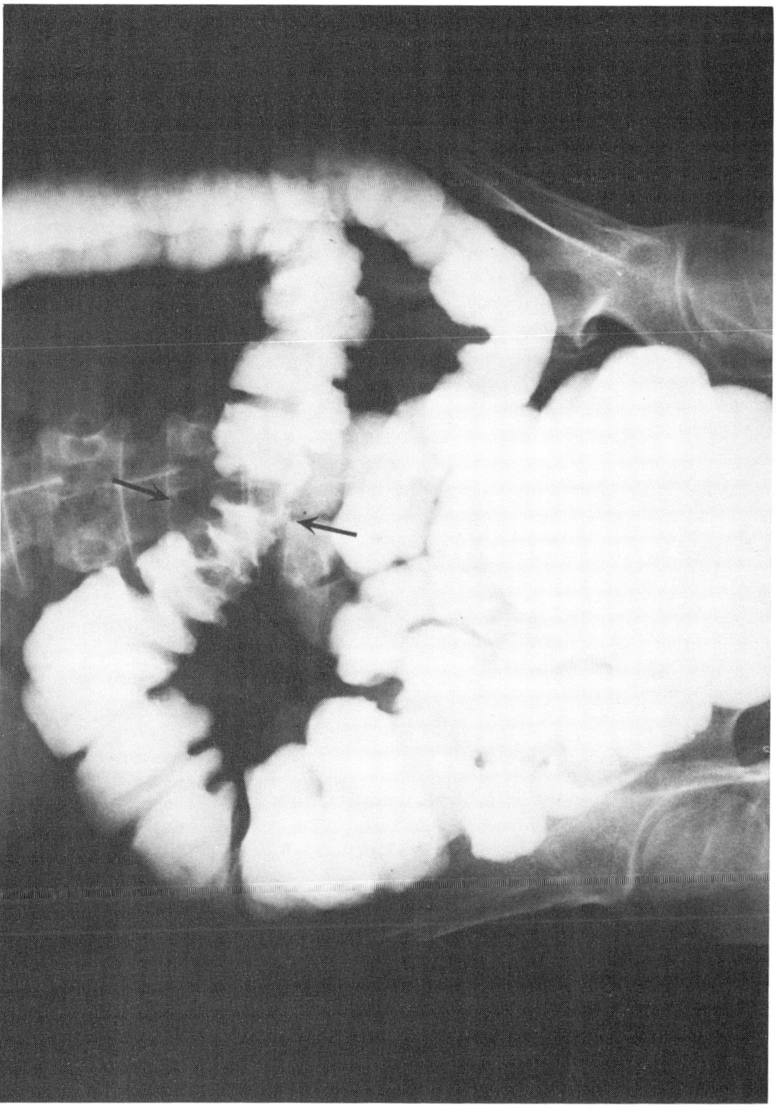

Figure 11. Patient was a 54-year-old white woman with a three-year history of intermittent crampy abdominal pain with diarrhea which was attributed to colitis. Barium enema done during a symptomatic phase showed thumbprinting of a short segment of proximal transverse colon. Laparctomy showed ischemia of colon and small bowel. Patient became asymptomatic after an endarterectomy of the superior mesenteric artery. (Published with permission from Dunbar JD, Nelson SJ.: *Am J. Radiol. Ther. Nucl. Med.*, 99:127–135, 1967.)

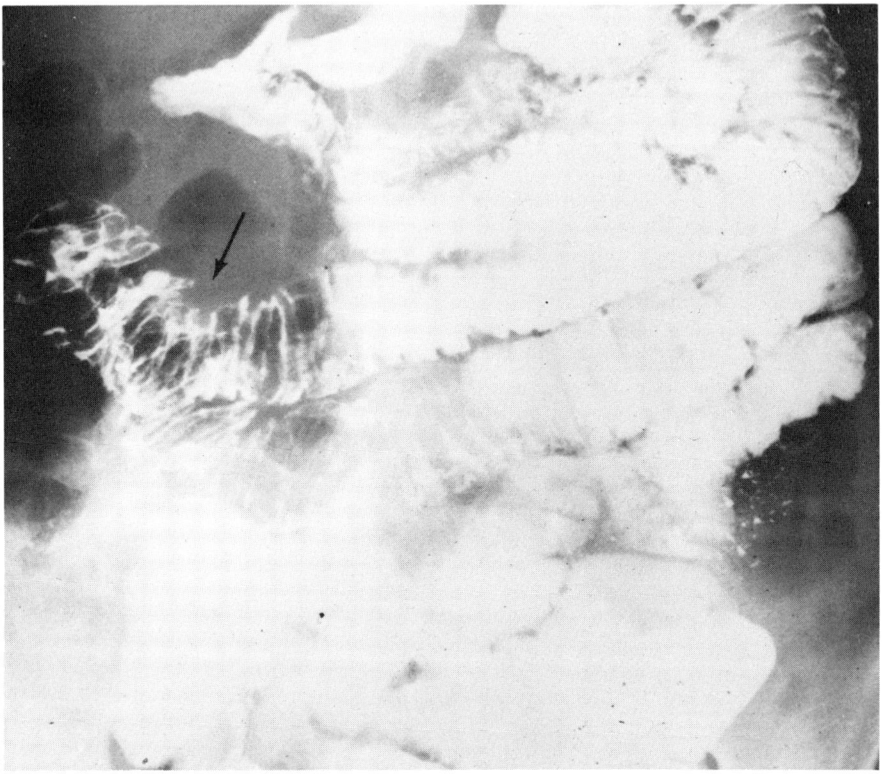

Figure 12. Small bowel film shows transverse ridging.

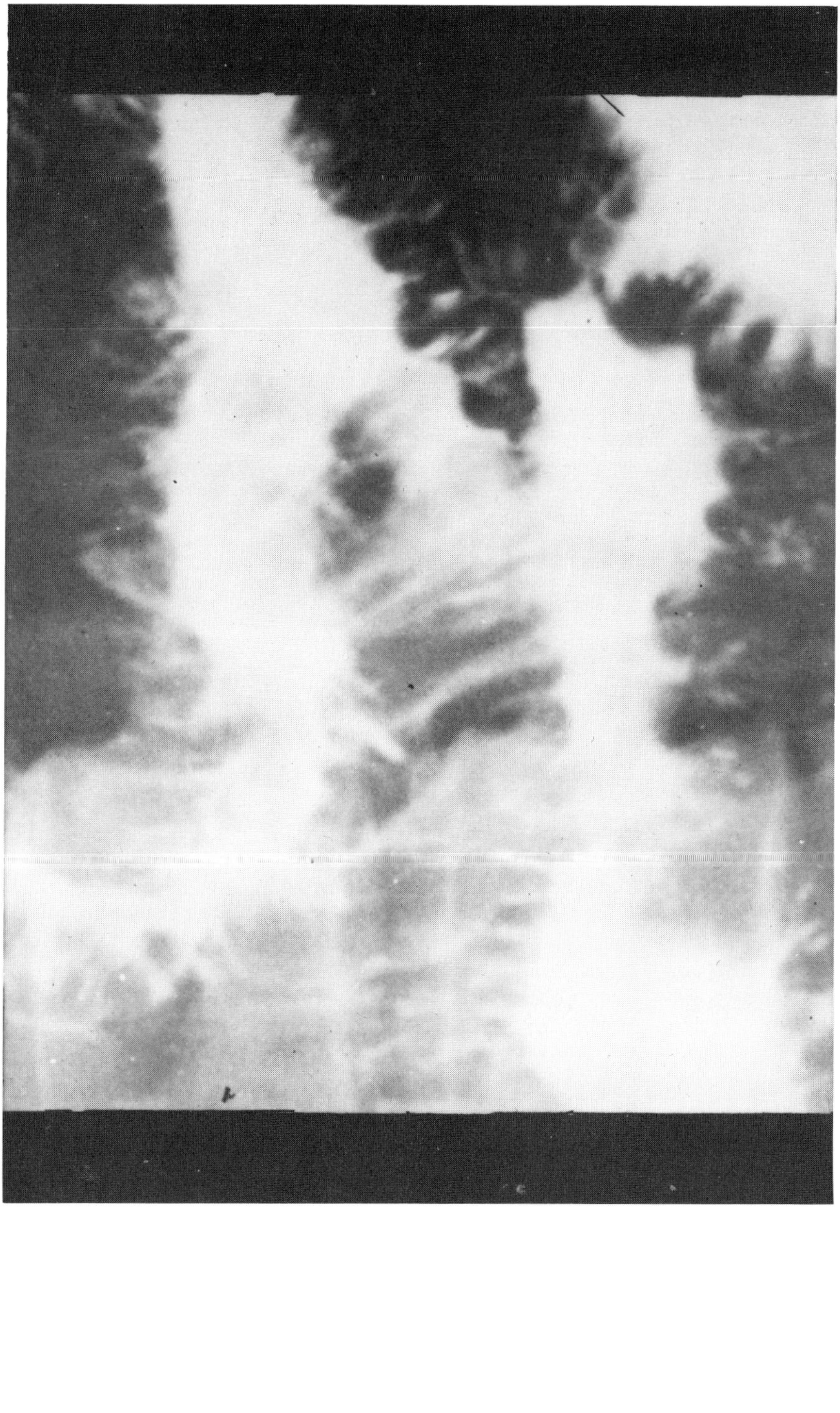

Figure 13. A patient with lupus arteritis shows thumbprinting, thickened folds, and transverse ridging on a small bowel spot film.

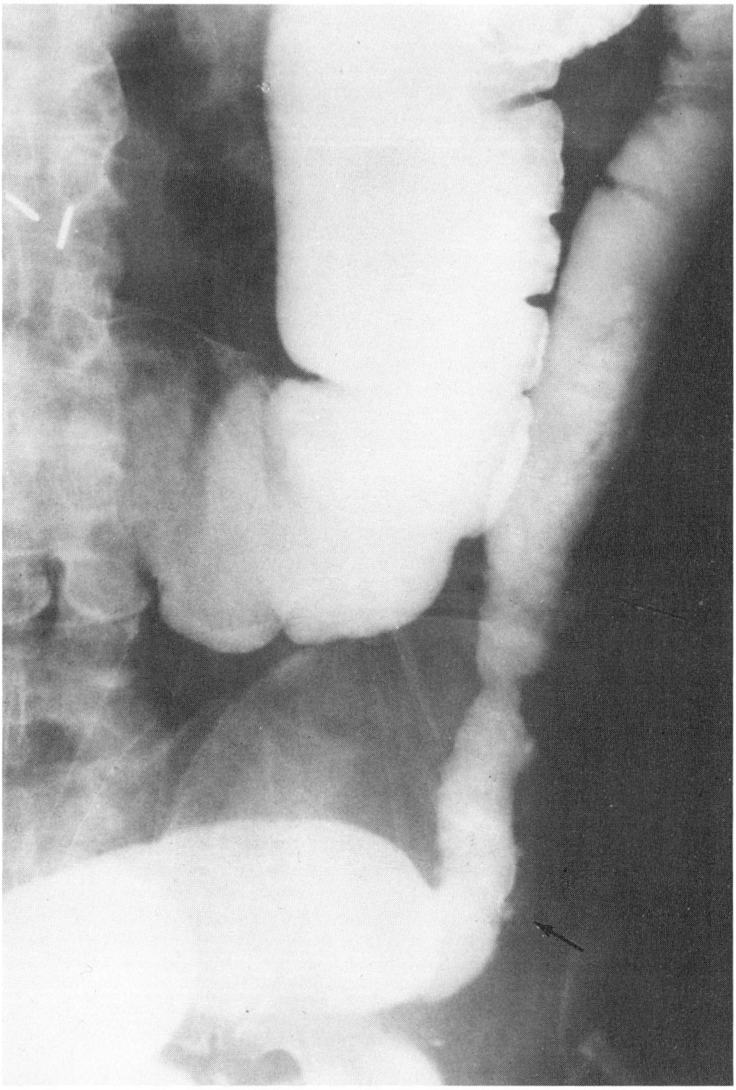

Figure 14A. A 54-year-old white man had bright red rectal bleeding 2 weeks after repair of a ruptured abdominal aortic aneurysm. Full-column barium enema film shows narrowing of descending colon and multiple ulcers (→).

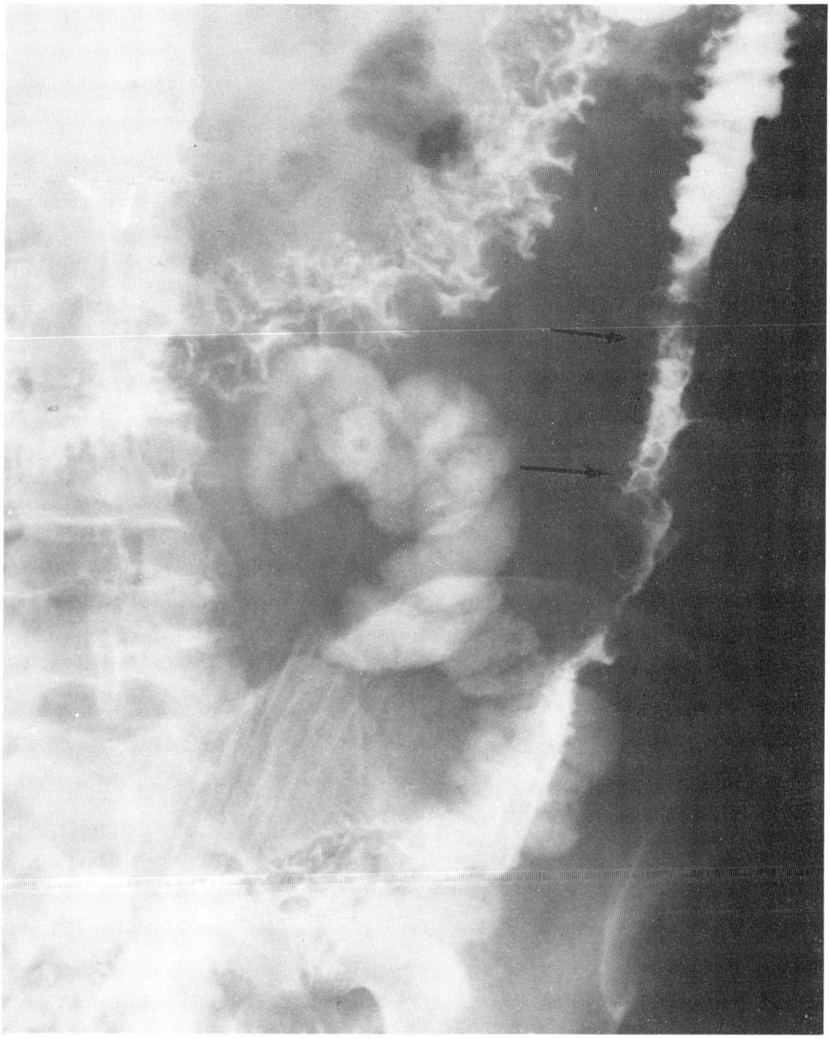

Figure 14B. Postevacuation film shows pseudopolypoid or cobblestone appearance (→).

The ulcerations are commonly superficial and generally resemble those of ulcerative colitis. Deep ulcers can occur and have been likened to an Erlenmeyer flask. Flask-shaped ulcers strongly suggest bowel ischemia, but unfortunately are seen in only about 10% of cases.[23] While uncommon, retroperitoneal abscesses occur and patients with continuing symptoms of ischemic colitis should have a repeat barium enema to disprove a walled-off perforation.[27] Rarely, deep ulcerations with intramural fistulae can occur (Figure 15) but this is much more common in diverticulitis, Crohn's disease, and malignant neoplasms.[11–15] Initial barium studies have been shown to correlate well with the extent of the disease.[8,22] Once the extent of the disease is defined on the initial barium enema, repeat studies are recommended every week to monitor healing.

The radiographic changes of colonic ischemia on barium enema studies are analogous to those in the small bowel seen on barium studies. Regardless of whether small bowel ischemia was diagnosed on small bowel barium studies, at angiography, or at operation, follow-up barium studies are recommended to monitor healing.

Healing Stage

The amount of damage to the bowel depends on the duration of the ischemia, the rapidity of its onset, and the adequacy of collateral blood supply. If damage is limited to the mucosa and submucosa, complete healing without residual deformity is the rule. If ischemia involves the muscular layer, fibrosis occurs, leading to stenosis. If all layers of the bowel wall are involved, gangrene results.

Early in the healing process, submucosal hemorrhages are reabsorbed, and the mucosal ulcers heal. In more severe disease, as the reparative process continues, fibrous tissue begins to form. Radiographically, this appears as flattening and rigidity of one border of the colon with the contralat-

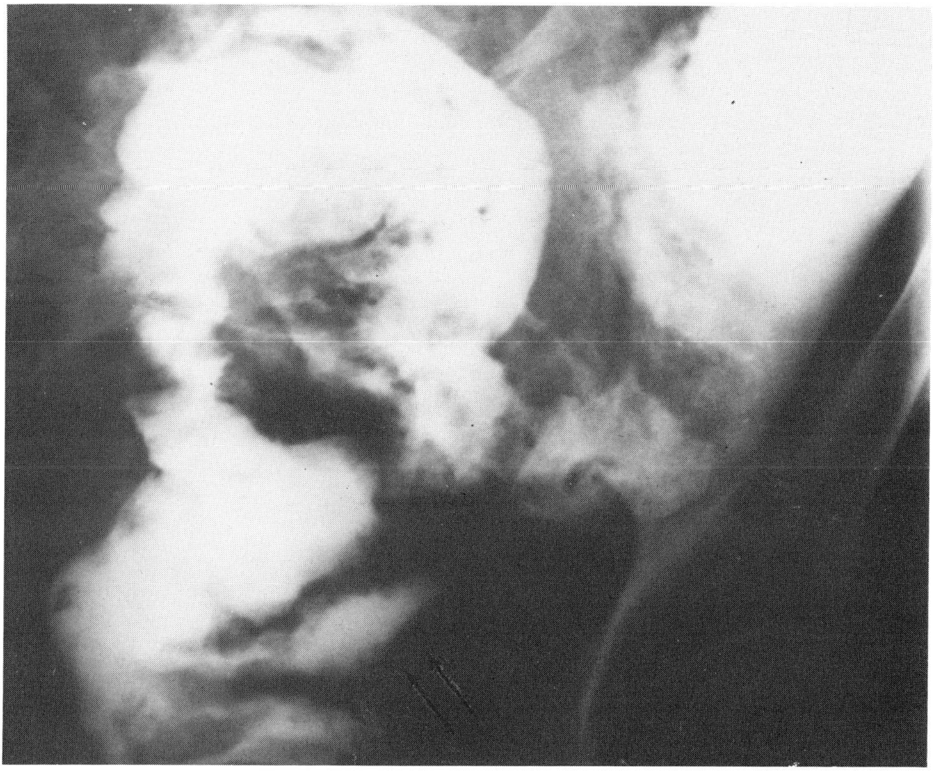

Figure 15. An elderly man had a two-week history of bloody diarrhea. Barium enema shows double lumen in the rectosigmoid. Mucosa had sloughed and formed an intramural fistula (→). Angiogram confirmed the presence of complete occlusion of the inferior mesenteric artery.

eral contour becoming pleated. Eventually sacculations or pseudodiverticula appear (Figures 16 and 17)[25–28] and with further fibrosis, the bowel lumen has a concentric narrowing with smooth tapered margins (Figures 18 and 19).[26–28] The stricture can be of any length, but is usually between 7 and 10 cm.[27] If a series of barium enemas show the ex-

(*Text continued on page 97*)

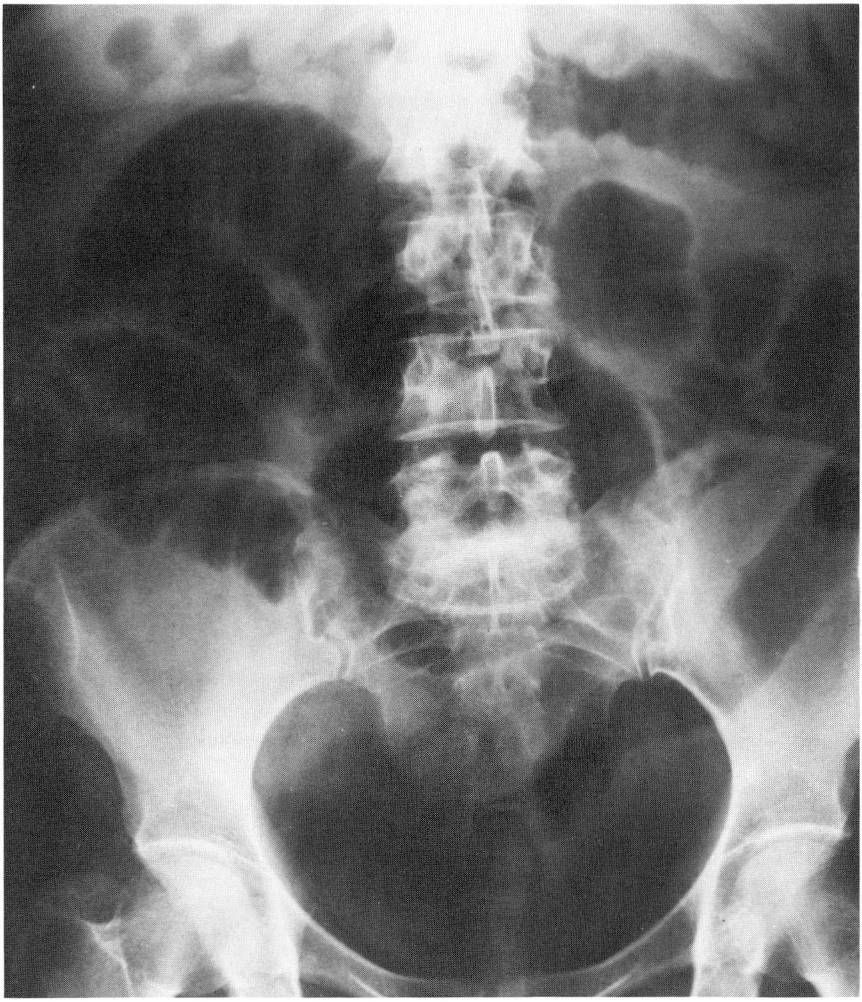

Figure 16A. Supine abdominal film (A) reveals dilatation of several loops of small bowel associated with gas in the colon and adynamic ileus pattern. Thumbprinting is seen in the transverse colon.

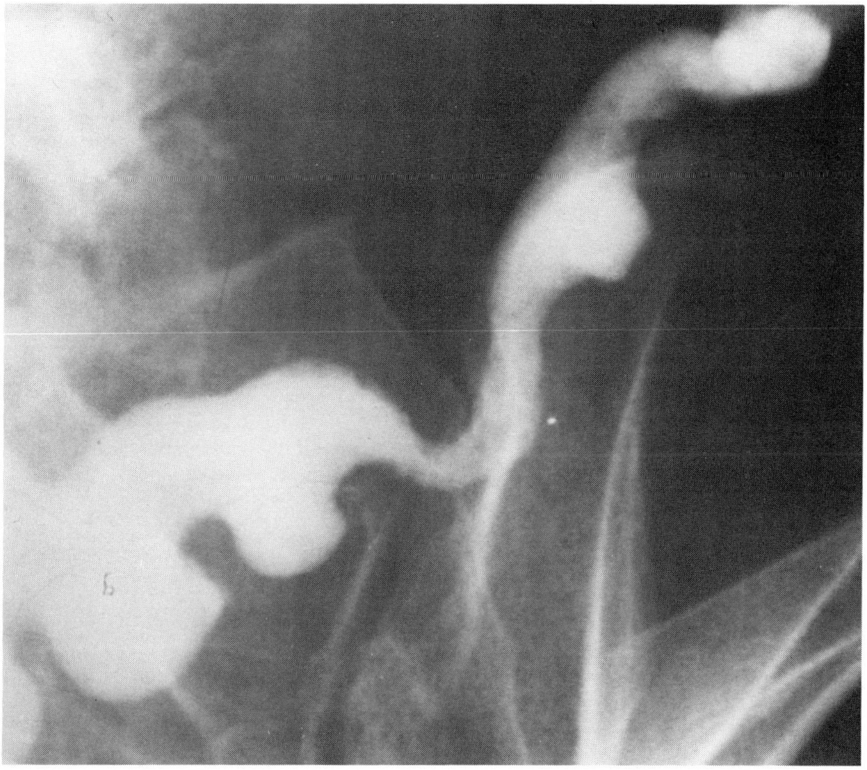

Figure 16B. (See also Figures 16C and D.) Barium enema two weeks later demonstrates mucosal irregularity with superficial ulcerations, thickened blunted mucosal folds with thumbprinting and pseudosacculations.

(Illustration continued on the following page)

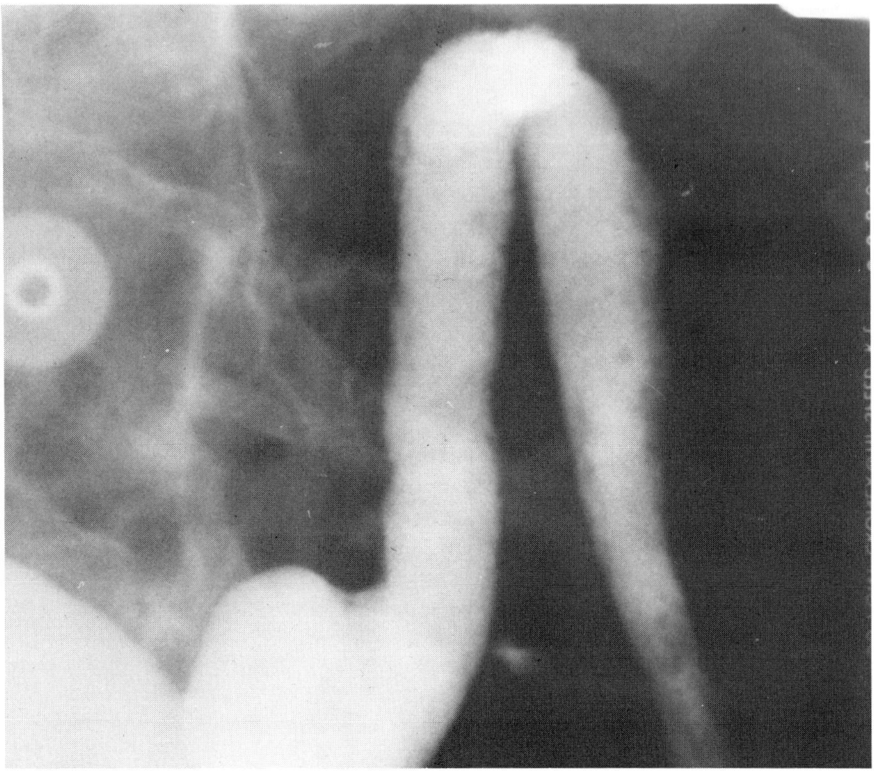

Figure 16C.

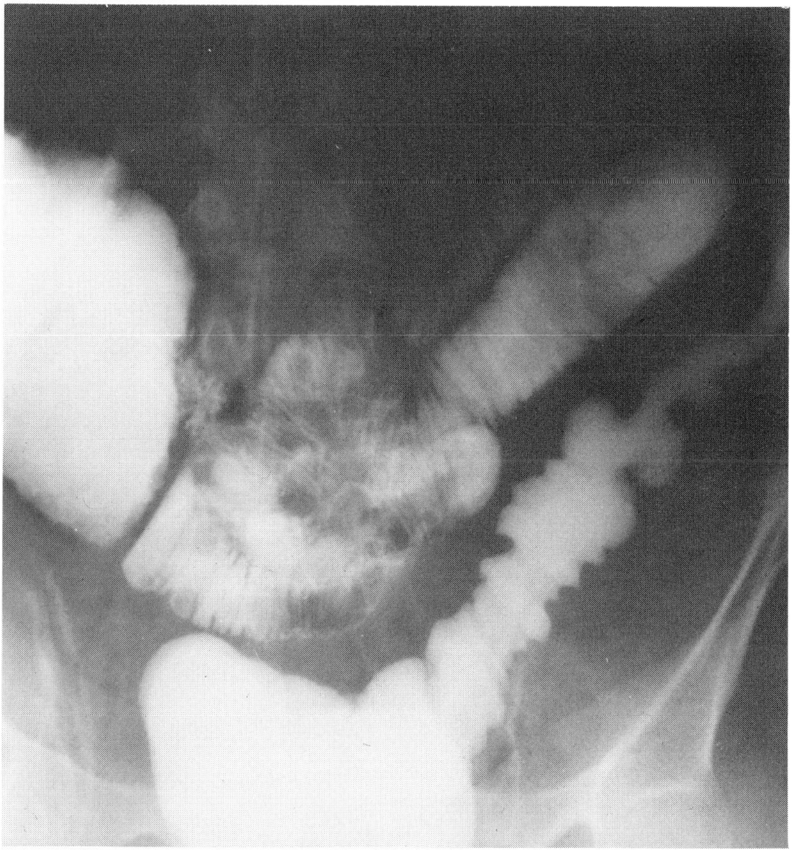

Figure 16D.

(Illustration continued on the following page)

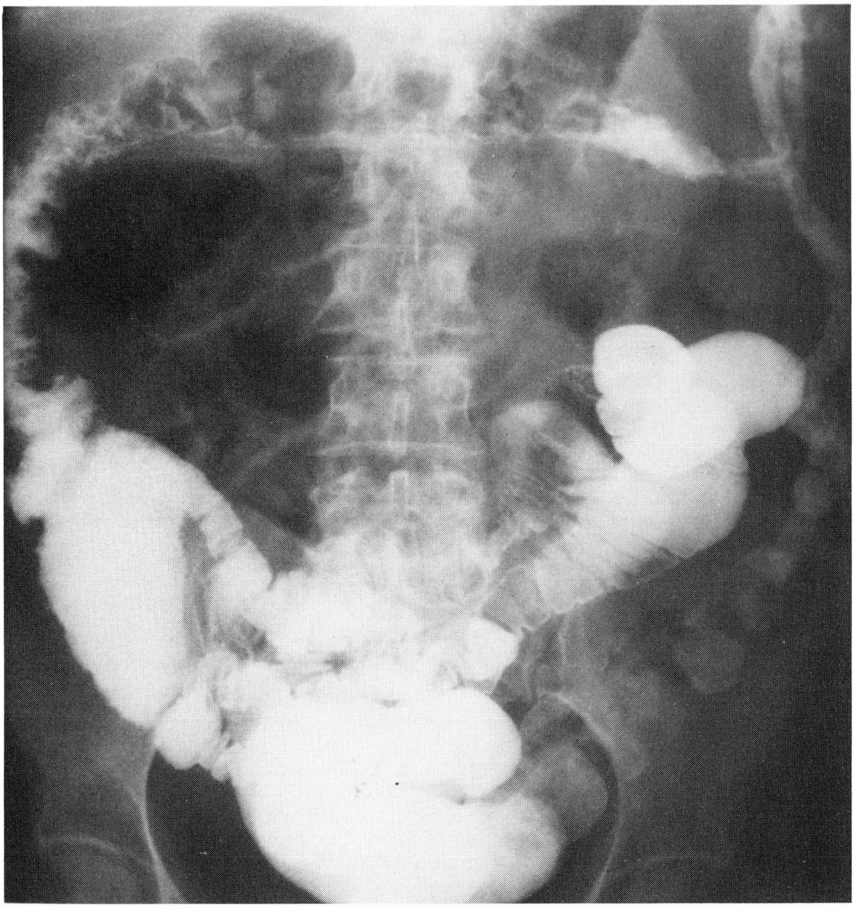

Figure 16E. Postevacuation film best demonstrates the extent of the process from the proximal to the mid-transverse colon to the sigmoid colon. This combination of findings is seen in the early healing phase.

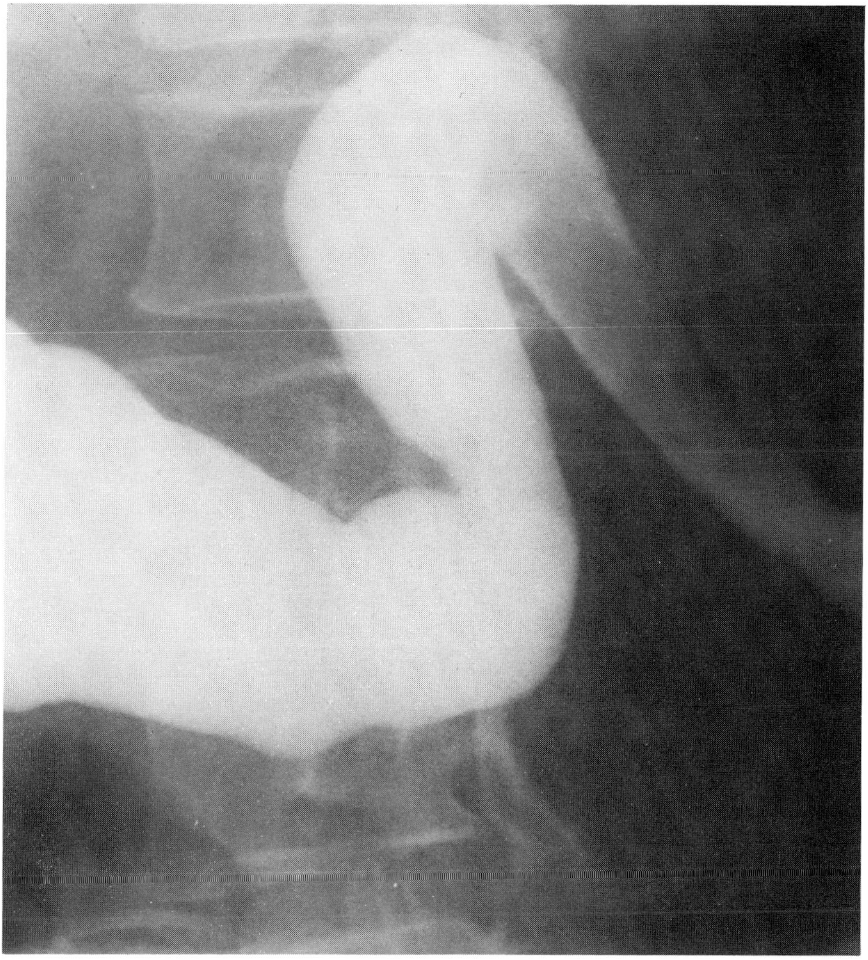

Figure 16F. Ten days later the mucosa has healed. Portions of the colon now have a smooth, tubular appearance.

(Illustration continued on the following page)

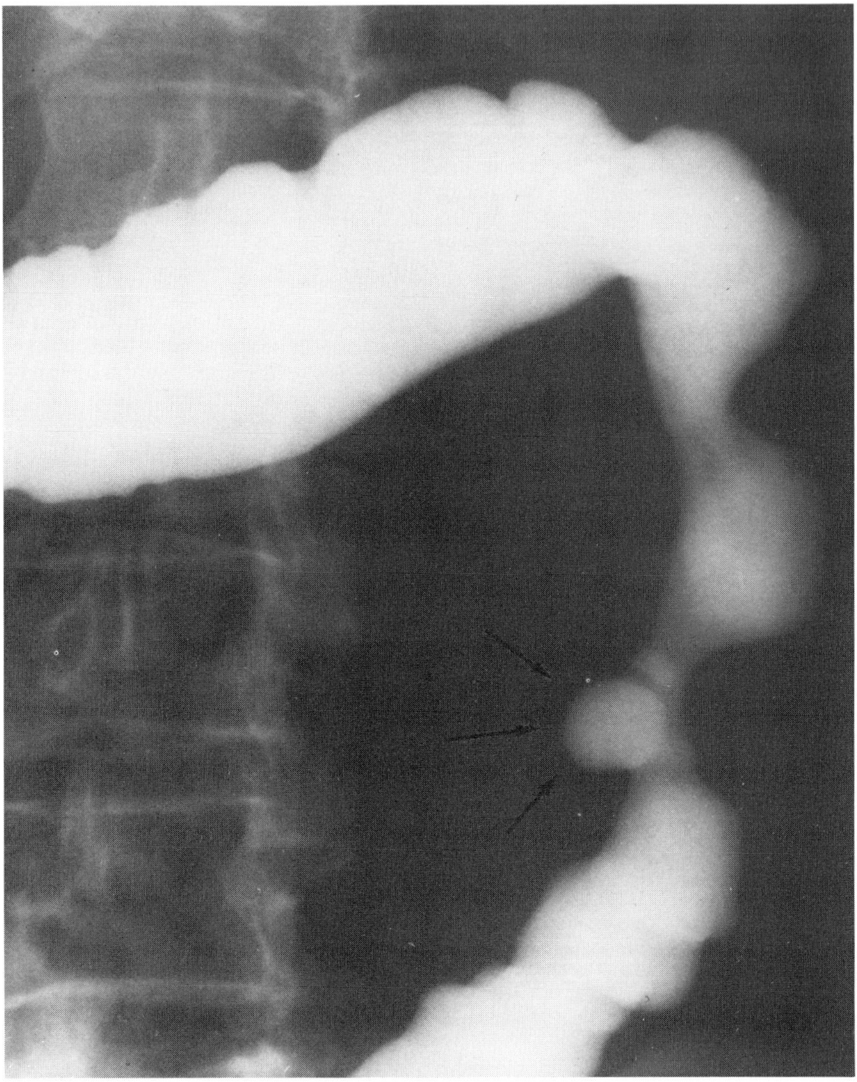

Figure 16G. One year later, three short, smooth strictures associated with pseudosacculation (arrow) are present in the descending colon. (A segmental colon resection was performed. The pathologic changes were compatible with healed ischemic colitis.)

pected sequence of events; ulcerations and submucosal hemorrhages followed by resolution of the ulcers with pseudosacculations progressive to stenosis, carcinoma can be excluded. With only a single study, however, differentiation of an ischemic stricture from a tumor may be difficult. A persistent abdominal mass, abrupt contour change, or pronounced local rigidity are all features of carcinoma and are not associated with benign strictures. Depending on its severity, the stricture may or may not be symptomatic, but generally it does not cause a significant degree of obstruction. The healing process is rapid, being complete in several weeks.

The Role of Angiography in the Evaluation of Intestinal Ischemic Disorders

The role of angiography in the evaluation of acute mesenteric ischemia remains controversial. However, it contributes to the evaluation and treatment of ischemia involving the superior mesenteric system. The mortality of acute superior mesenteric ischemia is high, ranging from 70–80%.[28] This is related to delay in diagnosis, progression of the infarction even after the cause of the decreased blood flow has been corrected, and the increased frequency of nonocclusive mesenteric ischemia. The latter now accounts for about 50% of all ischemic episodes, and untreated, carries a 90% mortality rate.[17,28]

The pathogenesis of nonocclusive mesenteric ischemia is related to splanchnic vasoconstriction.[9] This can be stimulated by several events, most commonly decreased cardiac output, hypovolemia, hypotension, dehydration, and vasopressor agent infusion. Most patients who exhibit this have a predisposing condition such as an acute myocardial infarction, refractory congestive heart failure, aortic insufficiency, or renal or hepatic failure. A significant number of patients have recently undergone major abdominal or tho-

(Text continued on page 102)

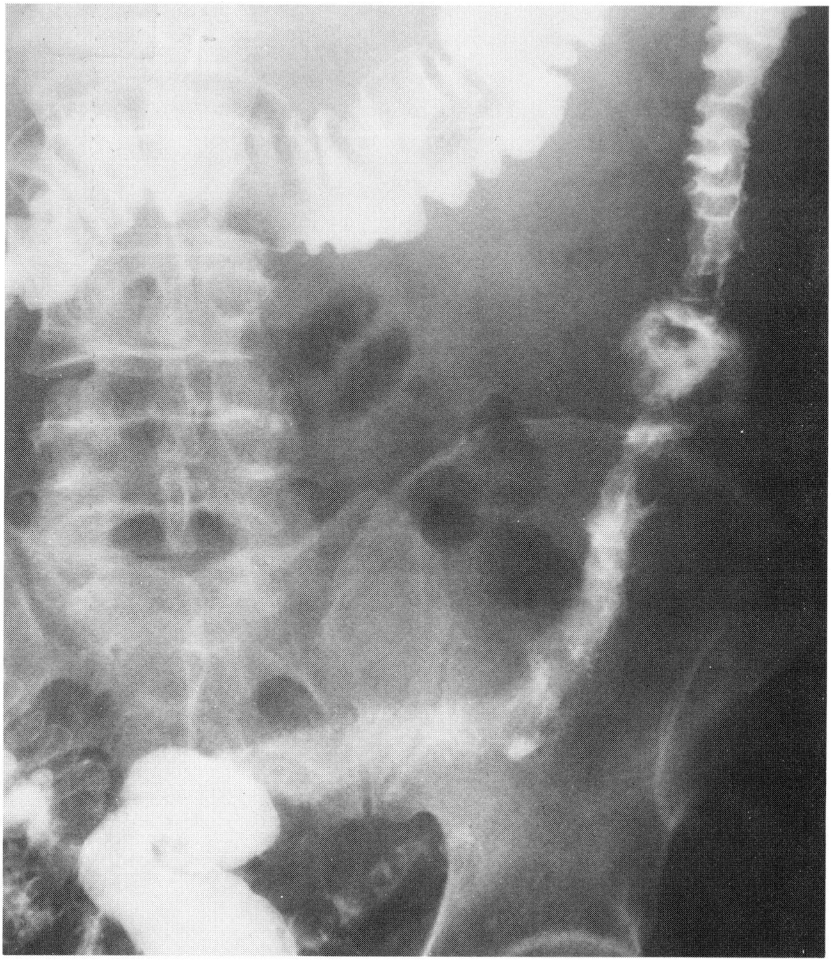

Figure 17A and B. Same patient as in Figure 14. Follow-up examination shows a few persistent ulcers but also the development of a sacculation (arrows) in the descending colon indicative of healing.

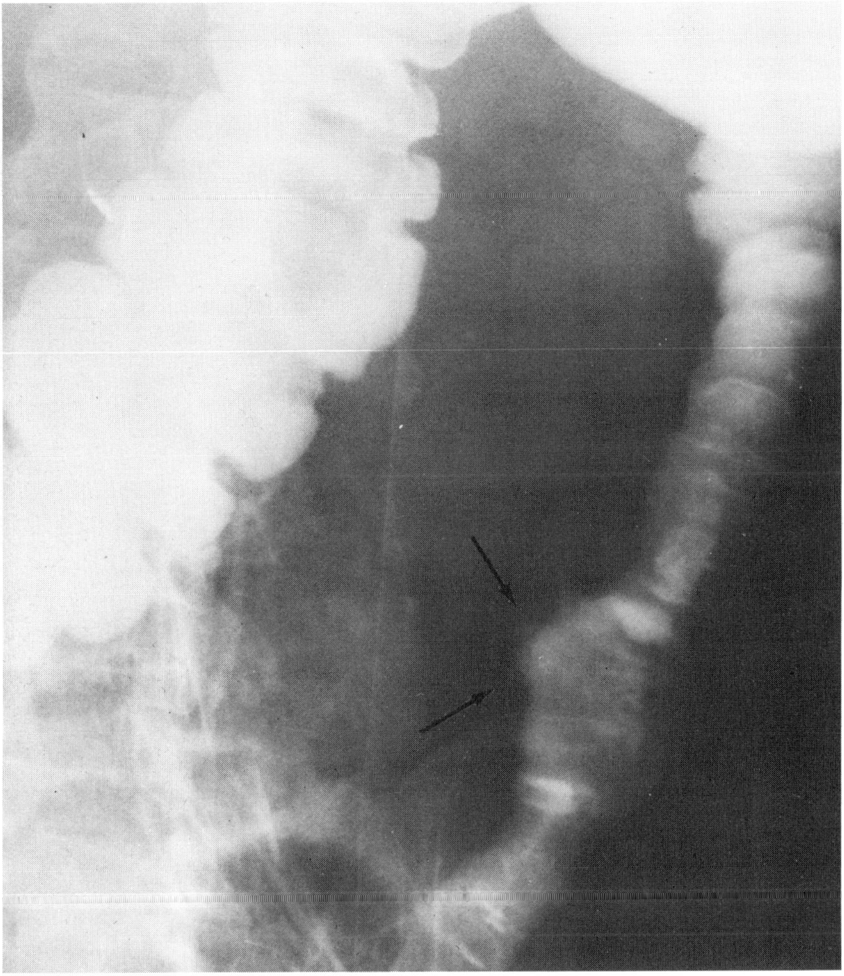

Figure 17B.

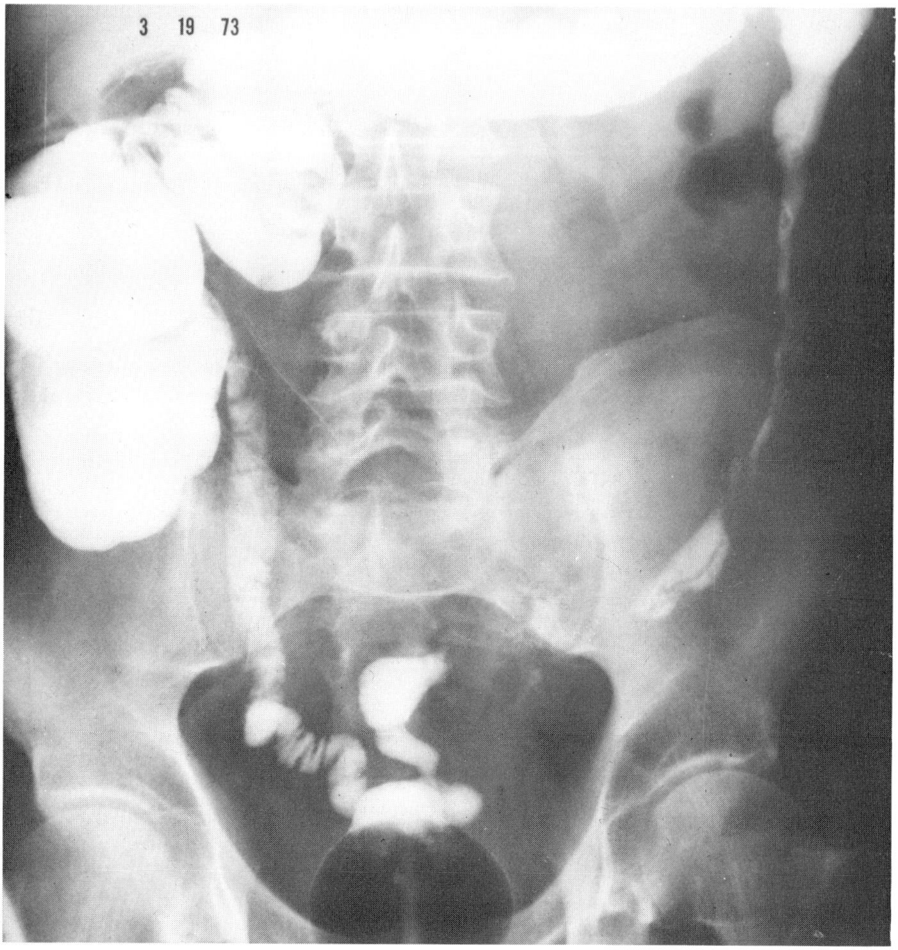

Figure 18. Same patient as in Figure 15. Follow-up barium enema several months later shows long segment of concentric narrowing in the descending colon. Surgical removal of stricture was eventually necessary.

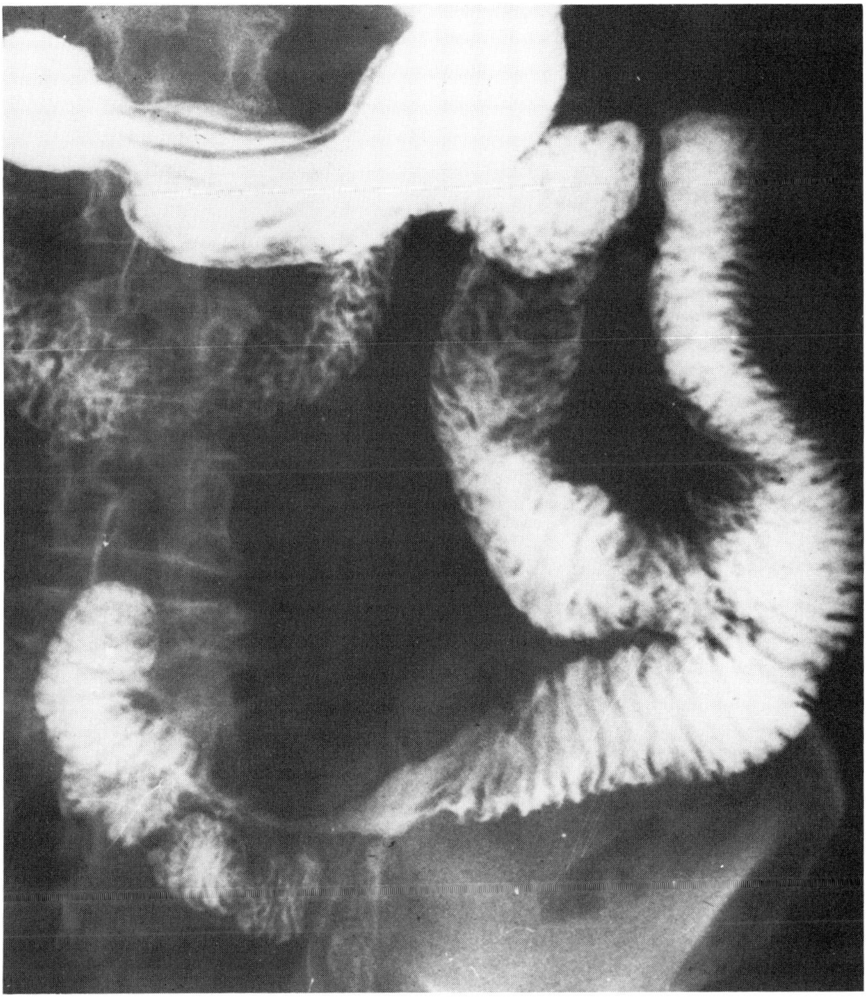

Figure 19. A 70-year-old white woman had an acute episode of severe upper abdominal pain with repeated vomiting three months before this examination. She refused surgery and her symptoms subsided. Radiographs demonstrate a 6 cm smooth, tapered narrowing of the jejunum with mild dilatation of the bowel proximal to this. The clinical history, roentgenographic appearance and time sequence are classic for segmental ischemia involving the jejunum (unproved). (Published with permission from Dunbar JD, Nelson SJ.: *Am. J. Radiol. Ther. Nucl. Med.*, 99:127–135, 1967.)

racic surgery. Often an immediate precipitating event is an arrhythmia or shock.

Boley et al. and others have shown that vasoconstriction occurring after temporary decrease in the blood flow to the superior mesenteric artery may persist for many hours after the cause of the decreased flow is reversed.[9,28,30] This may account for the late development of infarction in some patients, as well as for persistent ischemia in others. They also observed that the intraarterial injection of a vasodilator reduced the degree of mesenteric vasoconstriction.[28] Clinical trials and the subsequent success of these investigations resulted in the development of protocols for intraarterial vasodilator infusion, usually started in the angiography suite.

If acute superior mesenteric ischemia is clinically suspected, plain abdominal radiographs should be taken immediately. Supine and erect abdominal films as well as an upright chest film are recommended. If the patient is too ill to stand, decubitus abdominal films suffice. Positive findings on these initial radiographs have been reported in 20–60% of cases.[5,6] It should be cautioned that these findings might be seen late in the disease process and thus negative plain radiographs should not prevent an angiogram if clinical suspicion is high.

A femoral arteriotomy using the Seldinger technique is made, and a flush aortogram is performed with biplane filming. The aortogram is necessary for the detection of abdominal aortic aneurysms, aortic dissections, emboli to other major visceral arteries, diffuse arteriosclerotic changes, and the status of collateral vessels. This is followed by selective superior mesenteric artery injection.

Differentiation of emboli, especially an old embolus that has become partially organized, from thrombosis is difficult. Generally, emboli are rounded, sharply defined defects located at vessel bifurcations. They frequently are multiple and usually are seen at the branching points of the middle colic artery, the ileocolic artery, or one of the peripheral branches (Figure 20).[20–24,29] An embolus may occlude the

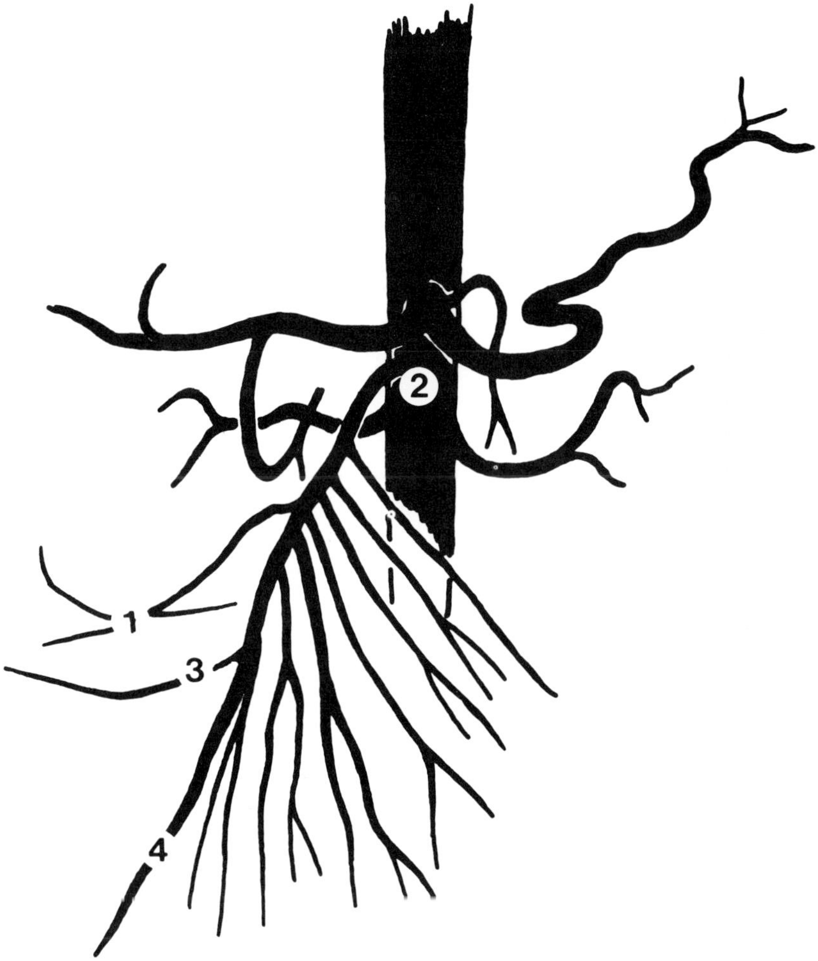

Figure 20. Emboli lodge in order of decreasing frequency in the middle colic artery (1), origin of the superior mesenteric artery (2), the right colic artery (3), and the ileocolic artery (4). (With permission from Nelson SJ, Christoforidis AJ.: *Am. J. Radiol. Ther. Nucl. Med.,* 104:505–521, 1968.)

entire superior mesenteric artery in a small percentage of patients. The major risk factors in developing emboli include atrial fibrillation, rheumatic heart disease, or a recent myocardial infarction (Figures 21 and 22). The patho-

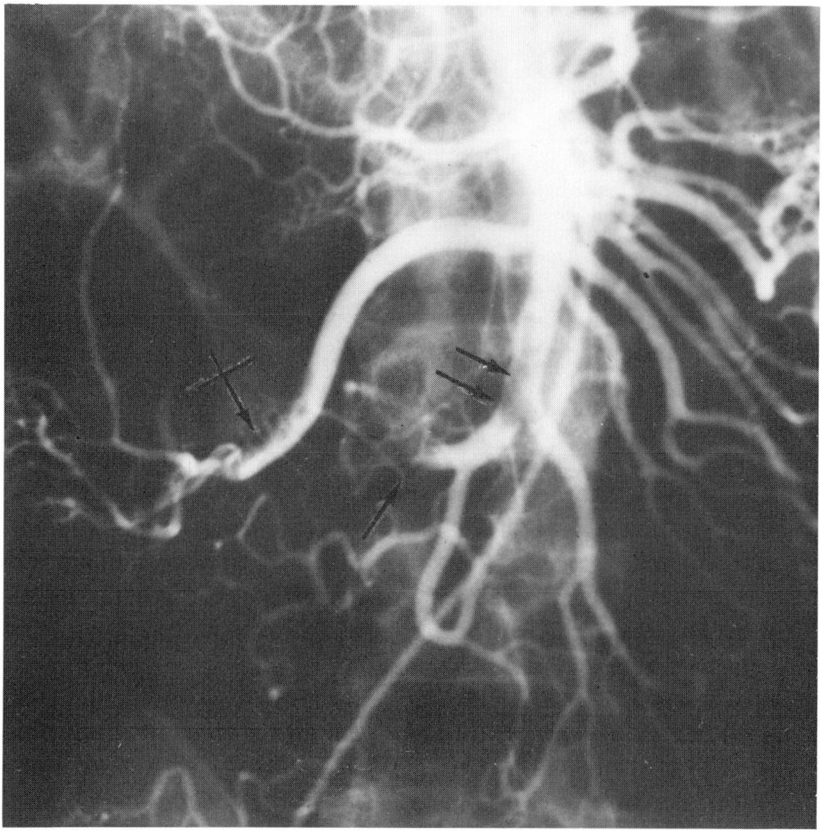

Figure 21A. Patient was a middle-aged man with rheumatic heart disease with acute onset of severe diffuse abdominal pain and bloody diarrhea. Superior mesenteric angiogram shows occlusion of the ileocolic artery just distal to its origin (→) and an embolus in the main trunk of the superior mesenteric artery (⇉) and in the right colic artery (↛). Radiographic changes are most likely secondary to emboli, possibly with secondary thrombus formation.

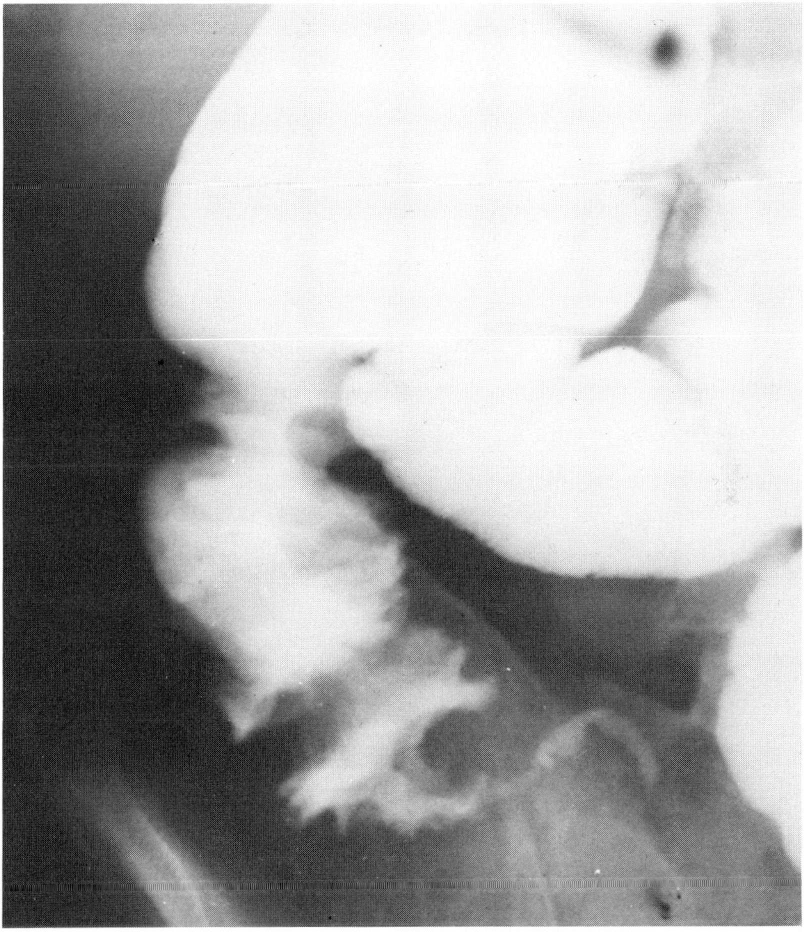

Figure 21B. Thumbprinting is well demonstrated in a selected film from a barium enema done a day after the angiogram.

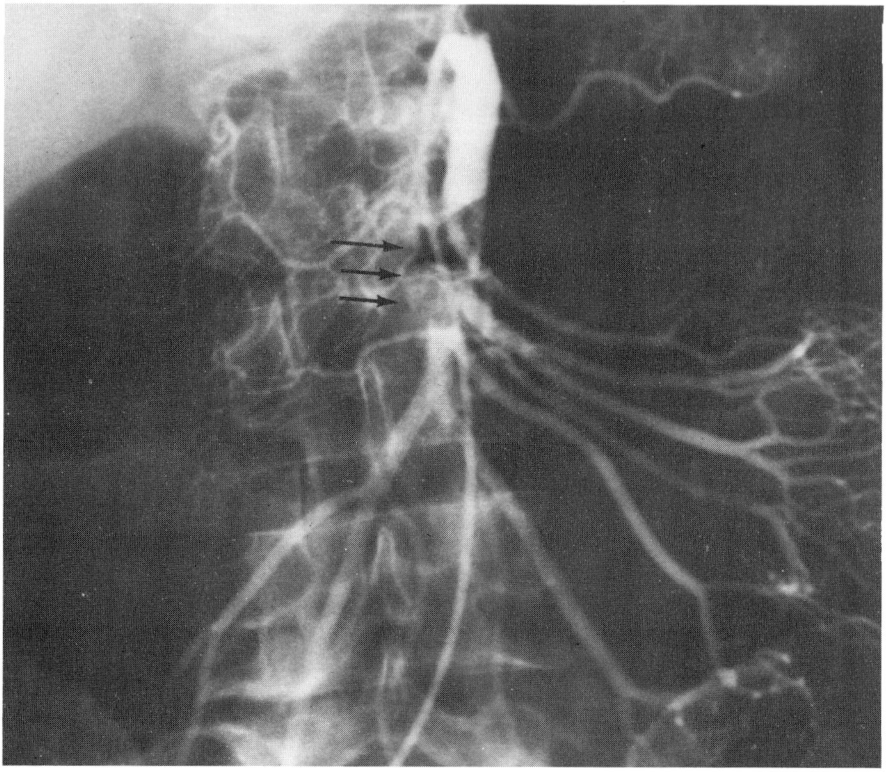

Figure 21C. Six weeks later, the superior mesenteric angiogram has returned to normal. (Published with permission from Dunbar JD, Nelson SJ: Nonangiographic manifestations of intestinal vascular disease. A.C.R. GI Syllabus.)

genesis of embolic and thrombolic disease differs. Emboli are commonly seen in patients without diffuse arteriosclerotic disease. Conversely, thrombi occur on a previously formed plaque, typically within one or two centimeters from the origin of the superior mesenteric artery (Figure 23).[29] Arteriosclerotic changes elsewhere in the vascular tree are common. The differentiation of an acute thrombus from an old thrombus is very important, since this may be

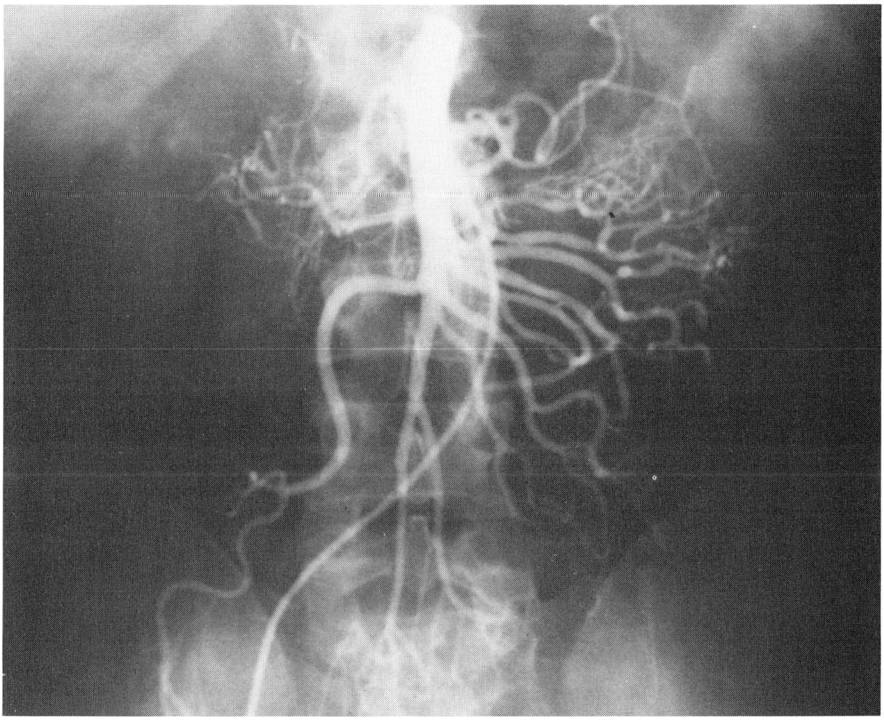

Figure 22. Patient was a 59-year-old man with rheumatic heart disease and severe abdominal pain. Angiogram shows an embolus in the superior mesenteric artery about 4–5 cm from its origin. Right colic artery was obstructed near its origin and did not fill on this study.

a prime factor in deciding whether a laparotomy is performed or expectant therapy is given. If the thrombosis is acute, no collateral vessels will be seen. Chronic occlusions will already have developed a large prominent collateral circulation.

Mesenteric arterial vasoconstriction can occur alone or may be superimposed on an acute embolic or thrombotic episode. Experimental and clinical investigations were undertaken by Boley and others to evaluate the angiographic changes in vasoconstriction. Reliable and reproducible cri-

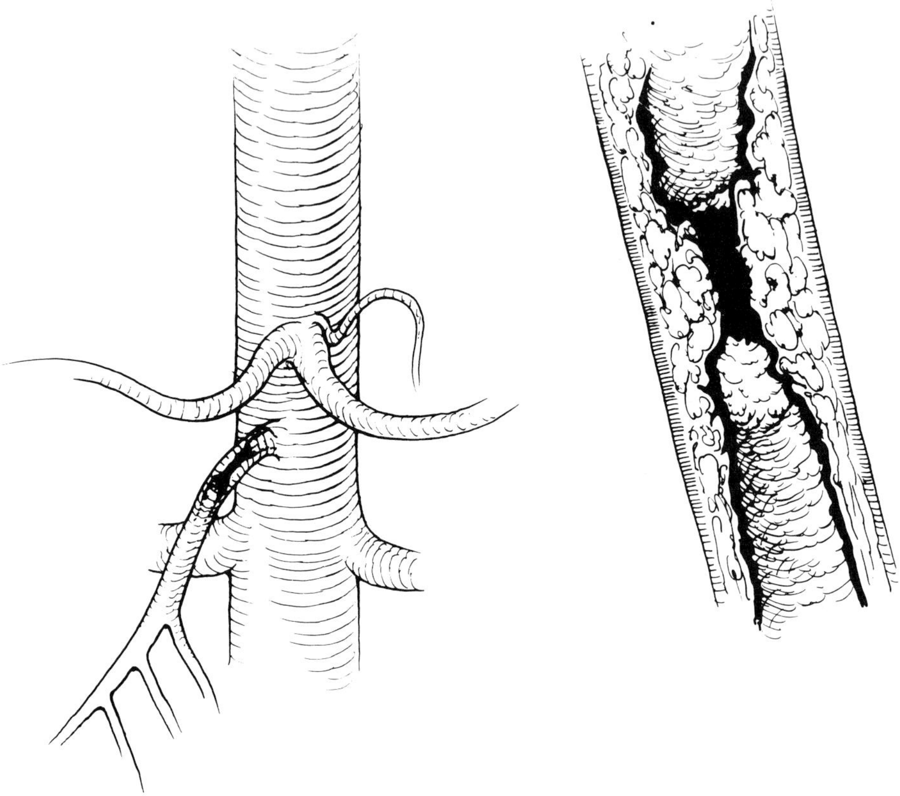

Figure 23. Thrombi most frequently develop in the origin of the superior mesenteric artery (left) at sites of atherosclerotic plaques (right).

teria for this diagnosis include: (1) narrowing of the origins of the major branches, (2) irregularity or beading of the branches, (3) spasm of the arcades; and (4) decreased filling of the intramural vessels (Figures 24 and 25).[30] Narrowing of a single branch vessel is occasionally seen in patients without mesenteric arterial vasoconstriction, but involvement of more than one branch vessel indicates ischemic vasospasm. A normal angiogram virtually excludes ischemic disease.

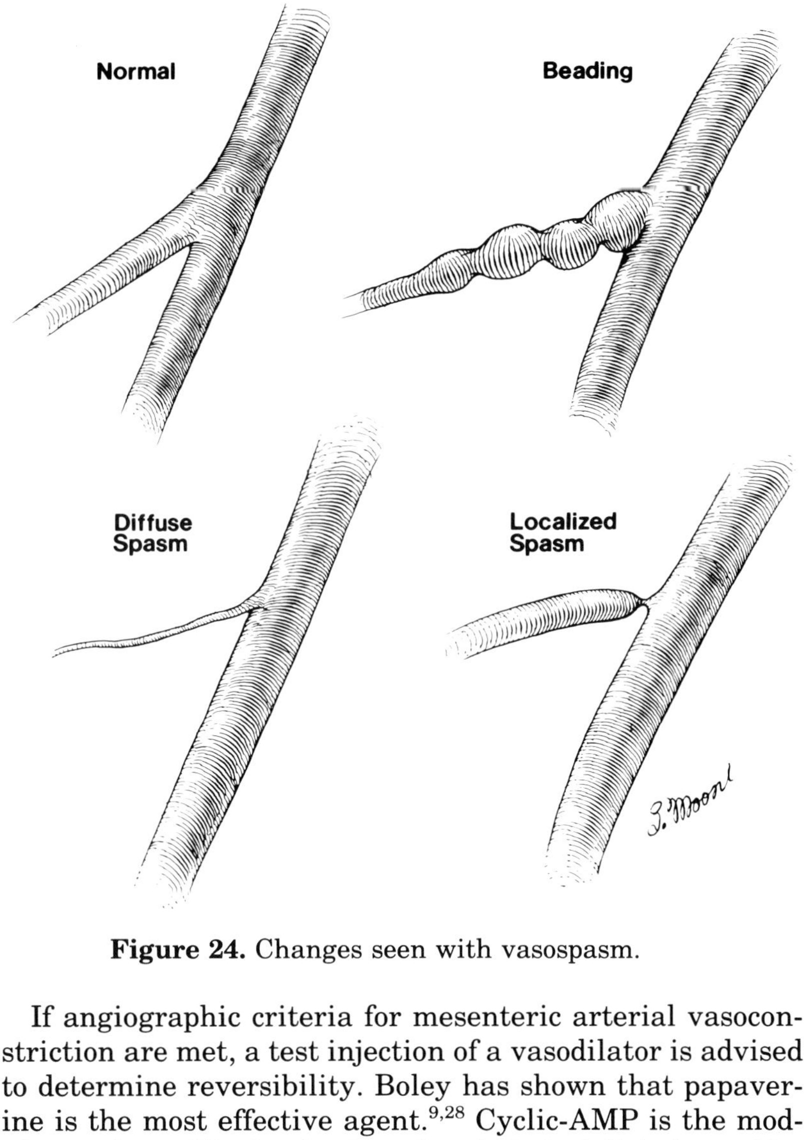

Figure 24. Changes seen with vasospasm.

If angiographic criteria for mesenteric arterial vasoconstriction are met, a test injection of a vasodilator is advised to determine reversibility. Boley has shown that papaverine is the most effective agent.[9,28] Cyclic-AMP is the modulator of vasodilation in the splanchnic bed. It is formed by the breakdown of ATP catalyzed by adenyl cyclase. This reaction is stimulated by many drugs, including glucagon, prostaglandins, epinephrine, and isoproterenol. Therefore,

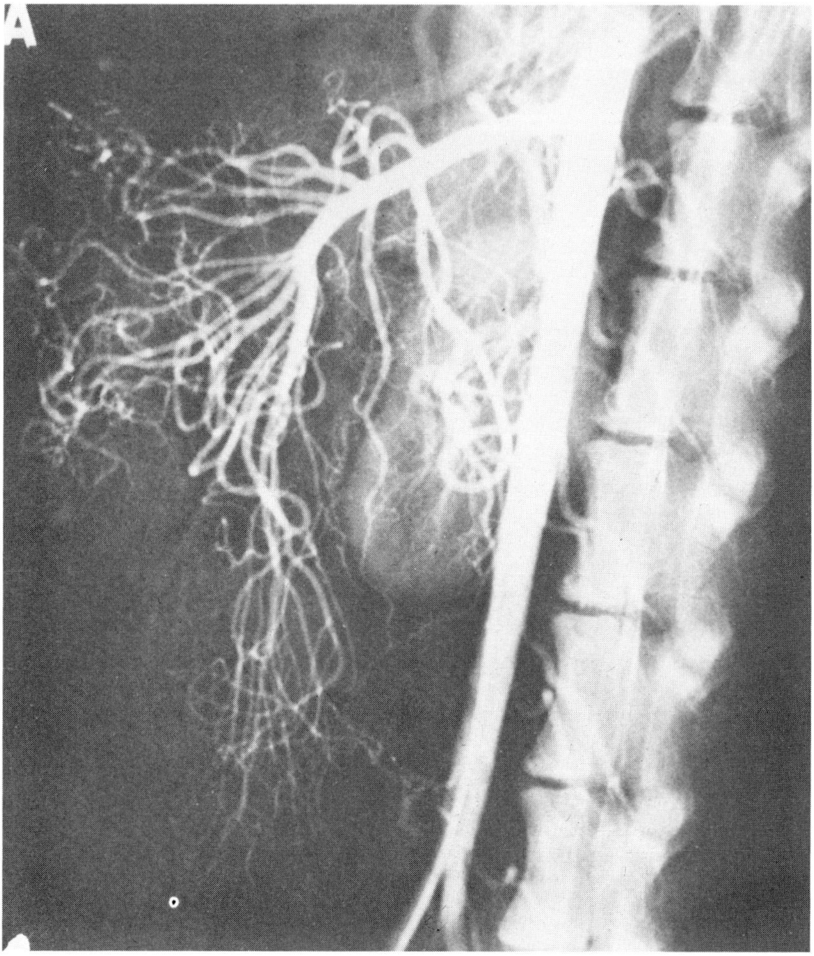

Figure 25. Experimental production of vasospasm in dogs. (A) Baseline normal superior mesenteric angiogram. (B) Arterial manifestations of vasospasm after intravenous Levarterenol infusion. Narrowing particularly at the origins of the jejunal branches is present. (C) Magnified view of (B). (Published with permission from Siegelman SS et al: *Radiology* 112:533, 1974.)

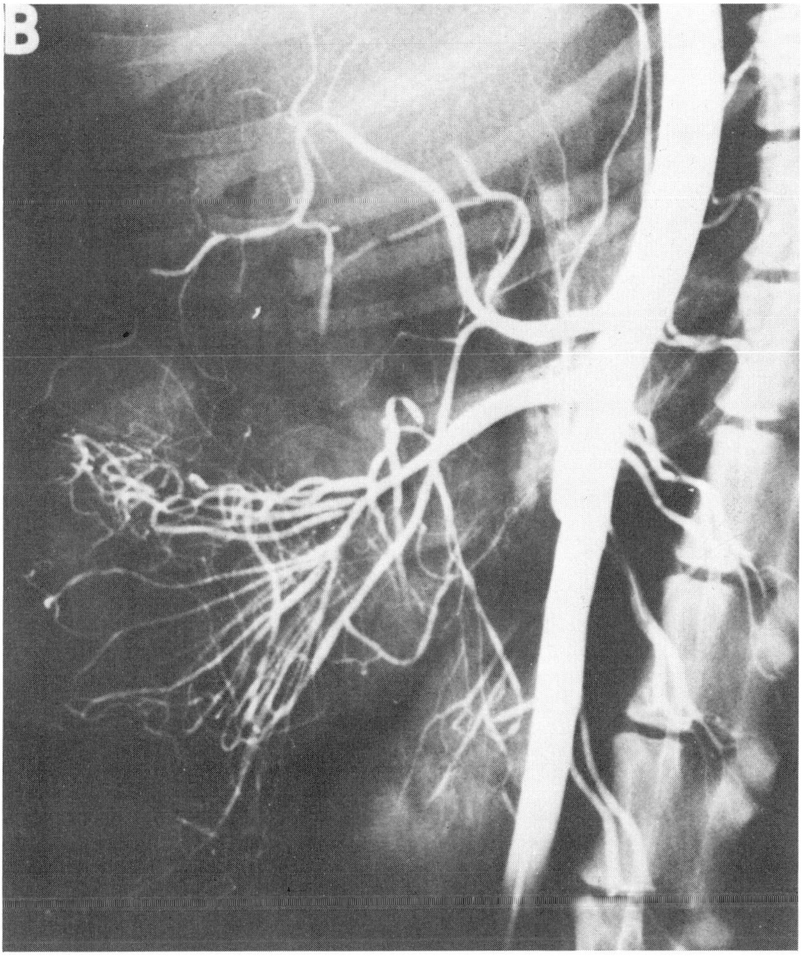

Figure 25B.

(Illustration continued on the following page)

any patient suspected of having mesenteric vascular occlusion should not receive these drugs. Cyclic-AMP is degraded to 5^1-AMP. This is inhibited by papaverine. Thus, intraarterial injection of papaverine causes dilatation of the arterioles by inhibiting the breakdown of cyclic-AMP.[28] Ninety percent of the drug is metabolized in the liver during a single pass so that large doses may be given.

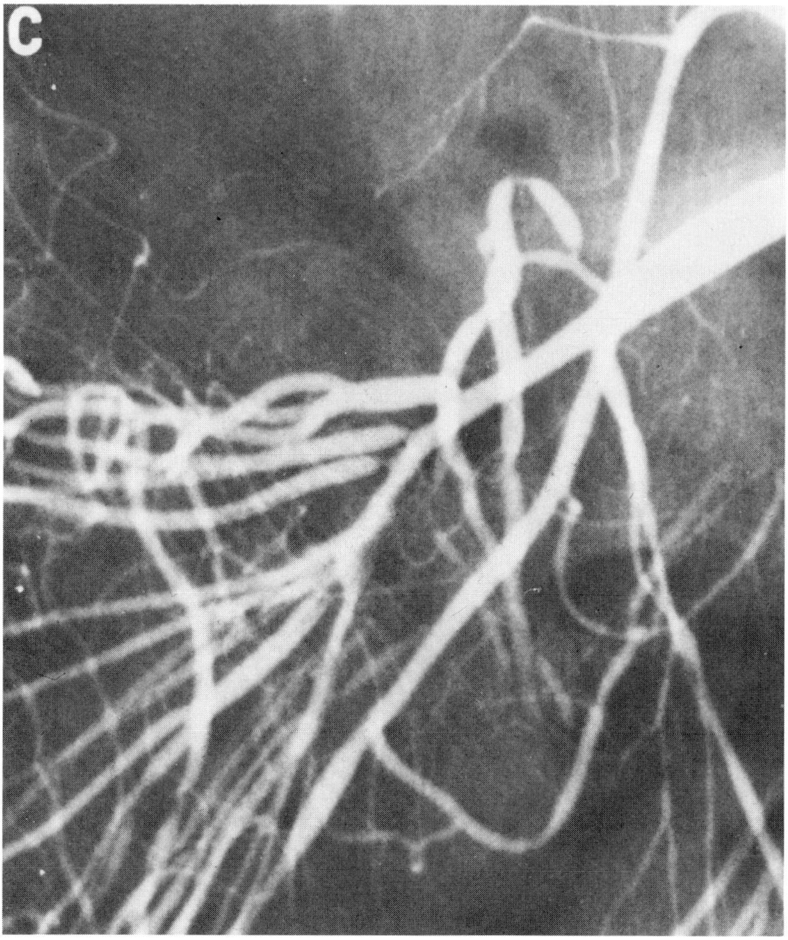

Figure 25C.

There have been encouraging reports of increased survival rates up to 54% with this method. Eighty-five percent of survivors are reported to have a normal, functioning gastrointestinal tract.[9,20] The complications of the infusion are minimal. The metabolism of papaverine in the liver is extremely rapid and is nearly complete after a single pass. The complications of any angiographic procedure are groin hematoma, dislodgement of an arteriosclerotic plaque with peripheral embolization, and possible potentiation of mesenteric artery vasoconstriction if the catheter is lodged too distally in a vessel. Occasionally a fibrin clot may form on a catheter, but this is unlikely to occur if an infusion pump is used.

In contrast to its role in the diagnosis and management of acute superior mesenteric ischemia, angiography contributes little in inferior mesenteric ischemia. Arteriosclerotic changes are frequent enough that occlusion of the inferior mesenteric artery is of little diagnostic significance. Furthermore, the patency of the inferior mesenteric artery has no prognostic significance. In one series, 65% of patients with an occluded artery and 66% of those with nonocclusive mesenteric ischemia recovered without operation.[7] Last, vasospasm has not been demonstrated so there is no rationale for the use of vasodilator therapy.

Angiography has not proved useful in the diagnosis of ischemic colitis after the acute phase.[32] Not only can the clinical presentation and barium studies of ischemic colitis and enteritis mimic acute ulcerative colitis or granulomatous colitis, but so may the angiographic features. The pattern of mild acceleration of the arteriovenous transit time, bowel wall thickening, and tortuous, dilated draining veins are present in healing ischemic disease as well as inflammatory disease. This is not surprising, since the bowel has only a finite number of ways to respond to a specific insult.

Other Methods of Detecting Ischemia

Several nuclear radiographic techniques for diagnosing mesenteric ischemia have been proposed. Zarins and Skinner[35] injected ^{99m}Technetium-labeled albumin microspheres measuring 30 microns in diameter into the aorta after experimentally inducing intestinal ischemia. Scintiscans were then performed. In their study, reactive hyperemia was a constant finding that correlated well with viability, and lack of reactive hyperemia correlated well with gangrenous bowel.[35] However, this method seems not only cumbersome but invasive, and offers no advantages over angiography.

Bardfeld wanted to devise a rapid, noninvasive method of diagnosing ischemic bowel disease. In his study, he injected ^{99m}Technetium-labeled autologous leukocytes into mongrel dogs with experimentally induced mesenteric ischemia. External scanning as early as one-half hour after injection showed positive uptake in the ischemic loops of bowel.[36] However, optimal uptake did not take place until two and one-half hours.

The detection of ischemic bowel disease by nuclear medicine studies remains experimental. Perhaps, methods will become available for clinical application sometime in the future.

Reports of echographically detectable intramural hemorrhage have been published.[37] The finding of a sausage-shaped, echofree mass with a linear echogenic center is nonspecific, however. This appearance has also been reported in bowel tumors and inflammation.

Summary

Radiology plays a vital role in the evaluation of any patient with abdominal complaints, including those with ischemic bowel disease. Plain abdominal films may show edematous, thumbprinted, or corrugated bowel mucosal folds, rigid and fixed intestinal loops, free intraperitoneal air, or occasionally intramural or hepatic portal venous gas. In an appropriate clinical setting, any combination of these findings is highly suggestive of intestinal ischemia. A nondiagnostic abdominal film series should not deter the performance of angiography or barium studies. These should be completed as early in the course of the disease as possible, since the prompt institution of therapy will obviously result in a higher salvage rate. The barium examination findings will parallel those on plain films, but will provide better detail as well as information on peristalsis. Angiography can detect emboli, thrombosis, or the spasm of nonocclusive mesenteric ischemia.

Occasionally, the clinical presentation will be confusing and the initial radiographic examinations may be diagnostically inconclusive. Such patients will benefit from barium studies repeated every five to seven days since a predictable pattern of change is often seen.

The greatest radiologic advances in the past decade have taken place in the technique of angiography. Angiographic criteria for the diagnosis of nonocclusive mesenteric ischemia have been reported. In some cases, the angiographer may commence therapy with intraarterial infusion of a vasodilator.

Experimentation in nuclear imaging may yield some clinically applicable methods of evaluation of mesenteric ischemia. Ultrasound and computed tomography do not have a useful role in diagnosing mesenteric ischemia. One can speculate that, based on the physical principles of magnetic resonance and position emission, perhaps one of these newer imaging techniques may play a role in diagnosis.

The authors gratefully acknowledge the aid of Drs. Sidney Nelson, John Johnson, Charles Mueller, Laura Knight, and John Dennis in contributing illustrations.

References

1. Nelson S: Pseudotumors. In *ACR-Gastrointestinal Disease First Series Syllabus*. Theros E (Ed), American College of Radiology 1973.
2. Dunbar JD, Nelson S: Nonangiographic manifestations of intestinal vascular disease. *Am J Radiol* 99:127, 1967.
3. Nelson S, Eggleston W: Findings on plain roentgenograms of the abdomen associated with mesenteric vascular occlusion with a possible new sign of mesenteric venous thrombosis. *Am J Radiol* 85:886, 1960.
4. Freimanis AK, Nelson SW: The chest roentgenogram in the diagnosis of acute abdominal disease. *Radiol Clin North Am* 2:3, 1974.

5. Miller W, Scott J, Rosato E, et al: Ischemic colitis with gangrene. *Radiology* 94:291, 1970.
6. Tomchik FS, Wittenberg J, Ottinger LW: The roentgenographic spectrum of bowel infarction. *Radiology* 96:249, 1970.
7. Scott JR, Miller WT, Uiso M, et al: Acute mesenteric infarction. *Am J Radiol* 113:269, 1971.
8. Wittenberg J, Athanasoulis C, Williams L, et al: Ischemic colitis. Radiology and pathophysiology. *Am J Radiol* 123:287, 1975.
9. Friman-Dahl: Roentgen examination in mesenteric thrombosis. *Am J Radiol* 64:610, 1950.
10. Boley S, Sprayregen S, Veith F, et al: An aggressive roentgenologic and surgical approach to acute mesenteric ischemia. In *Surgery Annual.* Vol 5, Nyhus LM (Ed), Appleton-Century-Crofts, New York 1973.
11. Eisenberg R, Montgomery C, Maegulis A: Colitis in the elderly: Ischemic colitis mimicking ulcerating and granulomatous colitis. *Am J Radiol* 113:1113, 1979.
12. Hubert F, Mayhall G, Harle T: Hepatic portal venous gas. A review and report on six cases. *Am J Med* 44:557, 1968.
13. Sherbon KJ: The radiology of ischemic colitis. *Radiology* 14:46, 1970.
14. Nelson S: Intramural hemorrhage. In *ACE-Gastrointestinal Disease Second Series Syllabus.* Theros E (Ed), American College of Radiology 1977.
15. Chino S, Johnson JC, Keith L: New clinical and radiographic signs in ischemic colitis. *Am J Surg* 128:640, 1974.
16. O'Hinger J: Nonocclusive mesenteric infarction. *Surg Clin North Am* 54:689, 1974.
17. Rosato E, Rosato F, Scott J, et al: Ischemic dilatation of the colon. *Am J Diag Dis* 14:922, 1960.
18. Ottinger L, Austen G: A study of 136 patients with mesenteric infarction. *Surg Gynecol Obstet* 124:251, 1967.
19. Kaminski D, Keltner R, et al: Ischemic colitis. *Arch Surg* 106:558, 1973.
20. Liebman P, Patten M, Manny J, et al: Hepatic-portal venous gas in adults: Etiology, pathophysiology and clinical significance. *Ann Surg* 187:281, 1978.

21. Nelson S: Extraluminal gas collections due to diseases of the gastrointestinal tract. *Am J Radiol* 115:225, 1972.
22. Boley S, Brandt L, Veith F: Ischemic disorders of the intestines. *Curr Prob Surg* 15:7, 1978.
23. Kilpatrick ZM et al: Ischemic proctitis. *JAMA* 205:64, 1968.
24. Moss A, Margulis A: Ischemic colitis with perforation. *Am J Radiol* 113:338, 1971.
25. Egger G, Hartzl M, Halter F, et al: Non-gangrenous ischemic colitis. Clinical and radiological diagnosis. *Fortsche Roentgenste* 115:432, 1971 (in German).
26. Marshak R, Linder A: Vascular Disease. In *Alimentary Tract Roentgenology*. Margulis AR, Burhenne HJ (Eds), The CV Mosby Co, St. Louis 1973.
27. Marshak R, Linder A: Ischemia of the colon. *Seminars in Roentgenology* 3:(1), 1968.
28. Marston A, Pheils M, et al: Ischemic colitis. *Gut* 5:1, 1966.
29. Williams L, Wittenberg J: Ischemic colitis: An useful clinical diagnosis, but is it ischemic? *Ann Surg* 184:439, 1975.
30. Boley S, Sprayregan S, Seigelman S, et al: Initial results from an aggressive roentgenological and surgical approach to acute mesenteric ischemia. *Surgery* 82:848, 1972.
31. Wittenberg J, Athanasoulis C, Shapiro J, et al: A radiological approach to the patient with acute, extensive bowel ischemia. *Radiology* 106:13, 1973.
32. Siegelman S, Sprayregen S, Boley S: Angiographic diagnosis of mesenteric arterial vasoconstriction. *Radiology* 112:533, 1974.
33. Anderson P: Ischemic colitis caused by angiography. *Clin Radiol* 20:414, 1969.
34. Reuter S, Kanter I, Redman H: Angiography in reversible colonic ischemia. *Radiology* 97:371, 1970.
35. Zarins C, Skinner D, James A: Prediction of the viability of revascularized intestine with radioactive microspheres. *Surg Gynecol Obstet* 138:576, 1974.
36. Bardfeld PA, Boley SJ, Sammartano R, et al: Scintigriphic diagnosis of ischemic intestine with Technetium-99m sulfur colloid-labeled leukocytes. *Radiology* 124:439, 1977.
37. Lee T, Brickman F, Avecilla L: Ultrasound diagnosis of intramural intestinal hematoma. *J Clin Ultrasound* 5:423, 1977.

6

Preoperative Preparation of the Patient with Intestinal Ischemia

Eric D. Anderson, M.D.

General Preparation

The basic principles of preparation of any patient for a major operative procedure can be readily enumerated. The task, however, may be quite difficult in the patient about to undergo an operation for intestinal ischemia. The visceral ischemic syndromes represent a wide spectrum of clinical presentations, but the preparation of each patient for surgery must be directed at the specific pathophysiologic derangement. For example, in the individual with chronic mesenteric insufficiency, timing of the operation is of minor importance. Of greater significance is attention to nutritional status and evaluation of any concomitant problems such as coronary artery or cerebrovascular disease. In a patient with acute mesenteric vascular occlusion and impending gangrene or peritonitis, however, time is of the essence. The potential lethality of the situation dictates rapid surgical intervention, and preparation for the operation must be initiated prior to completion of any diagnostic studies. Thus, a spectrum of urgency exists. The completeness and rapidity of preoperative preparation in each individual is dictated by the urgency of the operation.

Acute Mesenteric Vascular Insufficiency

The plan of treatment of the individual with suspected acute intestinal ischemia must be considered from the point of view of both operative and preoperative therapy. Preparatory measures are of such importance that they must frequently supplant diagnostic measures or precede determination of the exact cause of the ischemic event. This discussion of modes of therapy necessarily includes general therapeutic measures required, no matter what the cause may be, so that some overlap with other chapters is inevitable.

There are several different causes of acute intestinal ischemia. The final pathway leading to irreversible intestinal infarction and hemorrhagic necrosis, however, is always the same. The degree of involvement of the wall of the ischemic segment, the distribution of the lesion along the intestine, and the rapidity of the ischemic process vary widely with differing etiologies. It is the underlying pathophysiologic derangements that determine the measures required to prepare the patient for an operation.

Initial Resuscitation

Logically, resuscitation in any acutely ill patient begins with attention to the respiratory system. Oxygen should be administered immediately by face mask, or if the patient is moribund or in distress, endotracheal intubation and mechanical ventilation is required.

The next concern is to establish stable vital signs and

make immediate preparation for monitoring the status of the patient. All require the insertion of at least one large-bore intravenous cannula and the insertion of a central venous catheter. This allows for rapid fluid administration and permits measurement of central venous pressure. This may be inserted into either the subclavian or internal jugular vein. A radial artery catheter may also be inserted to allow easy access for procurement of blood samples and blood pressure monitoring. A Foley catheter should be inserted in the bladder of all patients to measure urine output.

A nasogastric tube should be inserted in all patients to decompress the stomach prior to the induction of anesthesia. This is important for several reasons. Emptying the stomach lessens the risk of aspiration and pneumonitis, a major source of postoperative morbidity. Avoidance of vomiting and relief of painful gastric distention are further symptomatic benefits. Gastric decompression improves ventilatory efficiency as well. A more subtle benefit is the fact that gastric suction prevents further distention of the small bowel from swallowed air. Any increase in intraluminal pressure over 30 mm Hg in either the small or large bowel results in progressive stepwise decreases in intestinal blood flow. There is also decreased arteriovenous oxygen difference, indicative of diminished oxygen extraction. In addition, the increased intraluminal pressure reduces flow not only to the distended segment, but also to the remainder of the small bowel. This diminished flow may persist for several hours after the distention is relieved. Preservation of blood flow will delay the onset of necrosis and lessen the risk of perforation and peritonitis.[1,2]

Rectal tubes have no place in intestinal decompression in these individuals. Long intestinal tubes (Cantor, Miller-Abbott) also are not indicated if acute intestinal ischemia is suspected. Attempts at passage of these long tubes lead only to further delays in diagnosis and definitive treatment.

Diagnostic measures are discussed elsewhere, but some that relate directly to resuscitative efforts are mentioned here. Initial laboratory work, prior to the operation, should include as a minimum: hemoglobin, hematocrit, leukocyte count, urinalysis, prothrombin time, partial thromboplastin time, serum electrolyte levels, serum amylase, blood urea nitrogen measurement, and determination of arterial blood gases. Other tests may be done as indicated, but should not be allowed to delay therapeutic maneuvers.

Fluid, Blood Volume, Electrolyte Therapy

The administration of intravenous fluids is a major component of the preoperative regimen. Major mesenteric vascular occlusions produce a myriad of systemic effects. Ischemia results in extensive abnormalities at the cellular level. Permeability to both bacteria and fluid occurs, resulting in a massive intracellular and extraluminal loss of plasma and fluid with resultant hypovolemia.[3]

The urgency of the operation determines the time available for fluid and electrolyte replacement. Most fluid losses are isotonic; therefore, serum electrolyte concentrations may be near normal, even with massive volume deficit. Resuscitation should begin with rapid administration of Ringer's lactate solution. Potassium may be added after urine flow is established. It is necessary to depend on clinical parameters to measure fluid requirements. These include central venous pressure, restoration of urine output, hematocrit, and pulse rate. In critically ill individuals, Swan-Ganz catheter placement and measurement of pulmonary capillary wedge pressure, and cardiac output may be required to adequately assess volume status.

Angiography should be delayed until intravascular volume is restored. Patients in shock will always show mesenteric vasoconstriction, even without intestinal ischemia.[4] Also, papaverine should be withheld initially, as this will increase the size of the vascular bed and worsen the hypovolemia. Vasopressors are not indicated for hypovolemic shock, especially if mesenteric ischemia is suspected.

Transfusion of blood may or may not be required. Despite the hemorrhagic infarction seen with mesenteric arterial occlusion, blood loss is usually not significant. However, in the individual with strangulation obstruction or mesenteric venous occlusion with infarction, there may be extensive sequestration of blood in the bowel wall, mesentery, or peritoneal cavity, requiring transfusion.[5] Blood replacement is best coordinated with measurement of volume restoration, as well as hemoglobin and hematocrit determination.

Antibiotics

Systemic antibiotics are an essential adjunct in the management of intestinal ischemia, and are always started preoperatively as soon as the diagnosis is established.

Acute mesenteric ischemia causes a loss of the structural and functional integrity of the cellular membranes and subsequent permeability of the bowel wall to bacteria. In addition, lowering of the oxygen tension as the intestine dies allows the emergence of anaerobic and microaerophilic organisms.[6] The antibiotic regimen selected should provide coverage for both Gram-negative organisms and anaerobes. The best coverage is provided by the combination of an aminoglycoside and an agent effective against anaerobes, especially *Bacteroides fragilis.* Clindamycin, metronidazole, or chloramphenicol fill this role. In a small percentage of cases, enterococcus is a pathogen. Ampicillin should be added in these instances. The third generation cephalosporin products now available, e.g., cefotaxime, moxalactam, may be useful as single agents. They provide a broad spectrum of coverage, and the potential nephrotoxicity of the aminoglycoside agents is avoided.

Cardiovascular

Acute intestinal ischemia is seen principally in elderly patients who frequently have underlying heart disease. Relief of congestive heart failure and, if possible, correction of cardiac arrhythmias must precede surgery. A baseline electrocardiogram is part of the initial evaluation. The decision to discontinue digitalis is difficult. Digitalis toxicity may contribute to some episodes of nonocclusive mesenteric ischemia. However, the drug is frequently required if the patient has congestive heart failure or atrial fibrillation with a rapid ventricular response.

Summary

Preparation for surgery must be rapid. Optimally, prior to the operation, at least half of the perceived intravascular volume deficit should be restored, and gross electrolyte abnormalities corrected. In addition, the patient should be clinically resuscitated from a shock state, as manifested by urine flow of at least 30 cc/hr and central venous pressure of 8–12 cm H_2O. Hemoglobin should be at least 10 gm/L, and typed and crossmatched blood should be available.

Of principal importance is the realization that these preparations must proceed concomitantly with any diagnostic studies and are initiated prior to the establishment of a diagnosis.

Chronic Intestinal Ischemia

Postprandial pain and weight loss are the most common findings in patients with chronic mesenteric vascular insufficiency. Clinically significant chronic intestinal ischemia is not seen without a decrease in total body mass. Classically, these individuals have weight loss to the point of emaciation and may resemble the patient with carcinomatosis. Other physiologic manifestations vary. They may be anemic, but occult blood is not always present in the stool. Malabsorption of fat and fat-soluble vitamin deficiencies may occur, but are not frequent.

Chronic mesenteric vascular insufficiency is most often the result of atherosclerosis. These individuals also have evidence of atherosclerotic occlusive disease elsewhere. Lower extremity arterial occlusive lesions are frequent. Coronary artery disease is common as well. Preoperative preparation is directed, therefore, not at urgent measures to prepare the patient for an emergency operation, but at restoration of the patient to a satisfactory nutritional status and careful assessment of the cardiovascular system.

Nutrition

Preoperative correction of caloric deficits is essential in the malnourished patient. Protein depletion markedly increases morbidity and mortality and has a profound adverse effect on pulmonary function.

Planning the nutritional regimen requires careful assessment of nutritional status. This is achieved by careful physical examination and a series of clinical and laboratory tests. Serum albumin, total iron binding capacity, total lymphocyte count, skin tests for immunologic competency, and anthropometric measurements are all useful parameters in assessing nutritional status.

Restoration of a satisfactory nutritional state in these individuals is best achieved by a course of parenteral alimentation. This technique requires central venous catheterization and requires a solution of hypertonic dextrose and amino acids. This provides suitable carbohydrates, protein moieties, and nutrients to achieve positive nitrogen balance. Optimum time for surgery is based on clinical improvement, weight gain, and improved nutritional parameters. Seven to ten days of nutrition are usually required preoperatively.

Cardiovascular

Careful assessment of cardiovascular function is essential. Coronary artery disease is common and is best managed if recognized prior to an operation. A history of myocardial infarction in the preceding six months is particularly ominous. Control of arrhythmias should be achieved prior to surgery if possible. Of prime importance is recognizing the fact that virtually all these patients have associated atherosclerotic disease and being prepared to rapidly care for any cardiovascular problem that may occur.[7,8]

Systemic Evaluation

Infection is another major source of morbidity. Perioperative antibiotics are useful and have been shown unequivocally to decrease the potential for infection in vascular reconstructive procedures.[9] Cefazolin, administered immediately preoperatively and for 24–48 hours following surgery, is the most commonly used agent. This antibiotic provides high sustained serum levels, and renal toxicity is virtually nonexistent.

Finally, preoperative assessment of pulmonary, renal, and hepatic function should be completed. Determination of serum creatinine, serum albumin, coagulation parameters, and preoperative pulmonary function tests are useful screening tests in this regard. The operation can be undertaken once nutritional status is restored and systemic evaluation is complete. These individuals are almost always elderly and while they tolerate a major operation well, they tolerate complications poorly. The goal of preoperative preparation is the prevention of postoperative morbidity.

References

1. Boley SI, Agrawal GP, Warren AR, et al: Pathophysiologic effects of bowel distention on intestinal blood flow. *Am J Surg* 117:228, 1969.
2. Tenrich PA, Treiber WF, Frank M, et al: Pathophysiologic effects of bowel distention on intestinal blood flow. *Curr Topics Surg Res* 2:59, 1980.
3. Merston A: Experimental aspects of acute superior mesenteric artery occlusion. In *Vascular Disorders of the Intestine.* Ch 19. Boley SJ et al. Appleton-Century-Crofts, New York 1971.
4. Klass AA: The treatment of superior mesenteric artery occlusion. A reappraisal. *Canad Med Assoc J* 93:309, 1965.
5. Nance FC: Strangulation in intestinal obstruction. In *Critical Surgical Illness.* 2nd ed, Ch 20. Hardy JD. WB Saunders, Philadelphia 1980.
6. Anderson CB, et al: Anaerobic infections in surgery. Clinical review. *Surgery* 79:313, 1976.
7. Cooperman M, Pflug B, Martin EW Jr, Evans WE: Cardiovascular risk factors in patients with peripheral vascular disease. *Surgery* 84:505–509, 1978.
8. Goldman L, et al: Multifactorial index of cardiac risk in noncardiac surgical procedures. *N Engl J Med* 297:845, 1977.
9. Kaiser AB, et al: Antibiotic prophylaxis in vascular surgery. *Ann Surg* 188:283, 1978.

7

Assessment of Intestinal Viability

Marc Cooperman, M.D.

The successful surgical management of patients with intestinal ischemia depends upon the surgeon's ability to determine accurately the viability of ischemic intestine. All nonviable bowel must be resected to prevent the sequelae of perforation and sepsis, but it is equally important to preserve all bowel that is viable. Because resection of large segments of bowel of questionable viability may result in the unnecessary creation of the short bowel syndrome, surgeons have performed second-look laparotomies to reassess questionable segments after a period of 24 hours. Unfortunately, this practice is associated with significant morbidity in seriously ill patients who must undergo a second general anesthetic and major operative procedure.

Until recently, surgeons have depended solely upon clinical criteria to assess the viability of ischemic intestine. The lack of uniform accuracy in purely clinical evaluations has led to a search for a reliable objective measurement of intestinal viability. Numerous methods have been tried, but have not met with widespread clinical acceptance. Recently, two methods, the detection of signals by Doppler ultrasound and the visual appearance of fluorescence after injection of fluorescein dye, have shown promise of supplementing the surgeon's subjective assessment.

Clinical Criteria

The criteria by which intestinal viability are assessed are bowel color, presence or absence of mesenteric pulsations, bleeding from the cut edge of the bowel, and the presence or absence of peristalsis. The problems with the use of these criteria are the need for subjective evaluation by the surgeon and the fact that changes indicating irreversible ischemic damage may take so long to develop that they cannot be observed at the time of operation.

Color changes depend both on the duration of ischemia and whether the cause is arterial or venous obstruction or both. Only when frank infarction has occurred and the bowel is thin-walled and green to black in color is the appearance totally reliable. Early arterial obstruction, particularly in the colon, may produce minimal changes in color immediately, with the bowel assuming a dusky hue only over time. Conversely, venous obstruction produces rapid changes in the appearance of the bowel, with the bowel and its mesentery assuming a hemorrhagic, suffused appearance. The degree of damage may appear much worse than it really is, and potentially viable bowel may be sacrificed unnecessarily.

Mesenteric pulsations may still be present in bowel in which irreversible ischemic changes have occurred. Conversely, the absence of mesenteric pulsations is not a reliable index of lack of viability. In cases of decreased cardiac output, whether due to hypovolemia or other causes, splanchnic vasoconstriction may result in the absence of palpable mesenteric pulsations, particularly in the distal arcades, in bowel that is still viable.

The limitations of judging viability by observing the amount of arterial bleeding from the cut edge of the bowel itself are obvious. Active arterial bleeding from the cut edge of resected bowel is a good indicator that the blood supply to the anastomosis is intact. However, an enterostomy cannot be justified in a segment of bowel of questionable viability to ascertain whether arterial bleeding occurs.

The presence of peristalsis suggests that ischemic bowel is viable. However, this finding also is not always reliable. Peristalsis may persist for a time after the onset of irreversible vascular compromise. Conversely, the absence of visible peristalsis does not mean that ischemic bowel will not survive.

All of these clinical findings have been shown, in both clinical and experimental settings, not to be reliable guides to intestinal viability.[1–7] As a result, numerous techniques have been developed in an attempt to replace subjective assessment of bowel viability with objective measurement.

In order to be clinically useful, a method of assessing bowel viability objectively should fulfill certain criteria. First, the method must be absolutely accurate, so that the surgeon may rely on the results, even if they appear to be inconsistent with the clinical appearance of the intestine. Second, use of the technique must not require significant added operating time. Third, the method should be as simple as possible to minimize the possibility of error in subjective interpretation of findings. Ideally, the equipment should be relatively inexpensive and readily available.

Numerous methods to objectively determine intestinal viability have been used in the laboratory. However, owing either to the lack of predictive accuracy or the complexity of the equipment or the time required, most have not been accepted for clinical use. Of the various techniques described, only Doppler ultrasound and fluorescein dye injection have found significant clinical application.

pH Determination

With the onset of ischemia, anaerobic glycolysis results in a drop in pH and rise in pCO_2. Changes in pH and pCO_2 have been investigated as predictors of intestinal viability in experimental animals. Studies have shown that ligation of the intestinal blood supply results in a prompt fall in the surface intestinal pH, with a corresponding rise in pCO_2. With revascularization, both the intestinal pH and pCO_2 rapidly return to normal levels.[8] However, neither the pH nor the pCO_2 of the ischemic intestine could be correlated with subsequent viability. Even in segments of intestine that ultimately became necrotic, restoration of blood flow resulted in return of surface pH and pCO_2 to normal levels.[8] Katz et al. also found that mucosal pH shifts were related only to the presence or absence of blood flow and were not predictive of viability.[9] Serosal pH values, taken alone, were also of limited predictive usefulness, but in combination with electromyography were helpful in predicting viability. In the presence of equivocal electromyographic activity, alkalotic serosal pH in the range of 7.95 to 8.40 is thought to indicate irreversible ischemic damage.[9] However, neither serosal or mucosal pH measurements have met with clinical acceptance in the assessment of intestinal viability, owing to their lack of predictive accuracy.

Tetrazolium Analysis

Tetrazolium analysis of intestinal mucosa is performed by grinding the tissue in a homogenizer and adding an amount of distilled water equal to the extract. Tetrazolium is then added to the mixture which is incubated at 37° C for two hours. As a result of the dehydrogenase enzyme system, tetrazolium is reduced to a compound called diformazan, which is blue. The amount of diformazan produced is determined with a colorimeter. Katz et al. showed that results of tetrazolium analysis correlated well with the degree of intestinal ischemia.[9] They observed a progressive linear drop with increasing occlusion times.

This assay, however, is not applicable clinically because biopsy of the ischemic intestine is required and performance of the assay requires two hours.

Electromyography

The normal electrical activity of the small intestine is reflected in regular slow waves that occur with a frequency of 12 to 15 per minute with an amplitude of 2 to 6 mV with spikes that reflect peristalsis. It has been shown that when the blood supply to the intestine is occluded, all electrical activity promptly ceases.[9]

The return of electrical activity after revascularization has been investigated as a guide to intestinal viability. In dogs, after two to four hours of vascular occlusion, electrical activity resumed within 10 minutes. Spike activity was increased, and slow wave activity was reduced in frequency. After six hours of vascular occlusion, no resumption of electrical activity was apparent during a 30-minute period of observation.[9] Bussemaker and Lindeman[10] also showed that the return of electrical activity was a good index of bowel viability. They found that the return of slow waves within 10 minutes indicated that the intestine was viable and stricture would be unlikely, so that intestinal anastomosis could be performed safely. The return of slow wave activity was more accurate in predicting viability than either the color of the bowel or the return of mesenteric pulsation.

Although the usefulness of electromyography has been demonstrated experimentally, this technique has not been put to widespread clinical use for several reasons. Special equipment requires both special preparation for its use and additional time for observation.[10]

Potential Difference

In the normal intestine, active transport of sodium results in a charge differential between the mucosal and serosal surfaces of the bowel. Because ischemia has been shown to abolish all active intestinal transport, including sodium, changes in potential difference have been examined as a guide to intestinal viability. Using rabbits, Gurll and Braxton[11] inserted potential difference bridges into ischemic loops of small intestine. They found no significant change in potential difference in ischemic but viable intestine compared to controls. In nonviable intestine the potential difference was significantly lower than in controls.

Despite its reported experimental accuracy, this technique is not suited for clinical use, since a stab wound into the ischemic loop of bowel is required for insertion of the potential difference bridge. Possible peritoneal contamination or subsequent leakage from the enterostomy make the technique clinically unsafe.

Intraarterial Dye Injection

Direct injection of trypan blue dye suspended in saline through the superior mesenteric artery has been shown experimentally to be a reliable predictor of intestinal viability.[12] Papachristou and Fortner created ventral ischemic loops of terminal ileum in adult Fischer rats. Fifteen minutes after revascularization, saline containing trypan blue was injected into the superior mesenteric artery. If homogeneous staining of the intestine occurred, the bowel was judged viable. Unstained portions were judged nonviable. The predictive accuracy for dye injection was 84%, much better than the 36% predictive accuracy achieved on a clinical basis.

Using the trypan blue test, two patterns of ischemia become evident. Most commonly, the entire loop of intestine fails to show dye staining, indicating irreversible ischemia. Alternatively, only small patches of unstained areas are seen with the majority of the loop taking up dye normally. These unstained areas are prone to perforation.

The major drawbacks to the use of this method clinically are the need to directly inject the superior mesenteric artery at operation and the lack of absolute accuracy of the technique.

Reactive Hyperemia Measured by Temperature Change

Reactive hyperemia is observed in viable ischemic intestine that has been revascularized. After restoration of blood flow, the blood supply is increased to ischemic intestine that is viable. This phenomenon does not occur in irreversibly ischemic bowel. Changes in surface temperature of the bowel wall have been used as an index of reactive hyperemia.

During experimentally induced ischemia in dogs, Bussemaker and Lindeman[10] found that the surface temperature of an ischemic bowel segment was significantly lower (5.7° C) than in adjacent normal bowel. Viability was indicated by reactive hyperemia causing a rise of 1° C or more above that in adjacent normal bowel. This temperature change occurred within 10 minutes of revascularization, and no further temperature rise was noted during an additional 20-minute period of observation. A 1° rise in surface temperature indicated that an anastomosis could be safely performed in the ischemic segment without fear of leakage or stricture. In another experimental study using ischemic segments in rats, this technique showed a 69% accuracy in predicting viability.[12]

Thermography has also been used successfully to assess the occurrence of reactive hyperemia and has been shown to be accurate in predicting viability. In dogs, Moss et al.[13] rendered segments of small intestine ischemic for periods ranging from 2 to 8 hours. Thermograms were made 10 minutes after revascularization. All dogs in which thermograms showed uniform reactive hyperemia survived and were subsequently found to have histologically normal bowel. If the thermogram demonstrated reactive hyperemia with areas of nonuniformity, survival was 67%, and histopathologic examination demonstrated severe residual ischemic damage in the survivors. If there was no thermographic evidence of reactive hyperemia, all animals died with intestinal infarction. Thermography was found to be significantly superior to direct recording of surface temperature in predicting survival.

Radioactive Microspheres

Another technique for the measurement of reactive hyperemia and the prediction of intestinal viability was reported by Moossa et al.[14] and Zarins et al.[15] After ischemic intestine had been revascularized, ^{99m}Technetium-tagged albumin microspheres were injected into the aorta. Counts were then made over both the ischemic segment and adjacent normal bowel. The ratio of the counts over the injured segment to those over a normal segment was taken as a measure of reactive hyperemia. A ratio greater than 1.0 indicated reactive hyperemia. Alternatively, rectilinear scintiscans of the ischemic segment may be compared to those obtained over normal segments to determine whether reactive hyperemia is present.

In an experimental study of ischemic small bowel and colon in dogs and monkeys, macroscopic assessment of intestinal viability was inaccurate in 12 of 18 monkeys and 15 of 26 dogs.[14] Reactive hyperemia was demonstrated by the injection of microspheres in revascularized ischemic bowel in all 16 surviving animals. Conversely, none of the 13 animals dying from intestinal infarction showed a hyperemic response. Of 13 animals developing either a perforation or stricture of the ischemic segment, none showed a uniform hyperemic response.

Zarins et al.[15] showed equal predictive accuracy with scintiscans. In a study of ischemic loops of small bowel in dogs, five showed hyperemic scintiscans, four normal scintiscans, and five ischemic scintiscans. All animals with hyperemic scans proved to have viable intestine, and all with ischemic scans died of intestinal infarction. Two of the four dogs with normal scans developed lethal ischemic complications.

These experimental studies clearly show that the demonstration of reactive hyperemia is an excellent indicator of viability. Ischemic intestine that fails to exhibit reactive hyperemia after restoration of blood flow is likely to progress to perforation, stricture, or frank infarction. The injection of technetium-labeled albumin microspheres is a reliable method of measuring reactive hyperemia and is superior to the subjective assessment of intestinal viability. Limitations to the clinical application of this technique, however, include the need for injection of microspheres into either the aorta or the superior mesenteric artery and the need for specialized scanning or counting equipment not routinely available in the operating room. Therefore, the clinical usefulness of this technique has not been assessed.

Doppler Ultrasound

The use of the Doppler ultrasound apparatus is a sensitive and accurate technique for measuring arterial and venous blood flow in both large and small vessels. It is capable of detecting flow in vessels as small as digital arteries, and therefore has achieved widespread use in the surgical treatment of peripheral vascular disease. This technique has been adapted to intraoperative use and has proved to be an accurate means of assessing intestinal viability. Extensive

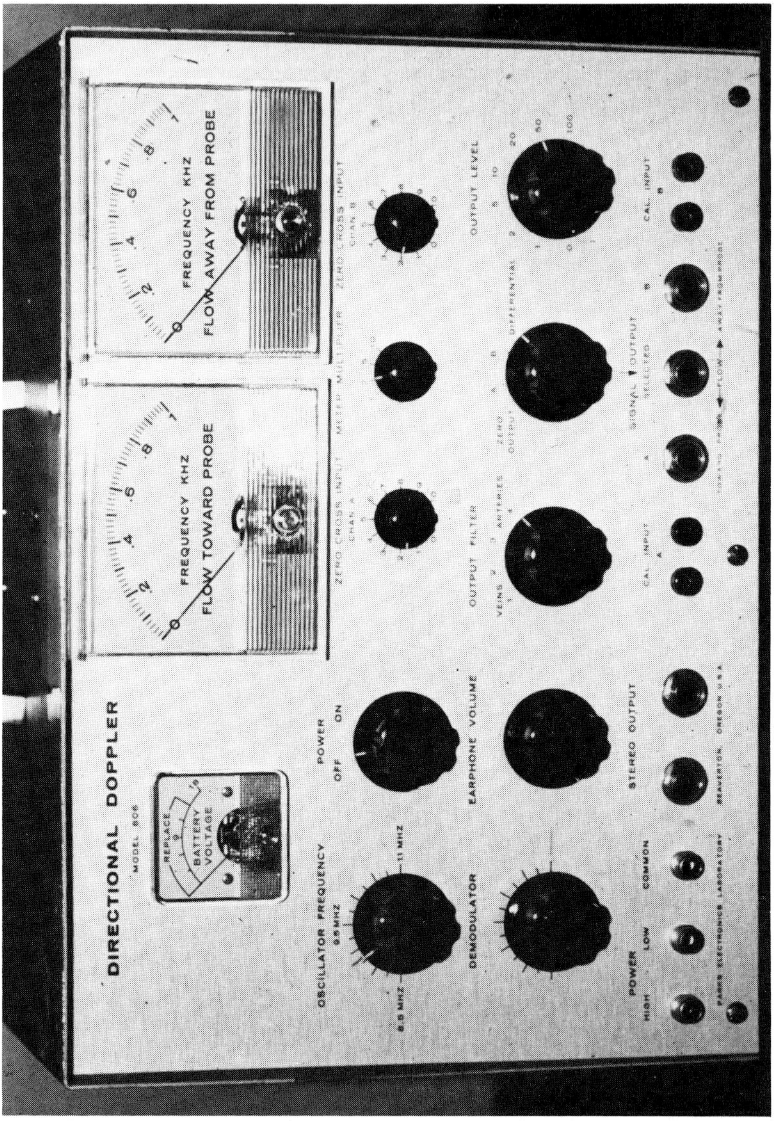

Figure 1. The Doppler ultrasound equipment is easily portable for operating room use.

clinical use has confirmed its reliability. Advantages of the technique include simplicity, minimal required time, relatively inexpensive equipment, and most important, high predictive accuracy.

A typical Doppler ultrasound device is shown in Figure 1, and the probe, sterilizable for intraoperative use, is seen in Figure 2. The equipment is light and easily portable. Probes must be gas-sterilized. Each probe contains two crystals, one of which acts as a high-frequency source and the other as a receiver. Arterial and venous flow signals are easily detected with a speaker or headphones or may be recorded graphically. Doppler ultrasonography is sufficiently sensitive that it is capable of detecting arterial flow

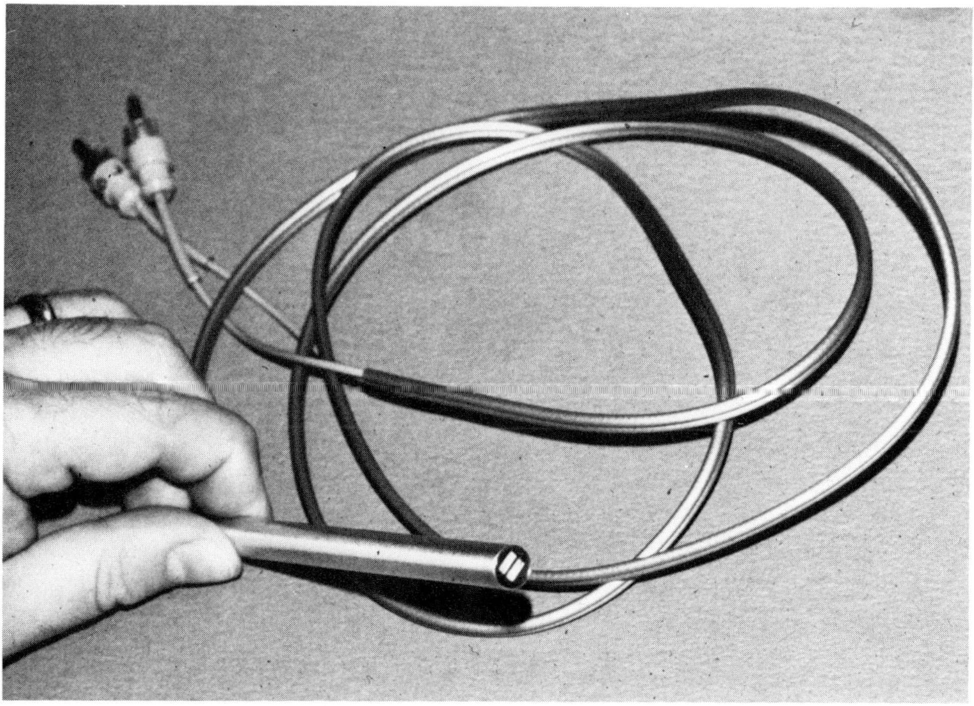

Figure 2. The Doppler probe may be gas-sterilized for intraoperative use.

within both the mesenteric vessels and the tiny vessels within the bowel wall itself. Arterial and venous flow signals are easily audible when the probe is placed on normal small or large intestine. In normal intestine, flow signals may be heard over the antimesenteric surface as well as over the bowel adjacent to the mesentery.

Wright and Hobson were the first to use Doppler ultrasound to predict intestinal viability.[16] Twenty-five centimeter segments of ischemic ileum were produced in dogs and allowed to remain ischemic for periods of 4 to 10 hours. Both arterial and venous flow were interrupted. After blood flow was restored, intestinal viability was assessed clinically and by applying the Doppler probe to the mesentery, the mesenteric-bowel junction, and the antimesenteric surface of the bowel. All animals were reexplored 24 to 48 hours later to evaluate the viability of the ischemic loops.

Loops of intestine subjected to 4 to 6 hours of ischemia rapidly improved in appearance after revascularization and appeared viable. Doppler examination demonstrated arterial flow in all, and viability was confirmed at reexploration. Twelve segments of bowel rendered ischemic for periods of 8 to 10 hours did not appear clinically to be viable. However, arterial flow could be detected in eight of the 12 by Doppler ultrasound, and all eight proved viable. Three of the four segments in which no Doppler arterial flow signals could be detected progressed to frank infarction.

Cooperman et al. confirmed the accuracy of this technique in predicting viability and showed that Doppler ultrasound could be used to select the site at which ischemic intestine should be resected and an anastomosis performed.[17] Twenty segments of ischemic small intestine were produced in dogs by ligating the arterial and venous supply. The Doppler ultrasound probe was then used to find the last audible arterial flow signal on the antimesenteric surface of the bowel wall. The dogs were reexplored after 24 hours and full-thickness biopsies of the bowel wall were performed at the last audible Doppler arterial flow signal and 1, 2, and 3 cm distal to it. Histologic examination showed all 20 segments to be normal at 1 cm distal to the last signal, while progressive degrees of necrosis were observed 2 and 3 cm distal to the last audible signal.

A second phase of the study was performed in baboons, in which a loop of intestine was rendered ischemic and resection with end-to-end anastomosis was performed. The point of resection was either at the last audible Doppler arterial flow signal on the antimesenteric border or 1, 2, 3, or 4 cm distal to it. All anastomoses performed at the last Doppler signal or 1 cm distal to it were normal one month later. Of the 15 performed at points 2, 3, and 4 cm distal to the last signal, 10 showed evidence of either stricture formation or disruption.[17]

Doppler ultrasound proved to be equally accurate in predicting viability in ischemic colon. Cooperman et al. used the site at which the last arterial flow signal could be heard on the antimesenteric surface of ischemic sigmoid colon in dogs to determine the point of resection.[18] All anastomoses performed either at, or 1 cm distal to, the last arterial flow signal healed normally. Fatal anastomotic disruption occurred in five of the 10 dogs in which anastomoses had been performed 2 and 3 cm from the last signal. At the time of resection, visual inspection of the ischemic colon showed no detectable differences between resection margins selected at the last Doppler signal and those 1, 2, and 3 cm distal to it. The margin of resection appeared clinically viable in all dogs.

Many clinical situations of intestinal ischemia are due to venous rather than arterial occlusion. Examples include volvulus, intussusception, and closed loop obstructions. Interruption of the intestinal venous return produces rapid and dramatic changes in the color of the bowel. The bowel and mesentery rapidly becomes dusky and hemorrhagic. Clinical judgment of intestinal viability in these instances is often inaccurate, and the surgeon tends to overestimate the severity of the ischemia. Cooperman, Martin, and Carey showed experimentally that Doppler ultrasound was a reliable predictor of intestinal viability in isolated venous occlusion.[19] Twenty loops of ischemic intestine were created in dogs by temporarily obstructing venous return. Doppler arterial signals within the bowel wall promptly disappeared following venous occlusion. In 10 segments, arterial flow signals returned after venous return was restored, and nine of the 10 were viable at reexploration 24 hours later. Conversely, of 10 segments in which arterial flow signals failed to return, only one proved viable.

Clinical experience with the use of Doppler ultrasound to evaluate intestinal viability has confirmed its usefulness and accuracy. The presence of arterial flow signals in a segment of ischemic intestine is an excellent predictor of survival; conversely, the absence of arterial signals within the bowel wall is certain evidence of irreversible ischemic damage. Cooperman, Martin, and Carey reported their experience during an 18-month period in 23 patients who underwent laparotomy with findings of ischemic intestine.[20] Intestinal ischemia was due to closed loop obstruction (9 patients), incarcerated hernia (5), arterioatherosclerosis (3), volvulus (2), trauma (1), low cardiac output (1), mesenteric venous thrombosis (1), and metastatic carcinoma (1). The small intestine was involved in 18 patients and the colon in five.

In this series of patients, the decision whether or not to resect the ischemic intestine was made solely on the basis of the Doppler ultrasound findings. After blood flow to the ischemic segment had been restored where possible, the viability of the bowel was initially evaluated by the surgeon according to standard clinical criteria, bowel color, mesenteric pulsations, and peristalsis, and a preliminary decision was made concerning the viability of the ischemic segment. A 9mHz Doppler probe calibrated to a Doppler flowmeter was then placed on the antimesenteric surface of the ischemic bowel (Figure 3). All probes had been gas-sterilized prior to use. A sterile water-soluble gel was used to enhance contact between the probe and the bowel wall. If arterial flow signals were detected throughout the entire ischemic segment, the bowel was considered viable and was

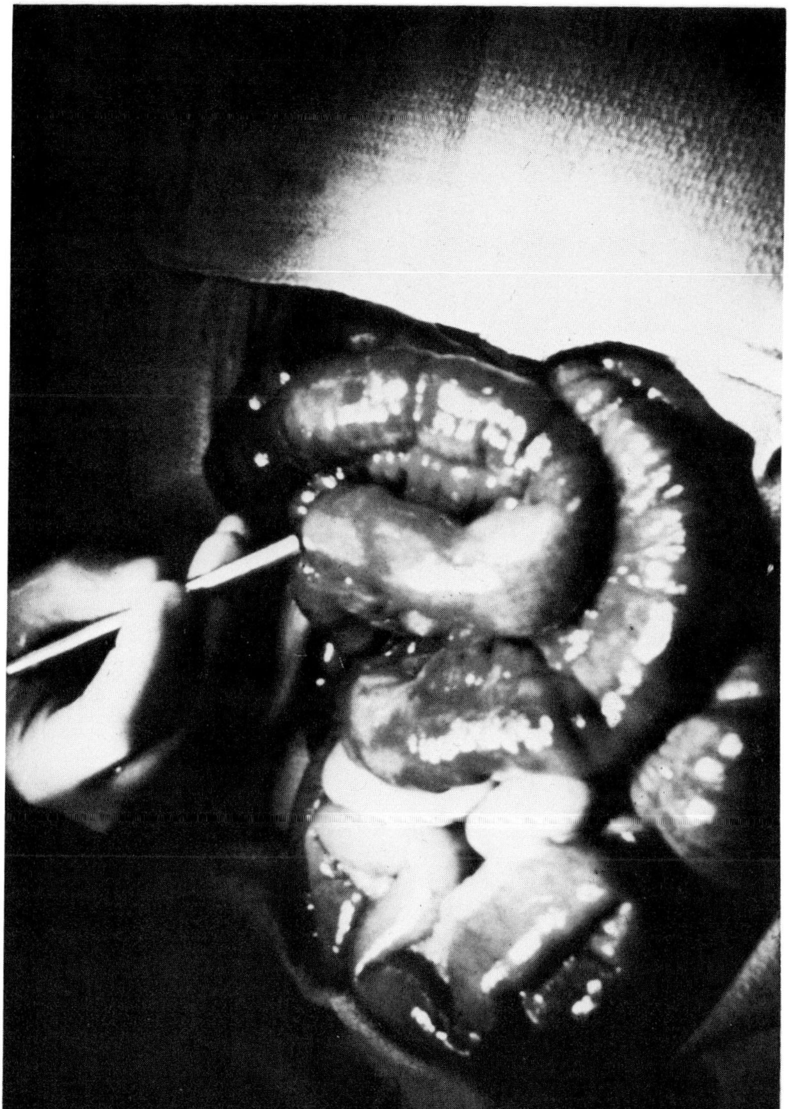

Figure 3. The Doppler probe is lightly applied at a 45° angle to the antimesenteric surface of the bowel. Despite the appearance of the bowel, audible arterial signals were present and resection was unnecessary.

not resected, regardless of its clinical appearance. Conversely, all segments with absent arterial flow signals were resected. Venous signals were not taken into account in determining viability.

There was little agreement between predictions of viability on clinical grounds and Doppler findings (Figure 4). The clinical judgment of the surgeon differed from the Doppler ultrasound findings in 48% of the 25 ischemic segments in these 23 patients. In all cases, the Doppler findings proved accurate. Four segments of intestine were judged viable both clinically and by Doppler ultrasound; all survived. Nine segments were judged nonviable, based on their appearance and the absence of Doppler signals. All were resected and showed either severe ischemia or fresh infarction. Ten segments of bowel were judged clinically to be nonviable, but transmitted Doppler arterial flow signals. All proved to be viable. Radiologic examination 2 to 3 months postoperatively demonstrated normal bowel without fistulas or strictures (Figure 5). Two segments were judged clinically viable, but transmitted no arterial flow signals. Both were resected and histologically demonstrated severe ischemic changes.

The clinical reliability of this technique has been confirmed by other investigators. O'Donnell and Hobson reported 3 patients with acute superior mesenteric arterial thrombosis in whom Doppler ultrasound findings accurately predicting intestinal viability[21] were confirmed by second-look laparotomies. Hobson et al. also reported the usefulness of Doppler ultrasound findings in predicting viability of the left colon and the need for reimplantation of the interior mesenteric artery during aortic reconstruction.[22] If arterial flow signals within the left colon remain audible when the inferior mesenteric artery is clamped, then it may be safely ligated. However, if arterial flow signals can no longer be heard, then the patency of the inferior mesenteric artery must be maintained or it must be reimplanted into the aortic graft.

Extensive additional clinical experience with the use of

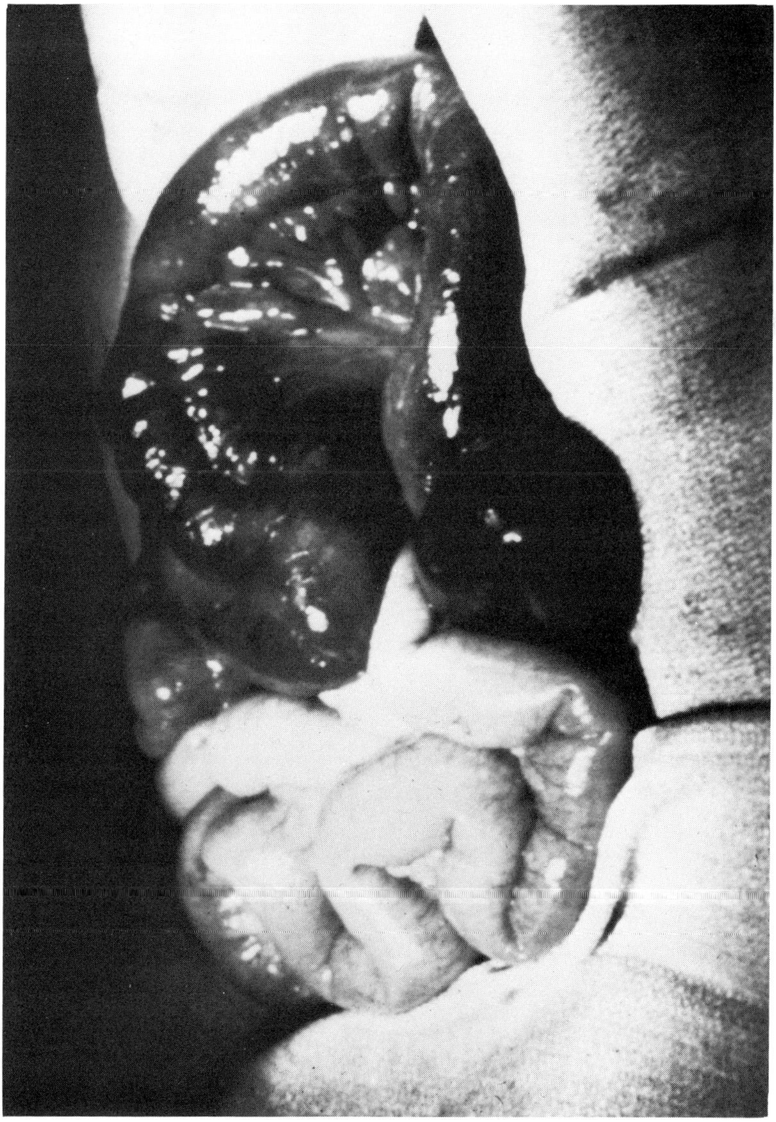

Figure 4. Ischemic intestine in a 28-year-old patient secondary to a closed loop obstruction. This picture was taken 20 minutes after release of the obstruction. On clinical grounds, the bowel did not appear to be viable; however Doppler signals were present and the bowel was not resected. The bowel proved to be viable.

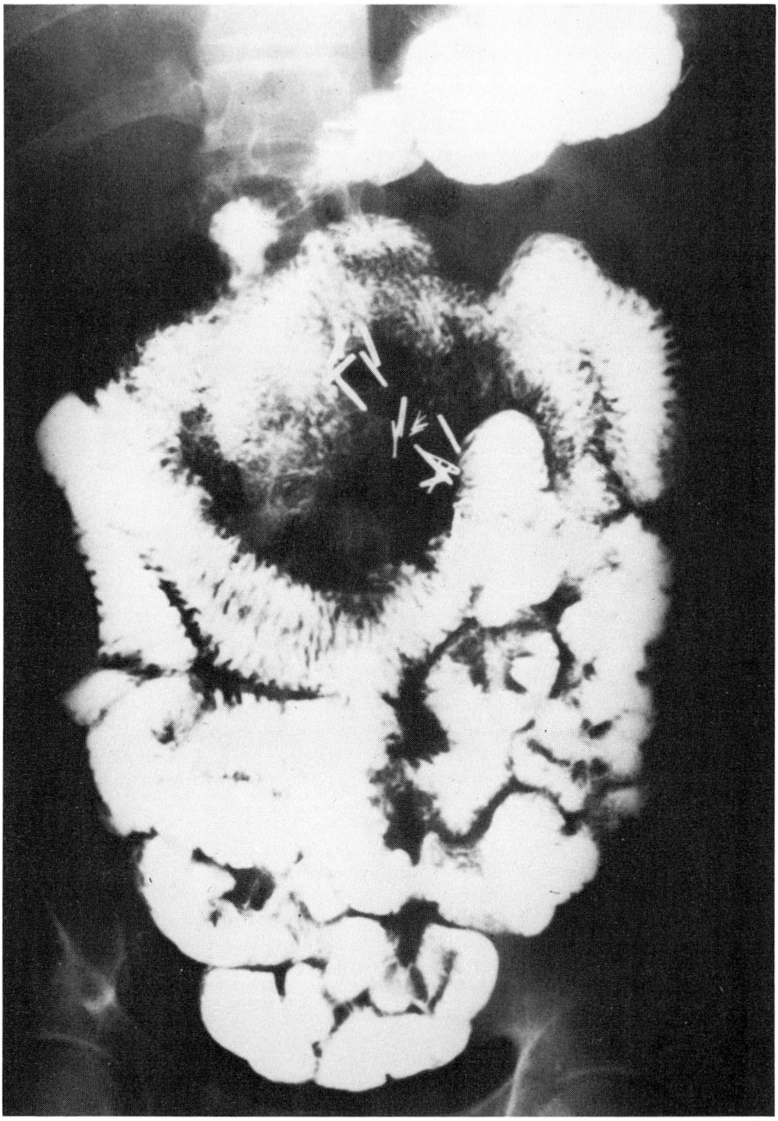

Figure 5. Small bowel barium study performed on the patient in Figure 4 two months postoperatively. There is no evidence of either fistulas or strictures.

Doppler ultrasound to predict intestinal viability has been gained by the author and others at Ohio State University Hospital since the initial report. It has continued to be uniformly accurate in evaluating the viability of ischemic intestine and has consistently proved to be superior to clinical assessment. A 9mHz Doppler pencil probe connected to the Doppler flowmeter is quite sensitive in detecting arterial flow within the small vessels of the intestine itself. It is useful to have several probes available, since they require gas-sterilization and may be used only once during a 24-hour period. Contact between the Doppler probe and the bowel wall is enhanced by the use of a sterile water-soluble gel. To date, there have been no infections attributable to the use of the Doppler equipment at Ohio State University Hospital. The probe should be lightly applied to the bowel wall at a 45° angle. Excessive pressure on the probe may compress the small vessels within the bowel wall and obliterate flow.

It is essential that only the presence or absence of arterial flow signals within the bowel wall itself be used as a criterion for viability. Arterial flow signals are readily distinguished from venous signals; whether or not venous signals are present is not helpful in determining viability. The probe should be placed on the antimesenteric surface of the ischemic bowel, the point at which the blood supply is most precarious. If the bowel is to be judged viable, arterial flow signals must be detectable within the bowel itself; flow signals over the mesentery do not predict viability.

Second-look laparotomies have not been necessary in our experience. None of the patients in whom Doppler arterial signals were present in a questionable segment of bowel required reoperation for intestinal infarction, nor have stricture or fistula formation been observed. The second-look laparotomy is not without risk; often a seriously ill patient must be exposed to a second general anesthetic and major operative procedure, which is appropriate only in the patient whose clinical postoperative course suggests peritonitis, intraabdominal abscess, or progressive intestinal ischemia.

If resection of ischemic intestine is necessary, the margins of resection may be selected using the Doppler apparatus in order to preserve maximum viable intestine. The point of resection should be located at the last audible arterial flow signals in the antimesenteric border.

Fluorescein Dye

Fluorescein dye has recently been successfully used experimentally and clinically to assess intestinal viability. Dye, intravenously injected, is rapidly distributed throughout the body's tissues, and it fluoresces when exposed to ultraviolet light. Approved by the FDA for clinical use, the dye has relatively few side effects, but it does impart a yellow color to the skin, which subsides in 36 to 48 hours. Rare anaphylactic reactions have been reported.

In a study of ischemic loops of small intestine experimentally produced in rabbits, Marfuggi and Greenspan injected fluorescein intravenously after revascularization.[23] If the intestine fluoresced when exposed to ultraviolet light from a Woods lamp, it was judged viable. This technique was 93% accurate in predicting viability, compared to the 80% accuracy of clinical evaluation.

Bulkley et al. successfully applied the technique clinically.[24] In 58 segments of ischemic intestine examined in 28 patients, fluorescein was 100% accurate in predicting intestinal viability. These authors found fluorescein dye to be superior to both clinical assessment and Doppler ultrasound examination.

The intraoperative use of fluorescein is technically simple. After blood flow to the ischemic bowel has been restored, all fluid is aspirated from the peritoneal cavity to prevent external staining of the bowel. Two ampules (1000 mg) are then administered intravenously. The operating room lights are turned off and the bowel is illuminated by a hand-held 3600 A Woods ultraviolet light. Based on its appearance under the ultraviolet light, the bowel is judged either viable or nonviable. Viable intestine demonstrates either a hyperemic, normal, or finely granular pattern, with normal to increased intensity.[24] If the bowel fails to fluoresce or demonstrates patchy fluorescence with areas of nonfluorescence greater than 5 mm in diameter, or if the intensity is diminished, the bowel is judged nonviable.[24]

Advantages of this technique include its simplicity, predictive accuracy, rapidity, and lack of need for expensive, complicated equipment. The major disadvantage is the requirement for subjective assessment of the degree to which the ischemic bowel fluoresces. If the operating surgeon is not experienced with this method, he may have difficulty interpreting borderline patterns of fluorescence.

In cases in which the fluorescence pattern is marginal, another method of determining viability should be employed. Doppler ultrasound is quite useful in these instances. If arterial flow signals are heard, the bowel need not be resected. If signals are absent, the segment in question is resected at the points where the last audible signals are present.

References

1. Bussemaker JB, Lindeman J: Comparison of methods to determine viability of small intestine. *Ann Surg* 176:97, 1972.
2. Glotzer DJ, Villegas AH, Anekamaya S, Shaw RS: Healing of the intestine in experimental bowel infarction. *Ann Surg* 155:183, 1962.
3. Jensen CB, Smith GA: Clinical study of 51 cases of mesenteric infarction. *Surgery* 40:930, 1956.
5. Moossa AR, Skinner DB, Stark U, Hoffer P: Assessment of bowel viability using technetium-tagged albumin microspheres. *J Surg Res* 16:466, 1974.
6. Wright CB, Hobson RW: Prediction of intestinal viability using Doppler ultrasound technics. *Am J Surg* 129:642, 1975.
7. Zarins CK, Skinner DB, Rhodes BA, Janes AE: Prediction of the viability of revascularized intestine with radioactive microspheres. *Surg Gynecol Obstet* 138:676, 1974.
8. Myers MB, Cherry G, Gesser J: Relationship between surface pH and pCO_2 and the vascularity and viability of intestine. *Surg Gynecol Obstet* 134:787, 1972.
9. Katz S, Wahab A, Murray W, Williams LF: New parameters

of viability in ischemic bowel disease. *Am J Surg* 127:136, 1974.

10. Bussemaker JB, Lindeman J: Comparison of methods to determine viability of small intestine. *Ann Surg* 176:97, 1972.
11. Gurll NJ, Maj MC, Braxton G: Potential difference as an estimate of intestinal viability. *J Surg Res* 18:611, 1975.
12. Papachristou D, Fortner JG: Prediction of intestinal viability by intra-arterial dye injection: A simple test. *Am J Surg* 132:572, 1976.
13. Moss AA, Kressel HY, Brito AC: Use of thermography to predict intestinal viability and survival after ischemic injury: A blind experimental study. *Invest Radiol* 16:24, 1981.
14. Moossa AR, Skinner DB, Stark V, Hoffer P: Assessment of bowel viability using ^{99m}Technetium-tagged albumin microspheres. *J Surg Res* 16:466, 1974.
15. Zarins CK, Skinner DB, James AE Jr: Prediction of the viability of revascularized intestine with radioactive microspheres. *Surg Gynecol Obstet* 138:576, 1974.
16. Wright CB, Hobson RW II: Prediction of intestinal viability using Doppler ultrasound technics. *Am J Surg* 129:642, 1975.
17. Cooperman M, Pace WG, Martin EW, Pflug B, Keith LM, Evans WE, Carey LC: Determination of viability of ischemic intestine by Doppler ultrasound. *Surgery* 83:705, 1978.
18. Cooperman M, Martin EW, Evans WE, Carey LC: Assessment of anastomotic blood supply by Doppler ultrasound in operations upon the colon. *Surg Gynecol Obstet* 149:15, 1979.
19. Cooperman M, Martin EW, Carey LC: Determination of intestinal viability by Doppler ultrasonography in venous infarction. *Ann Surg* 191:57, 1980.
20. Cooperman M, Martin EW, Carey LC: Evaluation of ischemic intestine by Doppler ultrasound. *Am J Surg* 139:73, 1980.
21. O'Donnell JA, Hobson RW: Operative confirmation of Doppler ultrasound in evaluation of intestinal ischemia. *Surgery* 87:109, 1980.
22. Hobson RW, Wright CB, Rich NM, Collins GJ: Assessment of colonic ischemia during aortic surgery by Doppler ultrasound. *J Surg Res* 20:231, 1976.
23. Marfuggi RA, Greenspan M: Reliable intraoperative prediction of intestinal viability using a fluorescent indicator. *Surg Gynecol Obstet* 152:33, 1981.
24. Bulkley GB, Zuidema GD, Hamilton SR, O'Mara CS, Klacsmann PG: Intraoperative determination of small intestinal viability following ischemic injury. *Ann Surg* 193:628, 1981.

8

Intestinal Ischemia in Infancy and Childhood

Denis R. King, M.D.

Although usually considered a problem of aging and the aged, ischemic diseases of the intestine are actually observed clinically from infancy to old age. Intestinal ischemia is a common problem in the everyday practice of pediatric surgery (Table I). The etiology of vascular insufficiency states in infants and children is quite diverse and includes congenital conditions such as malrotation with volvulus, acquired conditions such as intussusception, and iatrogenic conditions such as umbilical artery catheterization. Ischemic states characterized by mesenteric arterial inflow occlusion, nonocclusive vascular insufficiency, and venous outflow obstruction are all observed in pediatric practice. Various conditions associated with inadequate intestinal blood flow can be categorized according to the pathophysiology of the ischemic insult.

Table 1

Intestinal Ischemia: Age at Onset

Neonatal: 0–30 days
Jejunoileal Atresia
Spontaneous Gastric Perforation
Necrotizing Enterocolitis
Malrotation and Volvulus
Umbilical Artery Catheterization
Infancy: 1–24 months
Intussusception
Incarcerated Hernia
Childhood: 2+ years
Sporadic Occurrence

Arterial Inflow Occlusion

Jejunoileal Atresia

Mechanical intestinal obstruction is one of the most common neonatal surgical emergencies, and jejunoileal atresia with an incidence approximating one in every 1,000 live births remains the most frequent cause of bowel obstruction in infants.[1] Intrauterine intestinal infarction has been accepted as the cause of the majority of neonatal small bowel atresia since 1955, when Louw and Barnard reported their observations on experimental fetal mesenteric devascularization.[2] They subjected canine fetuses to late in utero ligation of the mesenteric vasculature and reproduced all the various atretic anomalies commonly observed in human infants. Intussusception, segmental volvulus, and internal hernias occurring in utero probably account for the occasional cases that are not primarily vascular in etiology.

Infants with jejunoileal atresia demonstrate many of the hallmarks of neonatal intestinal obstruction including polyhydramnios, bilious vomiting, abdominal distention, and failure to pass meconium. Supine and upright abdominal radiographs are usually diagnostic, documenting the presence of dilated intestinal loops with air-fluid levels indicative of mechanical obstruction (Figure 1A). If few bowel loops are distal to the duodenum, a high level of atresia (jejunum) is suggested. Many dilated bowel loops may be seen with either ileal or colonic disease, and a barium enema is required to evaluate the level of obstruction. A

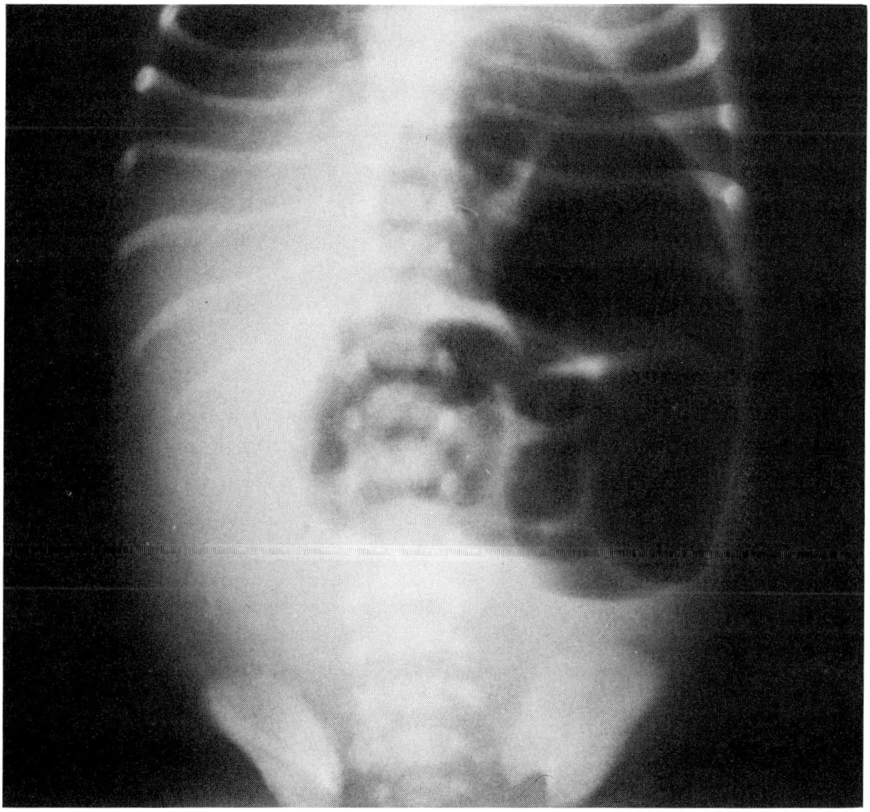

Figure 1A. This upright abdominal radiograph demonstrates dilated bowel loops with air-fluid levels indicative of mechanical intestinal obstruction.

(Illustration continued on the following page)

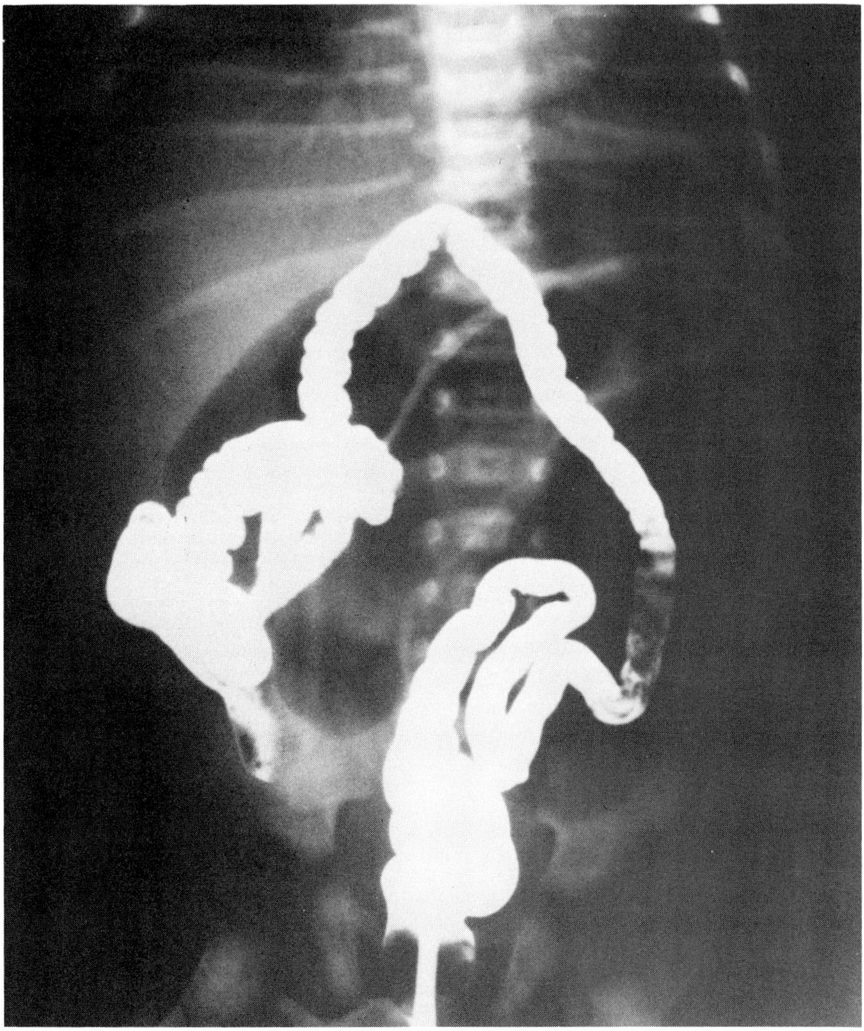

Figure 1B. This barium enema documents the presence of a normally rotated but "unused" colon typically observed in infants with jejunoileal atresia.

normally rotated microcolon is typically observed in infants with atresia of the small intestine (Figure 1B). Other possible radiographic manifestations are: (1) intraperitoneal calcification which is indicative of intrauterine bowel perforation and meconium peritonitis, and (2) diffuse gaseous distention with a relative paucity of air-fluid levels which suggests meconium ileus.

Surgical management should include resection of the grossly dilated bulbous portion of intestine immediately proximal to the atresia. Left in situ, this bowel segment produces ineffective peristalsis and results in anastomotic dysfunction. Multiple levels of atresia are observed in approximately 10% of patients, so the entire length of the intestine must be carefully evaluated. Distention of the bowel with normal saline beyond the atresia is easily accomplished intraoperatively, thus assuring an adequate distal lumen. Stamm gastrostomy is a useful addition to the surgical management of these infants who may require two to four weeks of nasogastric decompression before enteral feeding is tolerated. With the advent of effective parenteral alimentation, survival should be expected for the majority of infants (90%) with isolated jejunoileal atresia.[3]

Umbilical Artery Catheterization

Aortic catheterization via the umbilical artery is frequently performed in the neonatal intensive care unit to provide a convenient route for monitoring arterial pressures, blood gas tensions, and serum chemistries in sick infants. However, the complications of this procedure may be life-threatening, and are known to include aortic thrombosis, extremity necrosis, visceral infarction, and paraplegia.[4,5,6]

In a prospective study designed to evaluate the thrombotic complications of umbilical artery catheters, Neal et al. demonstrated a 95% incidence of aortic thrombus formation.[7] Seven of 12 infants autopsied (58%) had evidence of major vessel thrombosis, and in one patient the superior mesenteric artery was completely occluded, producing lethal midgut infarction. In a retrospective review of 165 neonates, Marsh et al. documented a 9% mortality resulting from the complications of umbilical artery-monitoring catheters.[6] Intestinal necrosis secondary to superior mesenteric artery thrombosis accounted for one of the 15 deaths. Although the incidence of visceral thrombosis is relatively low, infants with aortic catheters should be observed carefully for evidence of intestinal ischemia. The sudden onset of abdominal distention, tenderness, or hematochezia may be an indication for catheter removal and systemic heparin therapy.

Nonocclusive Vascular Insufficiency

Gastric Perforation

Spontaneous gastric perforation is an uncommon but recognized clinical entity characterized by acute respiratory distress and peritonitis early in the neonatal period. The cause of gastric perforation remains obscure, but retrospective analysis of large series of patients has prompted some authors to suggest nonocclusive vascular insufficiency. In 1969, Lloyd reviewed the clinical records of 87 infants with spontaneous gastrointestinal perforation,[8] and was impressed with the consistent clinical picture presented by many of these babies. He sought a concept that would clarify the pathophysiology of this condition.

One characteristic shared by 81% of the infants was the occurrence of a documented episode of cold stress, hypoxia, or shock during the neonatal period. Based on this observation, Lloyd postulated the "diving reflex" as the source of temporary selective mesenteric ischemia that resulted in spontaneous gastrointestinal perforation. This hypothesis implies that the newborn infant reacts much like a diving mammal in response to severe physiologic stress. As a result, splanchnic blood flow is restricted and diverted to the central circulation to preserve cardiac and cerebral function.[9] Under these circumstances, the gastrointestinal tract may sustain an irreversible hypoxic injury. Lloyd's initial observations were confirmed by Touloukian, who reported a 69% incidence of significant perinatal complications in a collected series of 95 patients with isolated gastric perforation.[10]

More than half of these patients are premature infants who exhibit perinatal distress. The first days of life pass uneventfully, but on the third or fourth day, the onset of massive abdominal distention and respiratory distress is abrupt. Lethargy, bilious emesis, and cyanosis are frequently observed. Recumbent abdominal radiographs may demonstrate the so-called "football sign" indicative of free intraperitoneal air, but upright abdominal films, which are preferable, usually reveal the massive pneumoperitoneum typical of gastric perforation. (See Figure 2.)

Nasogastric intubation, antibiotics, and aggressive fluid and electrolyte resuscitation are mandatory. Ventilatory insufficiency may result if the pneumoperitoneum is tense and diaphragmatic motion is impeded. Under these unusual circumstances, needle aspiration of the peritoneal cavity can be life-saving. Abdominal exploration should be performed through a generous transverse supraumbilical incision. The edges of the gastric perforation must be debrided back to well vascularized tissue and the stomach is closed in two layers. A Stamm gastrostomy should be placed if the size and vascularity of the gastric remnant are adequate. This obviates the necessity for prolonged nasogastric decompression and provides a convenient route for continuous tube feedings postoperatively if gastric reservoir function is seriously impaired.

The reported prognosis for infants with spontaneous gastric perforation is poor. But, with rapid diagnosis, aggres-

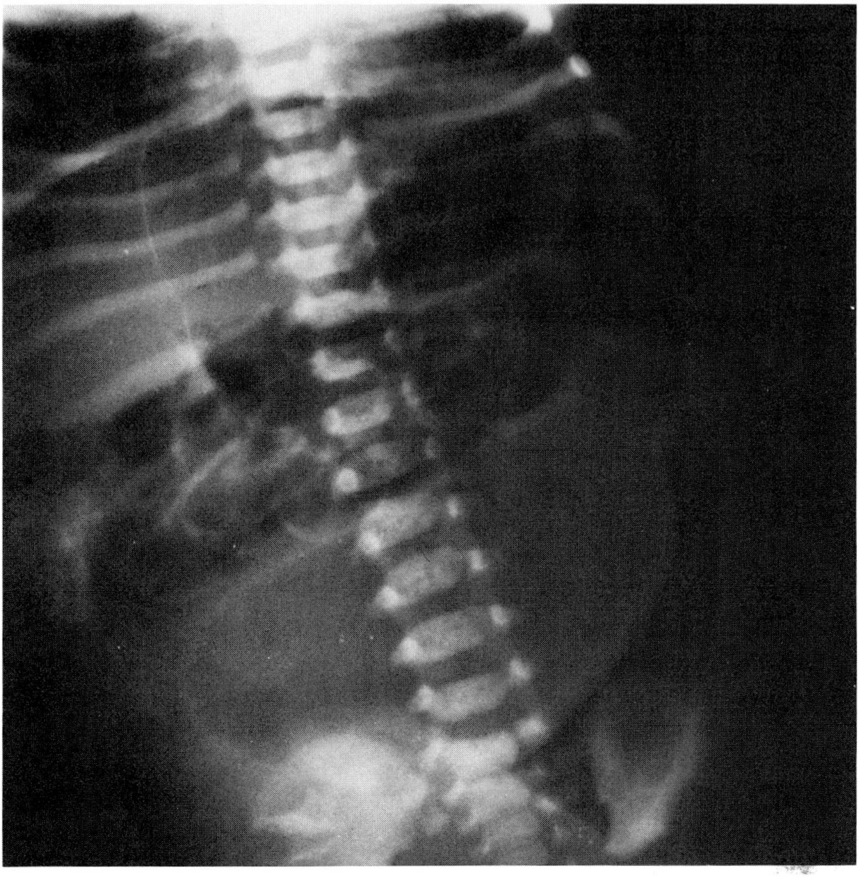

Figure 2. This falciform ligament (arrows) is well outlined on this recumbent abdominal radiograph indicating the presence of free intraperitoneal air.

sive resuscitation, immediate definitive surgery, and successful control of intraperitoneal sepsis, many babies will survive and live normal lives.

Necrotizing Enterocolitis

Necrotizing enterocolitis (NEC) was unrecognized in the neonatal nursery before 1960. As our ability to prolong the survival of the tiny premature infant improved, a whole new series of clinical problems appeared, many of which were the indirect result of life-sustaining therapeutic interventions. At present, necrotizing enterocolitis is estimated to affect up to 5% of all high-risk premature neonates, and in many centers it has become the single most common reason for emergency surgical intervention in the neonate.[11]

The precise etiology of necrotizing enterocolitis is not known, but it appears that the pathologic changes described in patients with NEC represent the final common pathway of response to significant physiologic stresses. Lloyd has popularized the "diving reflex" as one possible explanation of the pathogenesis of this disease. Other authors have documented the deleterious effects of hyperosmolar feedings on small premature infants and observed that necrotizing enterocolitis is rarely seen before oral feedings are instituted.[12] The possibility that necrotizing enterocolitis is caused by a transmissible enteric agent has been suggested by Book et al., who reported geographic and temporal clustering of cases and reduction of incidence of NEC by the implementation of infection control procedures.[13] Barlow et al. have emphasized the importance of breast milk in the prevention of enterocolitis.[14] No single theory explains the pathogenesis of all cases. This unique disease is currently considered to be multifactorial in origin.

The majority of patients with necrotizing enterocolitis are small premature infants who have sustained one or more catastrophic physiologic insults. Santulli et al. documented a perinatal complication rate of 95% in their patients, with respiratory distress syndrome, apneic episodes, cyanosis, low Apgar scores, and premature rupture of the membranes being most frequently noted.[15] NEC characteristically becomes evident during the first two weeks of life, and oral or gavage feedings have been established in most affected infants before the onset of symptoms. The initial clinical manifestations of NEC include mild abdominal distention, intolerance to feeding, and lethargy. Unfortunately, these nonspecific findings are distressingly common in any sick neonate. Analysis of the stool for reducing substances may demonstrate an abnormal fecal carbohydrate content (2+ or greater) which indicates impaired intestinal mucosal function. If the stools are also positive for occult blood, an anatomic rather than a functional disruption of mucosal integrity is suggested, and the possibility of necrotizing enterocolitis should be seriously considered. Intervention at this prediagnostic or incipient stage will generally prevent progression to overt NEC. If these subtle manifestations are not perceived, however, the subsequent development of prominent abdominal distention, bilious vomiting, and temperature instability herald the onset of clinical enterocolitis. Abdominal tenderness and grossly bloody diarrhea stools are common and localize the source of the symptoms to the gastrointestinal tract. Hypotension, tachycardia, and oliguria are frequent. Apnea and brachycardia are commonly observed. Failure to institute vigorous resuscitative efforts at this point invariably results in rapid clinical deterioration with metabolic acidosis, sepsis, and shock.

Laboratory data generally confirm the clinical impression and support the diagnosis of gram-negative sepsis. An elevated white blood cell count and thrombocytopenia, hallmarks of neonatal gram-negative bacterial infection, are present in most patients. Metabolic acidosis secondary to poor peripheral perfusion may be severe, and in the presence of advanced peritonitis with abdominal distention and restriction of diaphragmatic motion, a profound mixed metabolic-respiratory acidosis may be observed. Endotracheal intubation and respiratory support are frequently required. The earliest radiographic manifestations of necrotizing enterocolitis are nonspecific generalized gaseous distention of the intestine with scattered air-fluid levels and an increased distance between adjacent bowel loops. With progression of the intestinal involvement, pneumatosis intestinalis becomes apparent as small linear collections of subserosal gas (Figure 3A). Intrahepatic portal venous gas is less frequently seen (Figure 3B). Both findings are virtually diagnostic of NEC. The most ominous radiographic features are those associated with frank intestinal necrosis. These include a dilated intestinal loop unchanged in size

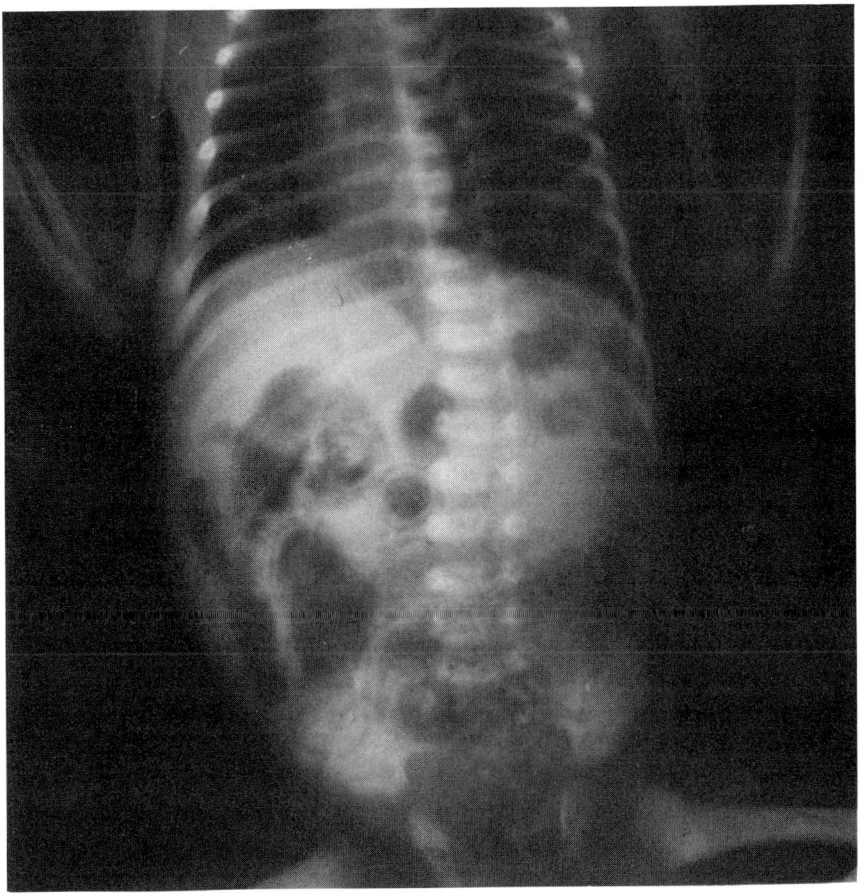

Figure 3A. Pneumatosis intestinalis (subserosal gas) is apparent in many bowel loops (arrows) indicating the presence of necrotizing enterocolitis (NEC).

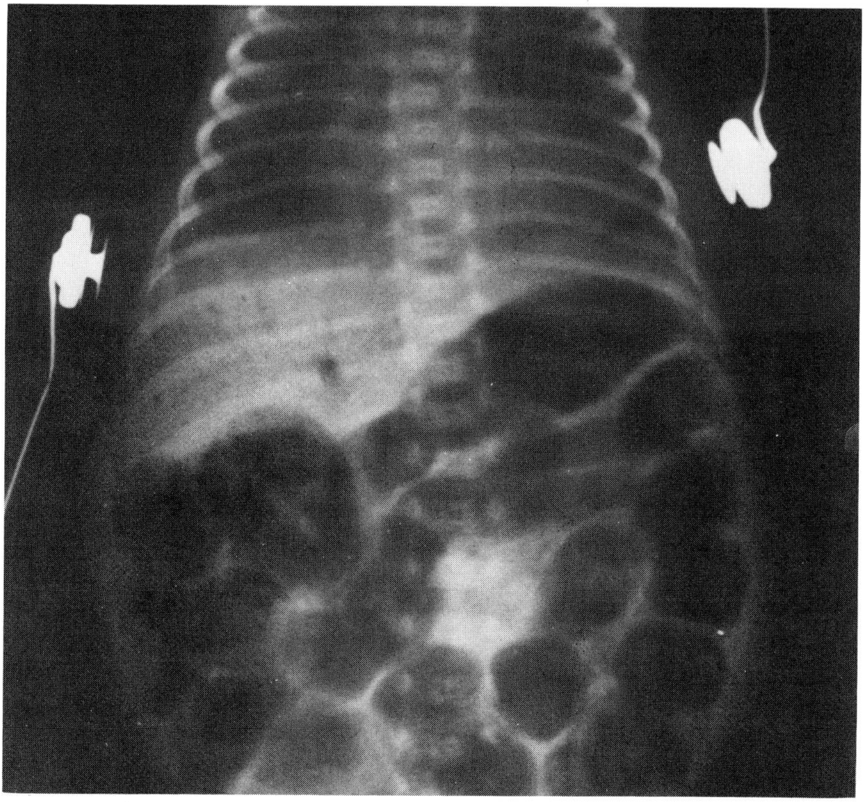

Figure 3B. Portal venous gas, virtually diagnostic of NEC, is observed less frequently.

or position that persists for 24 to 36 hours, increasing intraabdominal fluid accumulation, and free intraperitoneal air. The use of contrast studies is rarely indicated in patients with suspected NEC, since even the gentlest manipulation of the severely ischemic intestine may be followed by intestinal perforation.

The importance of combined medical and surgical evaluation and management of these babies cannot be overemphasized. The initial therapeutic approach for all infants with NEC should include vigorous resuscitation. Nasogastric decompression is instituted, and intravenous fluids are administered. Volume deficits should be rapidly repleted and ongoing third-space losses estimated and replaced. Mesenteric blood flow must be maximized if the anoxic damage to the intestine is to be reversed. Umbilical artery catheters should be removed. Broad-spectrum antibiotic therapy effective against the majority of gram-negative enteric organisms is initiated. Although the role of enteral antibiotics is far from clear, it has been our practice to administer Kanamycin (15 mg/kg/BID) by gavage. The potential advantages of this regimen appear substantial, and no significant complications have been observed.[16]

During the resuscitation and recovery periods, constant observation in a neonatal intensive care unit is advisable. The surgeon's responsibilities are to anticipate, identify, and immediately treat the catastrophic complications of NEC. Clinical observation, abdominal examination, and supine and decubitus abdominal roentgenograms are required at least every six hours. Free perforation, evidence of advancing peritonitis, and clinical deterioration despite therapy dictate the need for abdominal exploration.

If laparotomy is required, intraperitoneal fluid should be obtained for gram-stain and culture (aerobic and anaerobic). Intestinal involvement may be either local or diffuse, and the affected areas may be continuous or multifocal. Obviously necrotic segments of intestine should be resected. Primary anastomosis is not recommended in these critically ill infants with marginal intestinal blood flow and fecal peritonitis. Stomas should be constructed, the proximal bowel decompressed, and the peritoneal cavity copiously lavaged.

During the immediate postoperative period, continued vigorous fluid administration is frequently necessary in order to maintain cardiac output and obtain an adequate urine volume. Total parenteral nutrition is routinely started two to three days following operation, if the patient's clinical condition permits. Antibiotics should be continued for seven to 10 days, and oral feedings are not begun for at least two weeks. The well known propensity of these babies to develop strictures in the excluded bowel segments must be recognized, and restoration of gastrointestinal continuity should not be undertaken until the distal intestine has been found to be normal by careful evaluation of barium contrast studies.

The results of both medical and surgical treatment for necrotizing enterocolitis are somewhat disappointing, with most authors currently reporting an overall survival of 65 to 70%.[17,18] Successful treatment of NEC does not guarantee survival in these critically ill infants, as they not infrequently succumb to the primary process that produced the initial perinatal distress.

Venous Outflow Obstruction

Malrotation and Volvulus

Of all the conditions known to produce neonatal intestinal ischemia, malrotation with midgut volvulus is potentially the most devastating. Early recognition and urgent surgical management are required if intestinal viability is to be maintained. The abnormal embryogenesis that results in failure of complete rotation may occur as an isolated phenomenon, but it is also frequently associated with other congenital anomalies such as diaphragmatic hernia, omphalocele, gastroschisis, and prune belly syndrome.

Although malrotation with volvulus is a strangulating obstruction of the midgut that typically becomes apparent in the first thirty days of life (65%), many of the hallmarks of neonatal intestinal obstruction may be conspicuously absent.[19] If volvulus was not present in utero, polyhydramnios will not occur. Because of the proximal nature of the obstruction, abdominal distention is relatively uncommon, and since duodenal obstruction is incomplete, normal meconium is usually passed.

The majority of infants with midgut volvulus have sudden neonatal onset of persistent bilious emesis. If the duodenal obstruction is complicated by midgut ischemia, hypovolemia, hypotension, metabolic acidosis, and hematochezia rapidly become apparent.

Radiographic manifestations on routine abdominal views that suggest malrotation and volvulus are: (1) a double bubble characteristic of duodenal obstruction, (2) a relative paucity of intestinal gas, or (3) many dilated proximal bowel loops with air-fluid levels. A definitive diagnosis of malrotation is most reliably achieved by barium examination of the upper gastrointestinal tract (Figure 4A). In Simpson's report, 22 of 23 infants were accurately identified in this fashion.[20] Barium enema is considered less reliable (Figure 4B). Once the diagnosis is established, laparotomy should be performed expeditiously, since undue delay only increases the risk of intestinal infarction.

Operative management includes: (1) exploration through a generous upper abdominal transverse incision, (2) reduction of the volvulus with careful assessment of intestinal viability, and (3) Ladd's procedure. Only frankly necrotic bowel should be resected initially. This is particularly important if the ischemic injury is generalized. Our routine practice is to return both viable and marginally viable bowel to the abdominal cavity and reexplore in 24 hours. Definitive bowel resections are deferred until the "second-look" procedure. Primary anastomosis is not recommended after resection. Fixation of the colon to the left lateral abdominal wall is not routinely performed. If intestinal ischemia is insignificant, appendectomy is advised. The duodenum should be carefully evaluated because of the relatively high incidence (5%) of associated obstructing anomalies.[21]

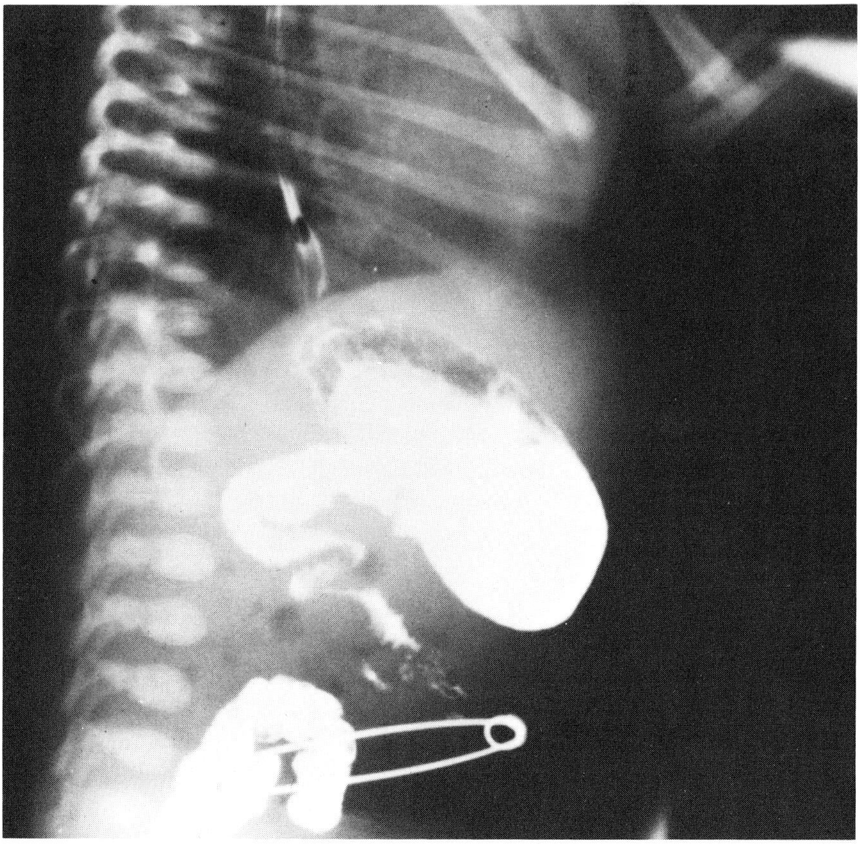

Figure 4A. Partial obstruction of the duodenum (note the corkscrew appearance) in this neonate confirms the diagnosis of midgut malrotation and volvulus.

The clinical outcome in infants with malrotation and volvulus is directly related to the severity of the intestinal ischemic injury. In the absence of bowel necrosis, survival is virtually assured. Early diagnosis is the key to successful management, and it must be emphasized that malrotation and volvulus should be considered in the differential diagnosis of all infants with evidence of proximal intestinal obstruction.

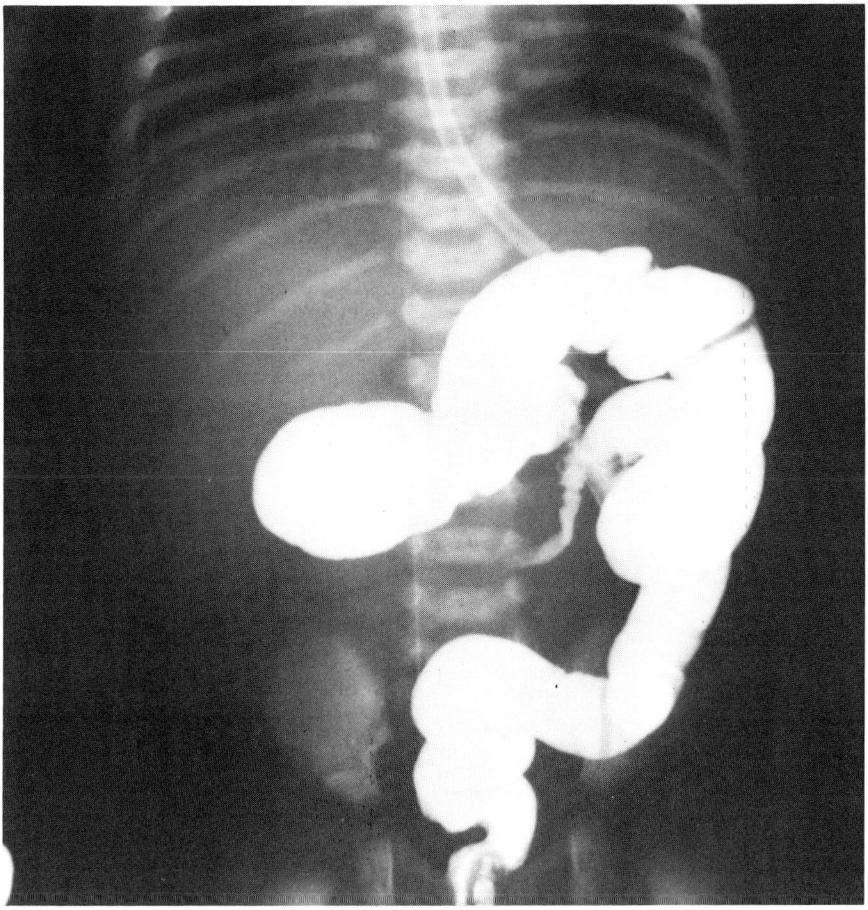

Figure 4B. This barium enema demonstrates the cecum and appendix in an abnormal mid-abdominal position consistent with malrotation of the midgut.

Incarcerated Inguinal Hernia

Indirect inguinal hernias are the most common of the surgically treated congenital anomalies, affecting perhaps 2% of all children. More than half the patients are in the first year of life, and elective repair can be safely accomplished. However, in a review of 2,764 consecutive patients, Rowe identified 351 children (12%) who required emergency management because of incarceration or strangulation.[22] The incidence of incarceration was highest in the first year of life, and both incarceration (17.2%) and irreducibility (29%) were more common in female infants. If the initial episode of incarceration was not followed by prompt repair, reincarceration of the hernia invariably resulted (100%).

All of the patients in Rowe's series were initially treated according to a standard protocol that included sedation with meperidine hydrochloride (1 mg/lb) and Trendelenburg positioning. Manipulation of the hernia was avoided. Successful nonoperative reduction of incarcerated hernias was accomplished within an hour or two in 281 patients (81%), who underwent subsequent prompt elective hernia repair. The remaining 68 children required emergency surgical management. Necrotic intestine necessitating bowel resection was found on only five occasions (1.4%) attesting to the safety of nonoperative management for the majority of infants.

Vascular insufficiency with tissue necrosis was most frequently observed (8 cases) in the testis on the affected side. Although incarceration is a relatively common phenomenon in children with inguinal hernia, strangulating injuries necessitating bowel resection are unusual. In the absence of clinical evidence of intestinal necrosis, the majority of affected infants can be safely managed with nonoperative reduction and urgent elective repair.

Intussusception

Intussusception is the most common cause of intestinal obstruction in infants with a reported incidence of two cases per thousand live births. Male preponderance (3:2) is noted in most large series and the majority of patients (85%) are less than two years of age.[23]

The archetypal patient is a previously healthy 10-months-old male infant who suddenly has recurring episodes of abdominal colic. During the episodes of pain, the infant is inconsolable, and pallor and diaphoresis may be observed. Nonbilious vomiting is common at the outset, but invariably progresses to bilious emesis if the diagnosis is not established and the intestinal obstruction not relieved. Hematochezia (currant jelly stool) is next observed, and this usually produces sufficient parental concern that a physician is consulted.

In most patients a tubular mass is palpable in the right upper quadrant or epigastrium. Mild direct abdominal tenderness over the intussusception may be noted, but rigidity and rebound tenderness are infrequent. Peritonitis is not present in the majority of children with intussusception. The cause of this condition in infancy is not well understood. The majority (95%) have no apparent anatomic abnormality in the ileocecal area, and once reduced, intussusception rarely recurs (2–5%). Most authors favor the explanation that hypertrophied lymphoid patches in the submucosa of the ileum are the initiating point of the intussusception. In unusual cases when a lead point is discovered (5–8%), Meckel's diverticula, polyps, and duplication cysts are most frequently noted. In older children, the possibility of lymphosarcoma must be considered.[24]

Once the intussusception has invaginated, strangulating obstruction of the involved intestine ensues. The mesentery is compressed between the layers of the bowel wall, producing venous and lymphatic obstruction. Edema in the engorged intussusceptum eventually produces tissue pressures sufficient to decrease arterial inflow with resulting necrosis of the leading edge of the intestine.

Intussusception is one clinical problem that can be readily diagnosed and in most cases successfully treated roentgenographically. Before fluoroscopy is undertaken, however, attention should be directed to correction of the physiologic deficits that accompany this form of strangulating intestinal obstruction. Intravenous rehydration, nasogastric suction, and antibiotic administration are initiated prior to any barium studies. Since Ravitch popularized hydrostatic reduction in the 1940s, the standard method of treating intussusception has been nonoperative reduction by barium enema. Hydrostatic reduction has been successful in 65 to 75% of the cases reported.[23,25] With strict adherence to the technical details of the procedure, bowel perforation and reduction of gangrenous intestine should be avoided. Abdominal palpation during reduction is unwise, since this can dramatically increase intraluminal pressure. Criteria for successful reduction include the free flow of barium into the small intestine, disappearance of the abdominal mass, and the relief of symptoms. If hydrostatic reduction is achieved, a 12-to-24-hour period of inpatient observation is advised. Laparotomy is required in the 25 to 30% of patients in whom attempts at hydrostatic reduction fail. The surgical incision used depends upon the position of the intussusceptum. Manual reduction is easily accomplished in the majority of surgical cases. Bowel resection is reserved for the few children with frankly necrotic intestine (5–10%). In the absence of gross peritoneal contamination or massive dilatation of the obstructed small bowel, primary anastomosis is encouraged.

The overall results of treatment of intussusception are excellent. Fatalities are virtually unknown and morbidity is low. Hydrostatic reduction is safe and effective in the majority of cases, and operative manipulation suffices for the others. Recurrence, complications, and late sequelae are distinctly uncommon.

References

1. Grosfeld JL: Alimentary tract obstruction in the newborn. In *Current Problems in Pediatrics.* Yearbook Medical Publishers Inc, Chicago 1975.

2. Louw JH, Barnard CN: Congenital intestinal atresia: observations on its origin. *Lancet* 2:1065, 1955.
3. Martin LW, Zerella JT: Jejunoileal atresia: proposed classification. *J Pediatr Surg* 11:399, 1976.
4. Bauer SB, Fewman SM, Gellis SS, et al: Neonatal hypertension: a complication of umbilical artery catheterization. *N Engl J Med* 293:1032, 1975.
5. Krishnamoorthy KS, Fernandes RJ, Todres ID, et al: Paraplegia associated with umbilical artery catheterization in the newborn. *Pediatrics* 58:443, 1976.
6. Marsh JL, King W, Barrett C, et al: Serious complications after umbilical artery catheterization for neonatal monitoring. *Arch Surg* 110:1203, 1975.
7. Neal WA, Reynolds JW, Jarvis CW, et al: Umbilical artery catheterization: demonstration of arterial thrombus by aortography. *Pediatrics* 50:6, 1972.
8. Lloyd JR: The etiology of gastrointestinal perforations in the newborn. *J Pediatr Surg* 4:77, 1969.
9. Scholander PF: Master switch of life. *Sci Amer* 209:92, 1963.
10. Touloukian RJ: Gastric ischemia: the primary factor in neonatal perforation. *Clin Pediatr* 12:219, 1973.
11. Kosloske AM: Necrotizing enterocolitis in the neonate. *Surg Gynecol Obstet* 148:259, 1979.
12. DeLemos RA, Rodgers JH, McLaughlin GW: Experimental production of necrotizing enterocolitis in newborn goats. *Pediatr Res* 8:380, 1974.
13. Book LS, Overall JC, Herbst JJ, et al: Clustering of necrotizing enterocolitis—interruption by infection-control measures. *N Engl J Med* 297:984, 1977.
14. Barlow B, Santulli TV, Heird WC, et al: An experimental study of acute neonatal enterocolitis: the importance of breast milk. *J Pediatr Surg* 9:587, 1974.
15. Santulli TV, Schullinger JN, Heird WC, et al: Acute necrotizing enterocolitis in infancy: a review of 64 cases. *Pediatrics* 55:376, 1975.
16. Bell MJ, Kosloske AM, Benton C, et al: Enterocolitis: prevention of perforation. *J Pediatr Surg* 8:601, 1973.
17. O'Neill JA, Stahlman MT, Meng HC: Necrotizing enterocolitis in the newborn. *Ann Surg* 182:274, 1975.
18. Wayne ER, Burrington JD, Hutter J: Neonatal necrotizing

enterocolitis: evolution of new principles in management. *Arch Surg* 110:476, 1975.
19. Stewart DR, Colodney AL, Daggett WC: Malrotation of the bowel in infants and children: a 15-year review. *Surgery* 79:716, 1976.
20. Simpson AJ, Leonidas JC, Krasna IH, et al: Roentgen diagnosis of midgut malrotation: value of upper gastrointestinal radiographic study. *J Pediatr Surg* 7:243, 1972.
21. Kiesewetter WB, Smith JW: Malrotation of the midgut in infancy and childhood. *Arch Surg* 77:483, 1958.
22. Rowe MI, Clatworthy HW: Incarcerated and strangulated hernias in children. *Arch Surg* 101:136, 1970.
23. Ravitch MM: *Intussusception in Infants and Children.* Charles C. Thomas Publisher, Springfield, Illinois, 1959.
24. Kobayashi A, Akiyama H, Kawai S, et al: Chronic intussusception associated with ileocecal lymphosarcoma. *Helu Paediatr Acta* 30:315, 1975.
25. Frye TR, Howard WHR: The handling of ileocolic intussusception in a pediatric medical center. *Radiology* 97:187, 1970.

9

Celiac Compression Syndrome

William E. Evans, M.D.

Lipshutz, in 1917, described anatomic distortion of the celiac axis thought to result from compression by surrounding structures.[1] Marjola, in 1963, reported a patient with abdominal pain and extrinsic compression of the celiac artery identified by arteriography. Division of a fibrotic constricting celiac ganglion resulted in relief of symptoms and created interest in the possible causal relationship between intermittent celiac compression and abdominal symptoms.[2] Since then, the existence of the celiac compression syndrome and the role of surgical treatment have been subjects of controversy.

Pathology

It is thought that the celiac compression syndrome, also known as the median arcuate ligament syndrome, is due to compression of the celiac axis just beyond its origin by the median arcuate ligament of the diaphragm and the nerve fibers of the celiac plexus. The mechanism by which this produces symptoms is poorly understood, but it is suggested that the compression results in decreased celiac flow and a resultant "steal" from the superior mesenteric artery.[3] Mitigating against the clinical significance of the celiac narrowing is the rich collateral supply to the stomach and the fact that celiac axis stenosis is often incidentally found in asymptomatic patients.

Clinical Presentation

Pain located in the epigastrium is the most common complaint. Frequently the pain is aggravated by meals and there may be a history of recent weight loss. Other symptoms are nonspecific, and often these patients have had an exhaustive negative examination, sometimes including laparotomy with negative findings.

Physical examination is usually completely normal, with the exception of the presence of an epigastric bruit that often suggests the diagnosis. Unfortunately, as pointed out by Gaspar,[3] epigastric bruits may be found in up to 31% of normal individuals. Often the bruit is increased on expiration as the descending median arcuate ligament increases the degree of celiac stenosis.

Diagnosis

The diagnosis rests primarily on the use of angiography and the exclusion of other diseases that produce upper abdominal pain such as peptic ulcer disease and biliary disease. All patients should have complete gastrointestinal examination with barium studies, upper endoscopy, and biliary evaluation. If no other cause for the pain is found, then angiography should be considered. Celiac axis compression will be demonstrated on the lateral projection as a narrowing of the upper portion of the vessel just beyond its origin. Collateral filling of celiac branches from the superior mesenteric artery may also be seen.[3]

Treatment

At operation, the abdomen should be completely explored to exclude other pathologic conditions. Treatment of celiac stenosis consists of careful division of all surrounding fibrous and nerve tissue. The aorta should be exposed for several centimeters to ensure that all bands have been divided. Frequently, however, the narrowing in the artery will persist after the constriction has been divided and either an aortoceliac bypass graft or dilatation of the stenosis is required to achieve a satisfactory anatomic result.

Results

The results of surgical treatment are difficult to evaluate since reported series are small and controversy exists as to whether or not the disease itself exists. The majority of reports cite encouraging initial results after operation; however, symptoms tend to recur.

Discussion

In 1965, Dunbar, Molnar, Beman, and Marable reported 15 patients with vague, atypical abdominal complaints attributed to compression of the celiac artery and emphasized the role of the median arcuate ligament as the compressive agent. Treatment in 13 consisted of division of the ligament with minimal, if any, disturbance of the celiac ganglion. All 13 were relieved of symptoms. Conclusions were summarized as follows: “Although no definite pathophysiologic explanation can be offered for the clinical symptoms in these 15 cases with compression of the celiac trunk, the satisfactory and often striking response to the decompression of the arteries suggests the direct correlation between the abdominal pain and the partial obstruction of the celiac artery."[4]

In 1966, Marable reported three additional patients with vague chronic postprandial digestive complaints relieved by division of the median arcuate ligament. Because no clear pathophysiologic mechanism could be identified, Marable raised the possibility of a nonphysiologic mechanism: "Serious thought must be given to the possible placebo effect of the operation. There is no doubt that the abnormality (compression of the celiac artery) is relieved by the operative procedure described. It does not necessarily follow, however, that relief of the abnormality is responsible for the relief of symptoms."[5] It is important to note this concern by one of the early and major proponents of celiac decompression.

In 1967, Snyder, Mahoney, and Rob reported 2 additional patients with vague abdominal pain associated with compression of the celiac artery relieved by decompression. These authors, like Harjola, emphasized the contribution of neurofibrous tissue of the celiac ganglion as the offending agent.[6]

The same year, Drapanas raised serious questions about the likelihood of a clear physiologic basis for the syndrome, pointing out that total and permanent occlusion of the celiac axis in the absence of other abnormalities of the intestinal vascular supply seldom results in symptoms. He also was struck by the fairly high association of psychologic illness in these patients.[7]

In 1968, Harjola summarized the available reports and concluded that symptoms might be caused by anatomic disproportion between the aortic hiatus and the celiac axis, by fibrosis of the celiac ganglion, or by a combination of both. He reviewed his experience with 13 cases. All had postprandial pain; diarrhea occurred in only one, and weight loss was not described. Nine were relieved of symptoms and three were improved, while in one symptoms were unchanged by operation. Harjola, however, as did Marable, raised some serious questions about his own data: "Our material produced only four cases of pure celiac stenosis: in other words, these patients had no other concomitant diseases of the upper part of the abdomen making it impossible to draw far-reaching conclusions concerning the effect of freeing the celiac axis on the patient's pain. However, all four patients with true celiac axis syndrome became asymptomatic postoperatively."[8]

In 1968, Marable reported his accumulated experience with 30 cases of surgical celiac artery decompression. Of 25 available for follow-up ranging from 12 months to 48 months, 18 (72%) were symptom-free. However, in discussing Marable's paper, Drapanas again raised serious question concerning the syndrome, closing his discussion by saying "Careful long-term follow-up is needed, for many patients will have return of symptoms despite correction of the stenosis."[9]

Also in 1968, Lord, Stoney, and Wiley reported a series of 12 patients with celiac compression. As in other series, pain was rather vague, occurring postprandially in only three. More than half had diarrhea and weight loss in contrast to patients in other series. Like Marable, they thought that constriction was the result of the median arcuate ligament impingement. In eight of the 12, release of the contriction failed to result in a vessel of normal caliber and in six, pressure gradients were unchanged by division of the ligament. In these eight patients, revascularization was carried out with resection of the constricting artery in six. Each specimen showed intimal thickening with deposition of large quantities of fibrous tissue.

Of the four patients with simple division of the ligament, three were asymptomatic 25 and 38 months postoperatively. All eight of the patients in the revascularization group were symptom-free from 13 to 35 months postrevascularization. The authors attributed the results to elimination of pressure gradients in the celiac artery with reestablishment of normal flow pattern.[10]

Curl, Thompson, and Stanley, in 1971, reported a single patient with hypoplasia of the celiac and superior mesenteric arteries associated with median arcuate ligament compression. Revascularization resulted in symptomatic relief. The authors were able to identify 13 additional patients in the literature treated by revascularization, and all were asymptomatic at the time of reported follow-up.[11]

These two reports raised the question of revascularization as a necessary component of successful treatment. Raised also was further controversy concerning etiology.

Later in 1971, Stanley and Fry reported 15 patients, 12 of whom underwent operations. In 10 the median arcuate ligament was divided. Seven of the 10 had good initial results; two were classified as poor, although they were somewhat improved; and one was unchanged. The two patients undergoing revascularization had complete relief of symptoms. No data concerning patients not operated upon were presented. Complicating interpretation of results in these patients was the presence of concomitant gastrointestinal disease in five, including peptic ulcer in one, chronic cholecystitis in two, and a history of pancreatitis in two. Unfortunately, the data do not permit evaluation of the effects of these abnormalities, but do raise some question concerning the origin of symptoms.[12]

Included in this report was the result of d-zylose testing in seven patients in an attempt to clarify the etiology of symptoms. In three, abnormalities of d-zylose absorption were identified, and in two of these release of the median arcuate ligament was followed by a return of the d-zylose absorption test to normal. Stanley and Fry raised the possibility that the median arcuate ligament syndrome may, for this reason, be ischemic in origin and represent a steal phenomenon, since the d-zylose test is related specifically to proximal small bowel absorption and the absorption of d-zylose is proportional to blood flow to the area.

In discussing this paper, Szilagyi raised several points of critical disagreement. First, he noted: "Clinical symptomatology is very vaguely defined." Second, he felt the pathophysiology had not been objectively explained, particularly as it related to the arterial narrowing created by the compression. He was skeptical about the d-zylose test, since it was primarily a measure of small bowel mucosal absorption. Third, he was concerned that no evidence based on pathophysiologic data appeared to exist to explain the improvement following operation. Fourth, he noted the rather peculiar geographic distribution of the syndrome, pointing out that not a single case had been identified at Henry Ford Hospital in Detroit, despite the addition of 45,000 new patients yearly. Fifth, he pointed out the rich collateral pathways of the celiac axis and the general lack of symptoms in patients with total occlusion of this vessel. Sixth, there appeared to be a large number of patients with X-ray evidence of compression who were totally asymptomatic. In conclusion, Szilagyi remarked: "The coexistence of the abdominal symptoms and celiac arteriolar narrowing must be regarded as a chance event of unproved pathologic significance."[12]

In 1972, Szilagyi summarized his objections including the "amorphousness" of the clinical manifestations, the lack of a single pathologic cause, and the anatomic demonstration by Michaels et al.[13] of the rich and extensive collateral pathways as all mitigating against this syndrome. He again stressed the lack of "a logically consistent biologically acceptable rationale for good surgical results." No pathologic change in the celiac ganglion could be demonstrated and certainly no data were available to convincingly establish vasospasm as an etiologic factor. Nor could he find evidence to support the superior mesenteric artery steal phenomenon. The high incidence of celiac compression in asymptomatic patients was again stressed. In Szilagyi's own series, 49% of 157 angiograms showed celiac narrowing. Patients included those with suspected intestinal angina, gastrointestinal complaints not suspected to be ischemic, and miscellaneous problems not primarily involving the gastrointestinal tract. The highest incidence of stenosis of 40% or more was found in the asymptomatic miscellaneous group, mitigating against the correlation between symptoms and degree of narrowing of the celiac artery. Conclusions were that the changes noted on angiograms simply represented normal anatomic variants. The only proof of the existence of this syndrome, according to Szilagyi: "is the almost infallible cure of the alleged symptoms by an operation that usually but not always corrects the deformity by incising or excising the adjacent neurofibrous tissue."[14]

It was the concern and the inconsistencies identified by Szilagyi that led to our review in 1973 of Marable's original patients in an attempt to establish the pattern of long-term results in patients with decompression of the celiac axis.[15]

Of 72 patients treated from 1963 to 1971, 59 were available for detailed follow-up. Ages ranged from 13 to 68 years (46 were less than 50 years of age). There were 10 men and 49 women. All had abdominal pain, usually varied and without a pattern that suggested another diagnosis. Weight loss occurred in one-third. In fewer than one-half did pain show a postprandial pattern. Diarrhea was rare. All had a long history of abdominal complaints, and 70% had had at least one previous intraabdominal operation. Forty-seven underwent median arcuate ligament release. In three, cholecystectomy was also performed. Twelve patients were treated nonoperatively.

At six months, 39 of 47 (83%) patients undergoing operation were free of symptoms. Eight (17%) had no change in symptoms postoperatively. In assessing long-term results, the three patients who had median arcuate ligament release and cholecystectomy were deleted from the group since results could not be attributed specifically to either operation.

Of the 44 patients observed from three to twelve years postoperatively, only 41% were asymptomatic, fewer than one-half of those originally thought to have been cured by the operation. Nine percent felt better, but all had recurrence of symptoms similar to those noted preoperatively. In 50%, symptoms were totally unaltered by operation. Of the 22 patients not relieved of symptoms, 13 ultimately underwent subsequent intraabdominal operations and eight were free of symptoms at the conclusion of the study.

Of the 12 patients not operated upon, nine were without symptoms at the conclusion of follow-up. Four had had psychotherapy, three were improved by the elimination of dairy products from their diet, and two were "cured" by symptomatic treatment. The other three continued to have symptoms.

In a discussion of this paper, Fry reported similar long-term results with 50% showing relief of symptoms at the conclusion of the follow-up. In contrast, Stoney, in the same discussion, indicated good long-term results in 35 of 43 patients, although the duration and method of follow-up were not defined. Wylie raised the question of selection since only one-half of our patients had postprandial pain. Stoney and Wylie[10] also reported only three of their 12 patients had postprandial pain. We await the detailed long-term results of Stoney and Wylie, which may shed additional light on this apparent discrepancy and permit further evaluation of revascularization as a method of treatment.[16]

Watson and Sadikali, in 1977, reported 20 cases of celiac axis compression. Fifteen (75%) were relieved of symptoms by decompression or by revascularization. Eight of 20 had preoperative weight loss of more than 10 pounds. Good results in this subgroup also occurred in 75%. It should be noted that only four of these 20 patients had been followed for more than three years. Mihas also in 1977, reported six additional patients with symptomatic celiac compression. Four were treated surgically with arterial reconstruction. None of these four patients was benefited more than temporarily by corrective surgery. One patient had abdominal exploration and vagotomy unrelated to the celiac axis and was symptom-free 10 months after operation. One patient became asymptomatic without benefit of operation.[17]

Brandt and Boley, in 1978, extensively reviewed the literature and concluded that: "it does not appear to us that there is conclusive clinical or experimental data which either establishes or excludes compression of the celiac axis as a cause of abdominal pain," and indicated that there was even less evidence that ischemia could be incriminated as a cause. They did, however, point out that some patients do appear to have been benefited by operation even though the pathophysiology is obscure. They proposed four criteria which they felt should be met prior to considering operation: (1) abdominal pain, preferably postprandial, (2) weight loss, (3) abdominal bruit, and (4) angiographic demonstration of compression.[18]

At present, data continue to be mixed and the result varied. Long-term follow-up by Fry and Evans[15] casts doubt as to the efficacy of the operation with 40 to 50% cure rates. Selection of patients may cloud the issue since series are small, but at present a cautious approach appears to be most judicious. A few patients may be candidates for operation, but they must be very carefully selected, preferably by a limited number of investigators. It does appear reasonable to correct the compression if all other causes of disabling abdominal pain have been eliminated and when the results of laparotomy fail to demonstrate other explanations for symptoms. It seems equally obvious that if this is to be done, careful physiologic data should be recorded in these highly selected patients in an attempt to provide a more scientific basis for claims of cure. Long-term results must be carefully accumulated to assure that early placebo effects of surgery are not masking symptom patterns which may recur at a later date.

References

1. Lipshutz B: A composite study of the coeliac axis artery. *Am Surg* 65:159, 1917.
2. Harjola PT: A rare obstruction of the coeliac artery. *Am Chir et Gynaic Fenniae* 52:547, 1963.
3. Gaspar MR, Barker WF: Peripheral arterial disease. Vol IV. In *Major Problems in Clinical Surgery*. WB Saunders Co, Philadelphia 1981.
4. Dunbar JD et al: Compression of the celiac trunk and abdominal angina. *Am J Roentgenol* 95:731, 1965.
5. Marable SA, Molnar W, Beman F: Abdominal pain secondary to celiac axis compression. *Am J Surg* 111:493, 1966.
6. Snyder WA et al: Symptomatic celiac artery stenosis due to constriction by neurofibrous tissue of the celiac ganglion. *Surgery* 61:372, 1967.
7. Drapanas T: Stenosis of the celiac artery. *Am Surg* 164:1085, 1966.
8. Harjola PT, Lahtihayre A: Celiac axis syndrome. *Am J Surg* 115:864, 1968.
9. Marable JA et al: Celiac compression syndrome. *Am J Surg* 115:97, 1968.
10. Lord R, Stoney R, Wylie EJ: Coeliac axis compression. *Lancet* 2:785, 1968.
11. Curl J, Thompson U, Stanley J: Median arcuate ligament compression of the celiac and superior mesenteric arteries. *Am Surg* 173:314, 1971.
12. Stanley J, Fry W: Median arcuate ligament syndrome. *Am Surg* 103:252, 1971.
13. Michaels NA: Collateral arterial pathways to the liver after ligation of the hepatic artery and removal of the celiac axis. *Lancet* 6:708, 1953.
14. Szilagyi DE et al: The celiac axis syndrome: Does it exist? *Surgery* 72:849, 1974.
15. Evans WE: Long-term evaluation of the celiac bowel syndrome. *Surgery* 76:867, 1974.
16. Stoney R: Personal communication.
17. Watson WE: Celiac axis compression. *Am Fut Med* 86:278, 1977.
18. Brandt LJ, Boley SJ: Celiac axis compression. A cerebral review. *Am J Dig Dis* 23:633, 1978.

10

Acute Mesenteric Arterial Occlusion

William L. Smead, M.D.
Patrick S. Vaccaro, M.D.

Despite remarkable advances in the understanding of the clinical pathophysiology of acute intestinal ischemia and an increase in the frequency of accurate diagnosis, this catastrophic event remains an unsolved problem. Careful analysis has resulted in the recognition of distinct clinical syndromes: superior mesenteric arterial embolism and thrombosis, nonocclusive mesenteric ischemia, and mesenteric venous occlusion. Of the cases of acute infarction diagnosed prior to death, approximately one-half are caused by superior mesenteric artery occlusion.

Historical Perspectives

To properly analyze recent advances in the treatment of acute mesenteric ischemia, it is important to review the problem from an historical perspective. Elliot's initial report of resectional therapy in 1895[1] influenced the management of this condition for over half a century, and mortality rates consistently exceeded 90%. The frequency of preexisting chronic mesenteric arterial lesions was emphasized by Dunphy as early as 1936, when he correctly observed that lethal bowel infarction was preceded by symptoms of intestinal angina in one-half of the patients.[2] Two decades later, Mikkelsen reemphasized the importance of abdominal angina and observed that multiple vessel occlusion was necessary to produce symptoms.[3,4]

In 1951, Klass clearly defined superior mesenteric embolization as a clinical syndrome distinct from that of mesenteric arterial thrombosis and first described attempts at embolectomy.[5] Later in the same year, Stewart reported the first embolectomy in concert with limited bowel resection, with survival.[6] Shaw and Rutledge (1957) reported the first successful embolectomy without concomitant bowel resection, and more important, outlined in clear detail the principles of management including second-look laparotomy that are still valid 25 years later.[7] The following year, Shaw reported the first two cases of successful thromboendarterectomy for acute thrombotic mesenteric occlusion.[8] Brittain's report in 1963 of four patients remains a benchmark achievement.[9] The principles of bypass techniques have been successfully applied to mesenteric ischemia and developed through the experience of Crawford, Morris,[10] and DeBakey, as well as Bergan and his associates.[11]

Despite these early successes and rapid advances in vascular surgical technique, acute mesenteric infarction remained a nearly uniformly fatal clinical problem. Only more recent developments in the use of adjunctive diagnostic and supportive measures have offered hope of changing the dismal picture. Irreversible infarction at the time of the initiation of therapy can be avoided only by precise, early diagnosis. Progression of the ischemic process despite revascularization may be amenable to improved adjunctive supportive measures. Boley and his associates have reported markedly improved results in both areas, using early selective arteriography to document the diagnosis and papaverine infusion to block persistent vasoconstriction, relieve tissue ischemia, and promote collateral flow.[12, 13] Developments in surgical nutrition and the management of multiple system failure promise to further improve results in the therapy of this lethal clinical problem.

Etiology

Of all causes of acute mesenteric ischemia, approximately half result from mesenteric artery occlusion, one-fourth from nonocclusive infarction, and one-fourth from mesenteric venous thrombosis, arteritis, and other miscellaneous causes. In Ottinger's series from Massachusetts General Hospital, embolism accounted for 55% of patients presenting with mesenteric occlusive disease, and thrombosis was documented in 45%.[14] Bergan, reporting the Northwestern experience, found embolism to be more than twice as common as thrombosis, embolism occurring in 69% of 48 patients.[11]

Superior mesenteric emboli represent approximately 5% of all peripheral emboli. The majority of emboli originate from mural thrombus secondary to myocardial infarction or as a complication of rheumatic valvular heart disease.[15–21] Less common sources have been reported, including the venous circulation and right heart via paradoxical embolism, left atrial myxoma, bronchogenic carcinoma, aortic atheroma, and valvular prostheses.

The most common cause of mesenteric thrombosis is clearly atherosclerosis, with most patients presenting with the prodromata of chronic intestinal ischemia.[2,8,9,16–18,20,22–25] Less common etiologies include arteritis syndromes, specifically polyarteritis nodosa,[26,27] lupus erythematosus,[28,29] and rheumatoid disease.[30,31] Coagulopathies have been implicated including those related to the use of birth control pills.[32] Atherosclerotic as well as infected aneurysms of the superior mesenteric artery have been implicated by multiple authors[33–36] by the mechanisms of thrombosis as well as peripheral embolization. Superior mesenteric arteriovenous fistulae produced by penetrating trauma and surgical misadventure have been reported as causes of intestinal infarction.[37,38] Fibromuscular dysplasia of both celiac and superior mesenteric arteries have produced abdominal angina and infarction when the disease is diffuse and may be associated with similar lesions in the carotid and renal artery distributions.[39] Finally reports of traumatic disruption of the superior mesenteric artery have described subsequent ischemic complications.[40,41]

Pathophysiology

Intestinal ischemia may result from generalized poor perfusion as in the shock syndromes or from focal morphologic or functional lesions, all of which lead to inadequate circulation at a cellular level. Regardless of the cause, the final common pathway leading to hemorrhagic necrosis begins with reversible metabolic alterations and progresses sequentially to irreversible infarction.

Sequential ultrastructural analysis of ischemic intestine has been reported by Brown et al.[42] describing changes in the rough and smooth endoplasmic reticulum within 10 minutes and more extensive damage by 30 minutes with fluid accumulation between cells and the basement membrane. Oxygen consumption at this point was decreased 28%, suggesting mitochondrial dysfunction. Aho et al.[43] describe clumping of nuclear chromatin, breakage of microvilli, and mitochrondrial swelling during early phases of ischemia. By two hours, the junctional complexes between cells broaden, and detachment may occur through membrane disruption. Within four hours, continued alteration of intracellular organelles occurs, including the rupture of lysosomal membranes and the release of autolytic enzymes which sets up the cycle of progressive cellular death. Significant changes in cellular function can be demonstrated before the morphologic changes that can be seen by standard light microscopy.

The conventional histologic picture of bowel ischemia is hemorrhagic necrosis, progressing from mucosal hemorrhage to mucosal necrosis with submucosal and interstitial edema to submucosal hemorrhage and finally to transmural infarction with necrosis of the muscularis propria and eventual perforation.[44] Impressive physiologic alterations accompany those morphologic changes. As the mucosal cells undergo necrosis, they lose the ability to produce mucus and may be digested by intraluminal enzymes, destroying the barrier to bacterial invasion and to various toxins.[45] Massive fluid and electrolyte shifts into the gut lumen may occur secondary to this cellular dysfunction.[22] As the ischemic process begins to involve the muscularis layer, hyperperistalsis occurs, which progresses to disordered motility and atony.[46] With transmural infarction, perforation may occur with subsequent peritonitis or abscess formation.

Multiple profound metabolic effects accompany intestinal infarction.[47] Hemoconcentration produced by massive fluid loss into the gut results in an increase in hemoglobin concentration and hemocrit early in the course, findings often reversed as intraluminal hemorrhage occurs later. Metabolic acidosis may be profound and reflects anaerobic metabolism in the gut wall from local ischemia as well as generalized hypoperfusion consequent to hypovolemia. Amylase levels may be low soon after the onset of ischemia, but are typically elevated late as infarction progresses. The enzymes lactic dehydrogenase (LDH), serum glutamic-oxaloacetic transaminase (SGOT), serum glutamic-pyruvic transaminase (SGPT), and creatine phosphokinase (CPK) are all markedly elevated late in the course of mesenteric infarction but in a nonspecific pattern.[47] The liberation of vasoactive 5-hydroxytryptamine (serotonin) from ischemic intestine may explain the remarkable peripheral platelet aggregation that occurs with this event, causing diffuse microaggregation and multiple organ system failure.[48–50] Catecholamines, histamine, and bradykinins are released in large amounts and contribute to eventual circulatory collapse.[50]

If an ischemic insult stops short of transmural infarction, healing may occur to produce normal bowel or intestine with varying degrees of morphologic and functional impairment. Mucosal involvement alone allows rapid regeneration and return of function. With deeper involvement of the submucosa, complete healing may occur, but protracted malabsorption has been described.[51] Injury to the muscularis propria results in later fibrosis producing stricture and partial or complete bowel obstruction. The factors which seem to influence most directly this spectrum of disease are the severity and duration of ischemia, an acute or chronic onset, the adequacy of collateral blood supply, and the status of host defenses.

Anatomy

The superior mesenteric artery (SMA) provides the major blood supply to the small intestine and proximal colon from the ligament of Treitz to the splenic flexure. A series of peripheral anastomotic arcades provides abundant collateral pathways. The most peripheral of these arcades is designated the marginal artery and gives rise to the vaso recti that supply the bowel wall directly. The marginal vessels are continuous with those of the celiac axis (CA) and inferior mesenteric artery (IMA). Within the bowel wall itself is a network of communicating submucosal vessels that can maintain the viability of short segments, even in the presence of extramural arterial occlusion. The collateral pathways open following major vessel occlusion in response to a fall in distal arterial pressure, and in the presence of gradual occlusion are generally adequate to maintain viability and function. As a general rule, at least two of the major vessels must be affected to produce symptomatic ischemia.[52] Even in the presence of three-vessel disease, the patient may be asymptomatic owing to hypogastric and other collateral flow. Vasomotor changes in the splanchnic circulation play an important role in total mesenteric blood flow and are mediated primarily through the sympathetic nervous system at alpha adrenergic receptors. Compromised central perfusion pressure and vasoconstriction may influence the adequacy of collateral flow and therefore the extent of ischemic damage.

In general, SMA thrombosis occurs at the origin of this vessel proximal to the middle colic artery origin. Intestinal infarction secondary to thrombosis, therefore, typically extends from the proximal jejunum to the midtransverse colon. On the other hand, superior mesenteric emboli generally lodge at the origin of a major branch distal to the middle colic and proximal jejunal branch origins. This additional opportunity for collateral flow leads to more limited infarction, sparing the proximal jejunum, hepatic flexure, and transverse colon (Figure 1).

Clinical Presentation

The clinical presentation of acute mesenteric ischemia invariably includes abdominal pain, but this symptom varies in nature, severity, and location. Typically, the pain begins as a steady, severe, poorly localized periumbilical pain that becomes progressively more severe and generalized as infarction becomes established. The duration of pain prior to diagnosis varies from a few hours to several days and is not necessarily related to reversibility. Embolic occlusion characteristically produces a more acute and fulminant picture than thrombosis, which may have an insid-

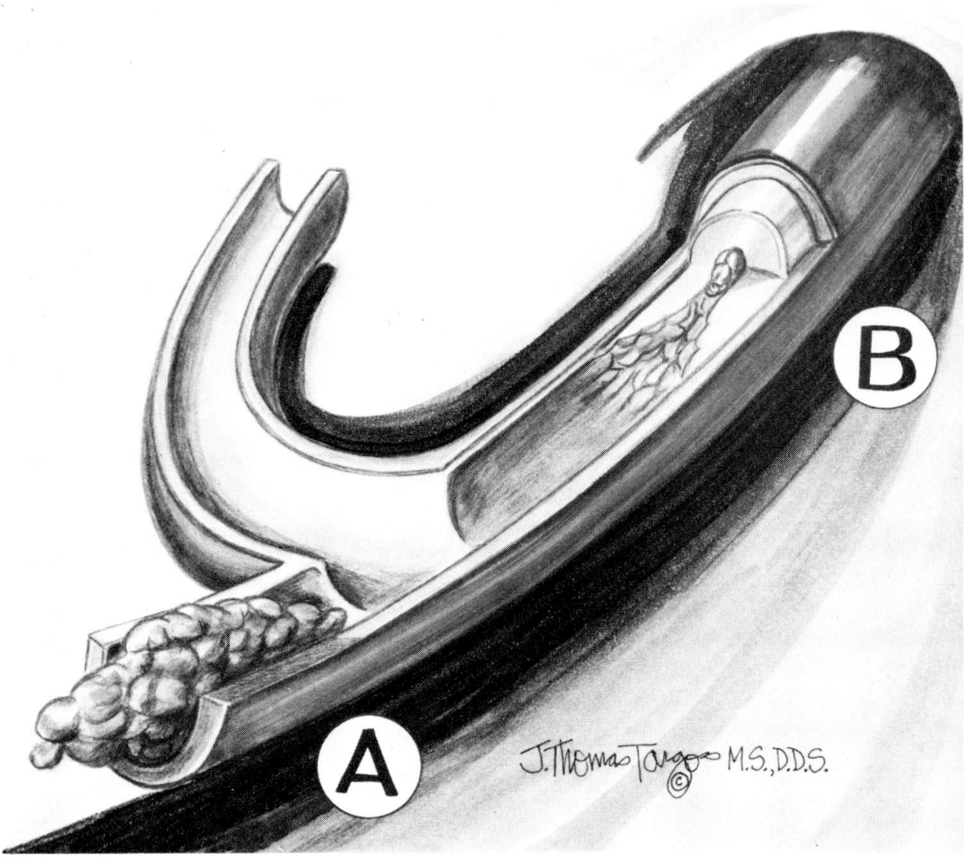

Figure 1. Superior mesenteric artery at middle colic artery origin. A = typical site for embolus; B = characteristic thrombosis at vessel origin.

ious onset. Classically, there is a marked discrepancy between the severity of pain reported and the objective abdominal signs on examination. Subjective complaints far exceed objective findings. Forceful gastrointestinal emptying is another characteristic symptom with vomiting in 56% of patients and diarrhea in 29%.[14] Mucosal hemorrhagic infarction produces gross or occult blood in 25–75% of cases.[14,20] With the development of transmural infarction, peritoneal signs can be perceived, first from transmural migration of bacteria, then from frank intestinal perforation.

The syndrome of mesenteric artery embolism is distinct, characterized by the sudden onset of catastrophic abdominal pain accompanied by gut emptying in a patient with cardiac disease prone to embolization.[11] One-third of the patients have a history of a previous embolic event, generally secondary to atherosclerotic or rheumatic heart disease.

The syndrome of mesenteric artery thrombosis, by contrast, is characterized by a more insidious course. Dunphy in 1936 noted that half the patients with intestinal infarction had gastrointestinal symptoms preceding the fatal event.[2] In the presence of chronic symptoms of intestinal angina, including weight loss and postprandial pain, a constant abdominal pain begins, produced by intense intestinal spasm and accompanied in a slowly progressive course by gut emptying and sepsis. The presence of other atherosclerotic occlusive diseases in the periphery should alert the clinician to the presence of thrombotic bowel infarction.

Mesenteric occlusion is generally a disease of the elderly with 75% of patients in one large study exceeding 70 years of age.[16] The mean age in Ottinger's study was 70 years with the peak age for patients with embolus a decade younger than those with thrombosis.[14] Hildebrand and Zierker, however, point out that mesenteric vascular disease is not necessarily confined to very elderly persons as over one-fourth of their patients were less than 60 years of age and two were infants.[52]

Laboratory Findings

Characteristic laboratory findings can be identified in patients presenting with intestinal ischemia but none are diagnostic and are, therefore, of limited value. Leukocytosis is a nearly uniform finding in all series. Ottinger, in 59 patients, found the white blood count to be less than 10,000/mm^3 in 10%, 10,000–20,000/mm^3 in 46%, and greater than 20,000/mm^3 in 44%.[14] The degree of elevation roughly corresponded to the extent and duration of infarction. In Boley's recent experience, more than 95% of patients have an elevated white blood count upon admission.[13] Approximately one-half display significant metabolic acidosis. Although serum amylase is elevated in 25–50% of patients, levels are often less than twice normal and are not diagnostic.[13,14] Massive elevations of LDH, SGOT, SGPT, CPK, and alkaline phosphatase are routinely seen in patients with far advanced ischemia.[11]

Roentgenographic Findings

Plain film roentgenographic diagnosis depends upon the recognition of specific bowel segments illustrating changes characteristic of infarction. In a large study from Massachusetts General Hospital, findings on plain film studies warranting a retrospective diagnosis of infarction occurred in only 19% of proved cases.[53] A small bowel pseudo-obstruction pattern, typically abnormal amounts of gas with dilatation and air-fluid levels, was identified in 36% and should bring the diagnosis to mind in patients with appropriate clinical signs. The splenic flexure cut-off pattern, characterized by a moderately dilated gas-filled transverse colon with minimal gas distal to the splenic flexure, was seen in 18% of cases and tended to be associated with extensive infarction. Fecal residue was absent to minimal in a majority of cases reflecting gastrointestinal emptying. The specific and nonspecific roentgenologic findings did not discriminate among the precise etiologies, although venous thrombosis produced the most striking bowel wall abnormalities. Embolism produced the highest incidence of roentgenologic changes justifying a presumptive diagnosis

(46%). Arterial thrombosis seldom led to specific diagnostic findings (11%) but frequently exhibited nonspecific changes. A normal examination does not exclude the diagnosis of mesenteric ischemia or infarction. In view of the nonspecificity of the findings described, perhaps the major value of plain film examination is the exclusion of other diseases that produce an acute abdominal catastrophe such as a perforated viscus or bowel obstruction.

Emergency arteriography has become an increasingly valuable technique for establishing a precise diagnosis and initiating effective therapy by the instillation of vasodilators. A flush aortogram with biplane filming is performed initially to detect the following associated problems: (1) aortic dissection, (2) aneurysmal disease, (3) thrombotic or embolic occlusions of other visceral vessels, and (4) the adequacy of collateral circulation.[12,13,54–56] Selective SMA arteriography is then performed to specifically evaluate embolus or thrombotic occlusion or vasoconstriction, and to assess the vascular bed distal to the obstructive lesion.

Superior mesenteric embolism typically produces the "meniscus sign" located just distal to the origin of the middle colic artery, at the origin of the ileocolic artery, or in a peripheral arcade depending on the size of the embolus.[11] The characteristic appearance of a sharp, rounded filling defect may change over time as thrombus accumulates proximally and distally. Often contrast may be seen to flow around the embolus prior to total occlusion.

Superior mesenteric thrombosis, in contrast, generally occurs within 1-2 cm of the SMA origin proximal to the middle colic artery. Total occlusion is the rule, and the distal arterial tree is usually well demonstrated via collateral perfusion. Chronic occlusion can generally be distinguished from acute thrombosis by the presence or absence of prominent collateral pathways from the celiac and inferior mesenteric systems. In the absence of collateral development, acute occlusion must be presumed and urgent measures undertaken.

Nonoperative Treatment

The initial management of the critically ill patient with acute mesenteric arterial occlusion is directed toward the achievement of hemodynamic stability. Massive volume replacement is frequently required, as transudation of fluid into the bowel lumen is one of the cardinal features of ischemic infarction. The use of the Swan-Ganz catheter with measurement of the pulmonary capillary wedge pressure facilitates accurate volume expansion in these patients with a typically high incidence of valvular or atherosclerotic cardiovascular disease. Cardiovascular support may be required despite adequate repletion of plasma volume; dopamine or dobutamine are the agents of choice as they have no splanchnic vasoconstrictor action. Control of cardiac dysrrhythmias may be crucial, but digitalis should be avoided if possible, as it may produce mesenteric vasoconstriction.[54] Significant metabolic acidosis must be corrected when identified by blood gas analysis. Broad spectrum antibiotics to cover both aerobic and anaerobic microorganisms are given intravenously in doses sufficient to achieve bacteriocidal levels early in the course of resuscitation.

Spontaneous recovery following acute mesenteric occlusion has been reported in the occasional circumstance in which collateral circulation develops rapidly with perfusion capable of supporting bowel viability.[57] There is, however, no specific or reliable method of identifying these patients early in the course of their disease. In large groups of patients the results of medical nonoperative therapy are dismal, with a nearly uniform lethal outcome.

Successful treatment of mesenteric embolism with the use of low molecular weight dextran has been reported by Serjeant.[58] The infusion of 500 cc 10% Rheomacrodex produced complete symptomatic relief. Two subsequent episodes characterized by abdominal pain thought to be embolic in etiology as well as a popliteal embolus were treated in a similar fashion, resulting in the patient's eventual discharge from the hospital. Low molecular weight dextran may be beneficial from many standpoints as a volume expander, a platelet inhibitor, and a facilitator of capillary microcirculation. A few isolated reports are available of survival with viable bowel in patients with documented acute mesenteric occlusion in whom the use of systemic heparinization and antibiotic coverage were chosen as primary therapy.[59,60] At the present time these pharmacologic approaches must be viewed as adjunctive measures complementing surgical therapy.

An aggressive approach highlighted by early arteriography, direct vasodilator infusion, and appropriate surgical management has been advocated by Boley and his colleagues.[12,13] Patients in high-risk groups with symptoms and signs suggesting acute mesenteric ischemia undergo intensive resuscitation with specific supportive and corrective measures. Emergency arteriography is performed to establish a definitive diagnosis and evaluate the collateral circulation. If embolism or acute thrombosis, or for that matter vasoconstriction, is identified, a single bolus of 25 mg of tolazoline hydrochloride is infused via the SMA catheter, after which a repeat arteriogram is performed to better visualize the peripheral circulation and document the vasoactivity of this arterial bed. Papaverine infusion is then initiated through the selective catheter at a rate of 30–60 mg/hr by a constant infusion pump. The duration of this vasodilator therapy varies with both the purpose of its use and the response of the patient. When this technique is used in conjunction with embolectomy or arterial reconstruction, the infusion has been maintained for 12–24 hours. An arteriogram is then repeated to confirm a satisfactory revascularization prior to catheter removal. If a second-look procedure is elected, arteriography is performed preoperatively and the infusion is continued until the status of the bowel is assessed directly. Obviously the status of the patient, including systemic and abdominal findings, is a major factor in this decision-making process. The proposed algorithm for patient management in Boley's study (Table I) discriminates on the basis of site of embolus and clinical state.[13] A similar schema can be constructed for the management of mesenteric thrombus.

The physiologic alteration that creates the rationale for this treatment approach is the mesenteric vasoconstriction that occurs in association with acute arterial occlusion. Laufman documented persistent vasoconstriction in the precapillary arterial circulation before and after release of experimental occlusion of the mesenteric artery.[61] Experiments by Boley demonstrated mesenteric vasoconstriction persisting several hours after relief of mesenteric arterial occlusion as brief as two hours.[62] Papaverine infusion was found to prevent this vasoconstriction and to relieve vasospasm once it became established. Therefore obliteration of this physiologic response becomes important in an effort to maximize intestinal perfusion even in the presence of a successful embolectomy or revascularization. Isolated reports of the use of serial epidural anesthesia[63] or direct splanchnic block[64] have appeared based on this same rationale, but the limited experience prevents any significant conclusions regarding their efficiency.

The selective infusion of thrombolytic agents such as streptokinase is currently investigational and, in combination with vasodilator therapy, may represent an attractive alternative.[13] A few scattered reports of successful outcomes and angiographic patency have been discussed. Certainly an extrapolation from other applications of this technique in the coronary circulation would suggest a role in selected patients.

Surgical Treatment

The initial problem encountered by the surgeon at exploration is the accurate assessment of intestinal viability in terms of longitudinal extent and depth of injury. Early in the course of disease, at a time when patient salvage is

Table I

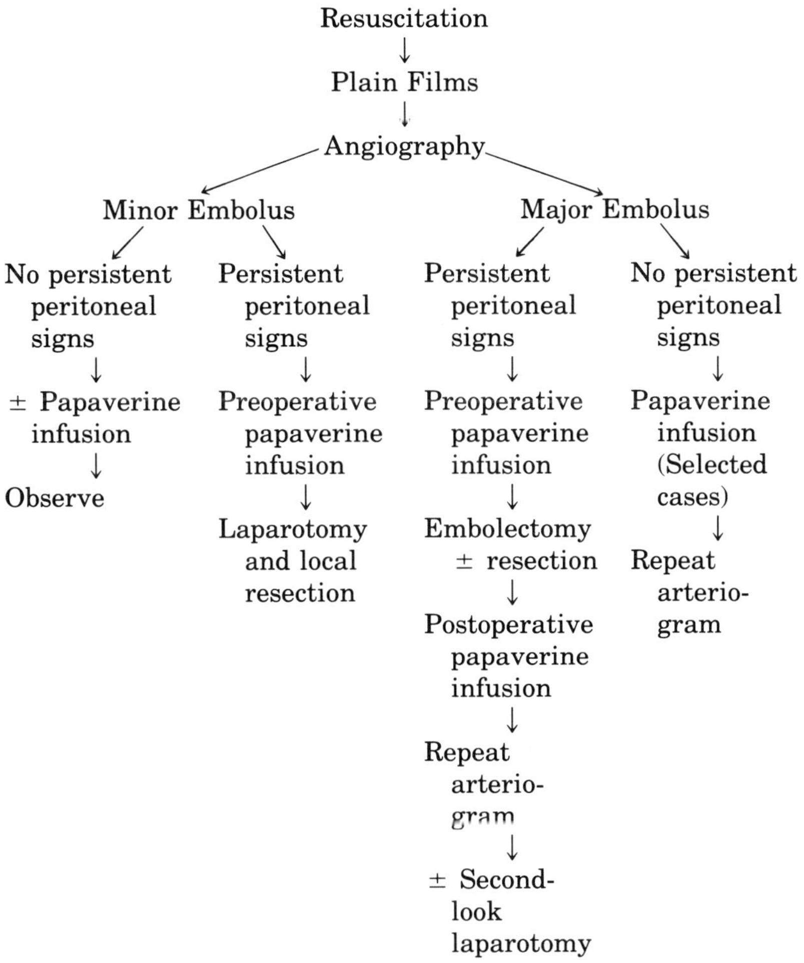

(Reprinted with kind permission: Boley SJ, Sproyregan S, Siegelman SS, Veith FJ: Initial results from aggressive roentgenologic and surgical approach to acute mesenteric ischemia. *Surgery* 82:848, 1977.)

greatest, findings at laparotomy may be deceptive. In the ischemic phase, the intestine appears progressively more avascular, becoming increasingly pale with a bluish tinge. Intense spasm and peristalsis are noted with rippling of the seromuscular surface. Faint peripheral pulses may be palpable, and even the experienced surgeon may miss the diagnosis, attributing these findings to systemic hypotension or vasospasm. As the ischemic process progresses to infarction, peristalsis ceases and the peritoneal surfaces lose their glistening sheen. Hemorrhagic infarction produces hemorrhage into the bowel wall and mesentery accompanied by massive tissue edema and intraluminal fluid accumulation. The picture of purulent peritonitis late in the course reflects permeation of bacteria through the bowel wall and profound bacteremia.

The initial examination should include an attempt to localize the occlusion, if arteriography has not been performed, by careful palpation of the main trunk of the SMA testing for a forceful pulsation. Exposure of the vessel may be required in questionable cases where collateral circulation may confuse the issue. If a pulse is palpable in the SMA, the obstructive mechanism is probably embolism. The absence of pulsation suggests mesenteric thrombosis. In general, embolic occlusion distal to the middle colic origin results in sparing of the proximal jejunum and right transverse colon (Figure 2). Thrombotic occlusion, typically occurring at the SMA origin, results in involvement of the bowel extending from the ligament of Treitz to the midtransverse colon (Figure 3). Distal occlusive lesions produce small segmental infarctions. More definitive techniques of documenting intestinal viability should await the completion of revascularization techniques.

Arterial Embolus

Once acute mesenteric arterial embolism is suspected on the basis of clinical presentation or preferably confirmed at arteriography, and initial resuscitation is in progress, preparation is begun for urgent surgical exploration. In addition to the entire abdomen, the groin and medial thighs

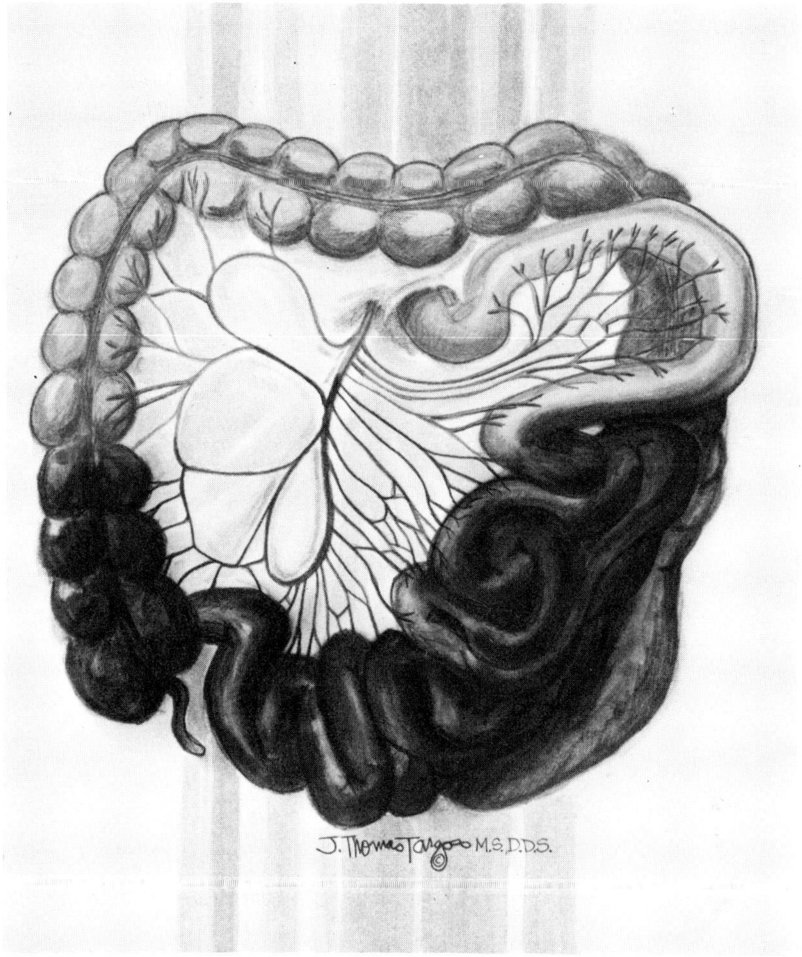

Figure 2. Characteristic distribution of intestinal infarction resulting from SMA embolism. Note sparing of proximal jejunum and right transverse colon.

should be prepared and draped into the surgical field in case the saphenous vein is required for revascularization. A long midline incision provides maximum exposure. The proximal SMA is approached by retracting the transverse

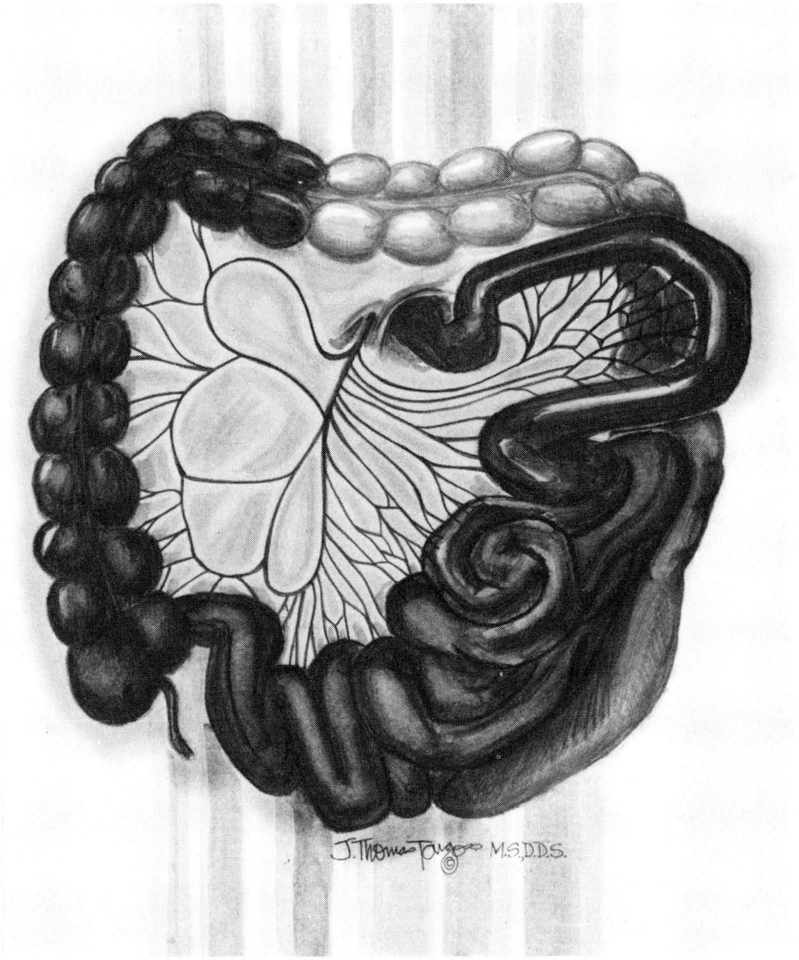

Figure 3. Characteristic distribution of intestinal infarction resulting from SMA thrombosis. Note involvement from the ligament of Treitz to midtransverse colon.

mesocolon superiorly and the entire small intestine inferiorly. The peritoneum is incised and the vessel dissected free from the dense, investing autonomic nerve fibers and branches of the superior mesenteric vein. The middle colic artery provides a valuable anatomic landmark. The SMA is freed for a distance of approximately 3–4 cm at this level and occluded proximally and distally with tapes or gentle vascular clamps. A longitudinal arteriotomy provides maximum exposure and ease of closure and facilitates the distal anastomosis, should bypass be required. The technique of embolectomy is standard, using the Fogarty balloon catheter to extract the embolus and any propagated thrombus from points proximal and distal to the arteriotomy. Flushing maneuvers further remove retained fragments of clot. After satisfactory inflow and backbleeding have been restored, the arteriotomy is closed with fine vascular technique. Vein patch angioplasty is only infrequently required for the repair of exceedingly small native vessels.

After an appropriate recovery interval, an assessment of intestinal viability is performed, and a judgment regarding the need for segmental bowel resection is made. Alternatively a decision may be made to proceed to a second-look procedure after a period of observation.

Resection as a primary method of treatment carries a prohibitively high mortality even when combined with vigorous parenteral alimentation in all patients except those with small peripheral emboli with short-segment infarction.

Arterial Thrombosis

Acute mesenteric arterial thrombosis is suspected at operation when the ischemic process involves the proximal jejunum and transverse colon and no pulse is palpable in the proximal SMA. Arteriography demonstrates SMA-origin occlusion without concomitant collateral enlargement. Initial attempts are directed at revascularization, after which bowel resection is performed as dictated by tests of intestinal viability.

Thromboendarterectomy has been used in the management of mesenteric thrombosis in small numbers of patients. Brittain and Earley reported an approach to the proximal SMA at its origin posterior to the pancreas, obtaining exposure anteriorly through the lesser sac.[9] Ottinger reported a larger experience with a "blind" endarterectomy using the same exposure as used for embolectomy.[14] Operative and early postoperative failure rates were high.

Most surgeons currently recommend aortomesenteric bypass under these circumstances.[10,11,24,54,65] Exposure is best achieved by retracting the transverse colon superiorly and the small bowel mesentery to the right, providing excellent exposure of the infrarenal aorta and the SMA. The aorta is dissected free from the renal vein to the IMA to allow convenient placement of a side-biting vascular clamp. The ligament of Treitz is taken down and the SMA is dissected free from the dense investing autonomic nerve fibers at a point immediately distal to the origin of the middle colic artery. A suitable segment of saphenous vein is harvested from the medial thigh, reversed, and interposed as a vascular graft using fine vascular technique. Care must be taken to avoid excessive graft length and kinking during this procedure. Distal thrombectomy of propagated clot is frequently necessary. Small residual clots in the periphery may be tolerated depending upon the adequacy of the collateral circulation, but under other circumstances, they may produce short-segment infarction requiring resection. Selective vasodilator therapy may minimize the impact of residual disease by maximizing collateral perfusion.[12] Vein appears superior to prosthetic materials in this acute circumstance as bacterial contamination is frequent.[11,14]

An alternative approach has been suggested by Wylie, Ehrenfeld, and Stoney.[10] They advocate antegrade bypass from the distal descending thoracic aorta exposed transabdominally by taking down the aortic diaphragmatic hiatus, and report higher patency rates with this technique. Others have anastomosed the ileocolic branch of the SMA to the right common iliac artery to accomplish retrograde perfusion.[54] This is clearly a technically demanding small vessel anastomosis where lower patency rates might be expected. Reassessment of intestinal viability is then carried out, using a variety of available techniques. Decisions regarding a second-look laparotomy or immediate resection are then made before the wound is closed.

Intraoperative Viability Testing

Following successful arterial reconstruction, an evaluation of intestinal viability is undertaken. Clinical assessment is notoriously inaccurate and may lead to resection of viable bowel or retention of nonviable intestine with subsequent perforation. Many techniques have been investigated. Measurements of serosal temperature and pH, electromyography,[66] the distribution of injected vital dyes or ^{99m}Tc-tagged albumin microspheres,[67] direct Doppler flow signal evaluation,[68] and fluorescein angiography[69] have been clinically helpful but variably reliable. Decisions regarding immediate intestinal resection are made on the basis of these studies, or alternatively, a second-look procedure is elected.

Second-Look Laparotomy

The first second-look procedure following intestinal revascularization was reported by Van Weel following wound dehiscence.[70] A more planned approach was first advocated by Shaw and Rutledge in their early report on revascularization.[7] Their rationale for early reexploration was: "not just to allow a clear definition between dead and live bowel to take place, but also to allow time for the institution of supportive measures, which may render more of the bowel viable" and maximize intestinal salvage. Few of their principles of management have changed in the subsequent quarter century. Zuidema reemphasized the usefulness of reexploration as experience increased.[71,72] However, Bergan in reviewing 49 successful mesenteric embolectomy cases in the literature found only seven instances in which second-look operations were performed, and in only two cases was further intestinal resection required.[11]

In Ottinger's study of 103 cases of acute mesenteric arterial occlusion, 36 patients were thought to be possible candidates for elective reexploration.[14] In 17 patients, no second-look procedure was performed, and retrospective analysis revealed that in four cases this approach may have been beneficial. In 19 patients, reexploration was planned, but was carried out in only 15 since four patients died during the interval period. In only four instances did reexploration fail to reveal disease requiring further surgical management. Of the entire group undergoing second-look surgery, only two survived hospitalization. Ottinger concluded from this experience that the decision to proceed to reexploration or not was usually correct when the indication was the question of intestinal viability.

To maximize benefit, a few basic principles of second-look surgery are best followed. The decision for planned reexploration is made at the original operation. Once that decision is made, laparotomy is performed regardless of the patient's condition. The usual interval is between 12–48 hours after the original operation. Clinical deterioration may prompt early reexploration, but rapid improvement and absence of complication should not alter the original planned approach.

Acute superior mesenteric arterial occlusion is a highly lethal syndrome. In an accumulated series of 274 patients from seven major centers up to 1972, the mortality rate for mesenteric infarction ranged from 88–100%.[11] The mortality rate at Massachusetts General Hospital reported by Ottinger showed only modest improvement from 92% in 1967[19] to 85% in 1975[14] despite careful attention to this problem. An aggressive diagnostic approach based on a high index of suspicion reported by Krensz and Manny improved these results only modestly to 77.5%.[73] Only the reports from Boley and his associates have shown any significant improvement in therapeutic results, with a mortality of 45% in patients with embolism treated with selective vasodilator infusion in addition to standard surgical therapy.[13]

In general, survival rates improve as the interval between onset of symptoms and diagnosis is lessened. The majority of successfully managed patients require minimal or no bowel resection, reflecting more limited or more reversible ischemia. The presence of signs of peritoneal irritation at the time of definitive diagnosis is a foreboding finding as it reflects transmural infarction and bacterial contamination.

Results of Therapy

Embolism

Clearly, expectant therapy of SMA embolism is unsatisfactory except in isolated patients with limited, peripheral embolization involving short segments with adequate collateral blood supply. The use of selective vasodilator infusion may further increase successful results in this small group of patients.[13] Resectional therapy alone is rarely successful except in similar circumstances of short-segment infarction.

Bergan summarized the 49 cases of successful SMA embolectomy reported up to 1974 and found a wide range in clinical presentation with time delays of 7–48 hours from onset of symptoms to operation.[74] Intestinal resection was required in only 13 cases and was usually limited in extent. Second-look laparotomy was performed in just seven instances, and in only two cases was further bowel resection required. Few large series of these cases are reported; a representative sample is shown in Table II.

Table II

Mortality-Mesenteric Embolism

Procedure	*Mortality (%)*
No operation	91–100
Bowel resection	50–100
Embolectomy	
Ottinger, Austen (1967)[19]	75
Ottinger (1978)[14]	74
Bergan et al. (1975)[11]	27
Boley et al. (1981)[13]	45

The use of selective vasodilator infusion in combination with embolectomy and perhaps limited bowel resection would seem to be a logical approach. Early reports from Boley are encouraging, with significant gains in survival noted in the combined treatment group (55%) compared to the standard treatment group (20%).[13]

Thrombosis

Nonoperative treatment of mesenteric thrombosis is nearly uniformly fatal. In the very occasional patient with short-segment infarction secondary to arteritis, limited resection may be successful when the basic disease process can be controlled medically. Only an aggressive multimodal approach to acute thrombotic occlusion including revascularization, limited resection, and selective vasodilator infusion has yielded significant survival. (See Table III.)

Complications

The most frequent complication of mesenteric revascularization, as with most vascular reconstructions, is throm-

Table III
Mortality-Mesenteric Thrombosis

Procedure	*Mortality (%)*
No operation	100
Bowel resection	90–100
Revascularization	
Ottinger, Austen (1967)[19]	100
Ottinger (1978)[14]	
Thromboendarterectomy	100
Bypass	75
Bergan (1975)[11]	100
Boley (1977)[12]	50

bosis.[11,14,19,22] Unrecognized, this event causes recurrent intestinal ischemia or infarction. Early thrombosis must be considered a technical complication and can be prevented by meticulous operative technique. Thromboendarterectomy has been associated with an unacceptably high failure rate, and has been abandoned in most centers in favor of bypass procedures.[10,11,14] Early thrombosis following embolectomy should be avoided by careful technique in arteriotomy closure or the use of patch angioplasty. Selective infusion of vasodilators may further decrease the incidence of early failure by promoting high flow-through in a maximally dilated outflow vascular bed.[12,13] Recurrent embolization is certainly possible and must be kept firmly in mind. Prolonged anticoagulation may be crucially important in preventing late thrombosis, not only from recurrent arterial embolism, but also from thrombosis.[14] Whatever the cause, urgent reexploration and revascularization is mandatory if intestinal salvage is to be achieved.

Early hemorrhage from the arteriotomy site has been reported on multiple occasions.[14,19] Certainly, technical imperfection may be responsible, but this cannot often be identified. Gastrointestinal hemorrhage is a frequent postoperative problem originating from mucosal slough and ulceration caused by the ischemic process.[14] Anticoagulation has been implicated by Boley, who reports a 40% incidence of hemorrhage requiring transfusion in patients receiving heparin in the immediate postoperative period.[13,54]

Shock and sudden death have been reported following revascularization and remain largely unexplained. In most instances, this event results from cardiovascular instability which is multifactorial in origin. Preexisting cardiac disease can be identified in the majority of patients with acute mesenteric ischemia, whether embolic or thrombotic in etiology. Massive fluid shifts occur between the intravascular and extravascular compartments, often compromising perfusion. Toxins, Gram-negative endotoxemia, and hyperkalemia have been further implicated.[46,75] In general, metabolic acidosis, toxemia, and blood/plasma loss are manageable problems. Precise monitoring using the Swan-Ganz catheter, arterial pressure lines, and urinary output greatly facilitate patient management through these treacherous times.

Diarrhea is characteristic of the recovery phase of revascularized ischemic intestine, resulting from loss of normal reabsorptive capacity.[13,14] Protein-losing enteropathy secondary to segmental ischemic enteritis has been described.[13,51] When the ischemic process extends to involve the muscularis propria, late ischemic stricture may develop, usually becoming symptomatic six to eight weeks following the insult.[14] This pathologic condition becomes manifest by partial or complete obstruction, resulting in further obstruction or diarrhea. The short gut syndrome and its attendant complications will, of course, result if massive intestinal resection is required for transmural infarction.

When early arteriography and selective vasodilator infusion is performed, the usual low incidence of catheter complications is observed, but rarely causes significant problems.[12,13] No systemic effects of papaverine infusion have been noted, as 90% of the drug is inactivated on one pass through the liver. Catheter occlusion can be prevented by continuous infusion; dislodgement requires replacement under fluoroscopic control.

Conclusions

Acute mesenteric arterial occlusion remains one of the most lethal of all diseases despite remarkable advances and contributions from pathology, radiology, medicine, and surgery. Recent advances reflected in improved survival statistics suggest an increasing role for arteriography and selective infusion of vasoactive drugs in the perioperative period. New techniques for evaluating intestinal viability promise to improve intestinal salvage and decrease morbidity. Technical advances in revascularization and the prevention and detection of complications will certainly further increase survival rates. Advances in cardiovascular monitoring and support, parenteral nutrition, and management of multisystem failure can be predicted to contribute to improved results as well. A definite, probably fixed, mortality rate will remain in these aged patients with cardiovascular instability, and a significant incidence of irreversible infarction will continue to be encountered at initial evaluation.

References

1. Elliott JW: Operative relief of gangrene of intestine due to occlusion of mesenteric vessels. *Ann Surg* 21:9, 1895.
2. Dunphy JE: Abdominal pain of vascular origin. *Am J Med Sci* 192:109, 1936.
3. Mikkelsen WP: Intestinal angina—Its surgical significance. *Am J Surg* 94:262, 1957.
4. Mikkelsen WP, Zaro JR, Jr: Intestinal angina. Report of a

case with prospective diagnosis and surgical relief. *N Engl J Med* 260:912, 1959.
5. Klass AA: Embolectomy in acute mesenteric occlusion. *Ann Surg* 134:913, 1951.
6. Stewart GD, Sweetman WR, Westphal R, Wise RA: Superior mesenteric artery embolectomy. *Ann Surg* 151:274, 1960.
7. Shaw RS, Rutledge RH: Superior mesenteric artery embolectomy in the treatment of massive mesenteric infarction. *N Engl J Med* 257:595, 1957.
8. Shaw RS, Maynard EP III: Acute and chronic thrombosis of the mesenteric arteries associated with malabsorption: A report of two cases successfully treated by thromboendarterectomy. *N Engl J Med* 258:874, 1958.
9. Brittain RS, Earley TK: Emergency thromboendarterectomy of the superior mesenteric artery: Report of four cases. *Ann Surg* 158:138, 1963.
10. Crawford ES, Morris GC Jr, Nyhus HO, Roehm JOF Jr: Celiac axis, superior mesenteric artery, and inferior mesenteric artery occlusions: Surgical considerations. *Surgery* 82:856, 1977.
11. Bergan JJ, Dean RH, Conn J Jr, Yao JST: Revascularization in treatment of mesenteric infarction. *Ann Surg* 182:430, 1975.
12. Boley SJ, Sproyregan S, Siegelman SS, Veith FJ: Initial results from an aggressive roentgenologic and surgical approach to acute mesenteric ischemia. *Surgery* 82:848, 1977.
13. Boley SJ, Feistein FR, Sammartano R, Brendt LJ, Sproyregan S: New concepts in the management of emboli of the superior mesenteric artery. *Surg Gynecol Obstet* 153:561, 1981.
14. Ottinger LW: The surgical management of acute occlusion of the superior mesenteric artery. *Ann Surg* 188:721, 1978.
15. Bergan JJ: Recognition and treatment of intestinal ischemia. *Surg Clin North Am* 47:109, 1967.
16. Pierce GE, Brockenbrough EC: The spectrum of mesenteric infarction. *Am J Surg* 119:233, 1970.
17. Purdue GD, Smith RB: Intestinal ischemia due to mesenteric arterial disease. *Am Surg* 36:152, 1970.
18. Galloway JMD, Walker PA, Moore GE: Mesenteric arterial occlusion as a vascular emergency. *Br J Surg* 56:431, 1969.

19. Ottinger LW, Austen WG: A study of 136 patients with mesenteric infarction. *Surg Gynecol Obstet* 124:251, 1967.
20. Hollman GL, Jordan GL, Cooley DA: Massive intestinal infarction: Survival after resection and superior mesenteric embolectomy. *Am J Surg* 112:770, 1966.
21. Marston A: Mesenteric arterial disease: the present position. *Gut* 8:203, 1967.
22. Bergan JJ, Dry L, Conn J, et al: Intestinal ischemic syndromes. *Ann Surg* 169:120, 1969.
23. Glotzer DJ, Shaw RS: Massive bowel infarction. *N Engl J Med* 260:162, 1959.
24. Morris GC Jr, DeBakey M, Barnhard V: Abdominal angina. *Surg Clin North Am* 46:919, 1966.
25. Fry WJ, Kraft RO: Visceral angina. *Surg Gynecol Obstet* 117:417, 1963.
26. Cohen RD, Conn DL, Ilstrup DM: Clinical features, prognosis, and response to treatment in polyarteritis. *Mayo Clin Proc* 55:146, 1980.
27. Travers RL, Allison DJ, Drettle RP, Hughes GRV: Polyarteritis nodosa: A clinical and angiographic analysis of 17 cases. *Seminar Arth Rheum* 8:184, 1979.
28. Hoffmann BI, Katz WA: The gastrointestinal manifestations of systemic lupus erythematosus. A review of the literature. *Seminar Arth Rheum* 9:237, 1980.
29. Rothfield N: Clinical features of systemic lupus erythematosus. In *Textbook of Rheumatology*. Kelly WN (Ed.). WB Saunders, Philadelphia 1981. pp 1106–1132.
30. Schmid FR, Cooper NS, Ziff M, McEwen C: Arteritis in rheumatoid arthritis. *Am J Med* 44:56, 1961.
31. Scott DGI, Bacon PA, Tribe CR: Systemic rheumatoid vasculitis: A clinical and laboratory study of 50 cases. *Medicine* 60:288, 1981.
32. Brennan MF, Clarke AM, MacBeth WAG: Infarction of the midgut associated with oral contraceptives. *N Engl J Med* 279:1213, 1968.
33. McClelland RD, Duke JH: Successful resection of an idiopathic aneurysm of the superior mesenteric artery. *Ann Surg* 164:167, 1966.
34. Hoehn JG, Bartholomew LG, Osmundson PJ, et al.: Aneurysm of the mesenteric artery. *Am J Surg* 115:832, 1968.

35. Thomas TV: Nonmycotic aneurysms of the superior mesenteric artery. *Am Surg* 35:492, 1969.
36. Case Record of Massachusetts General Hospital #24–1969. *N Engl J Med* 280:1346, 1969.
37. Gonshirt LW, Weaver FE, Olander GA: Mesenteric arteriovenous fistula. Review of the literature and report of a case. *Vasc Surg* 1:82, 1967.
38. Varner JE, Oliver RI: Superior mesenteric arteriovenous fistula. *Ann Surg* 170:862, 1969.
39. Ripley HR, Levin SM: Abdominal angina associated with fibromuscular hyperplasia of the celiac and superior mesenteric arteries. *Angiology* 17:297, 1966.
40. May AG, Lipchik EO, DeWeese JA: Repair of injured visceral arteries. *Ann Surg* 162:869, 1965.
41. Shirkey AL, Gusset DC, Jordan GL: Superior mesenteric artery division and intestinal function. *J Trauma* 7:7, 1967.
42. Brown RA, Chio C, Scott HJ, et al: Ultrastructural changes in the canine mucosal cell after mesenteric arterial occlusion. *Arch Surg* 101:290, 1970.
43. Aho AJ, Arstila SI, Akonen J, et al: Ultrastructural alterations in ischaemic lesion of small intestinal mucosa in experimental superior mesenteric artery occlusion. Effect of oxygen breathing. *Scand J Gastroenterol* 8:439, 1973.
44. Laufman H, Nora PF, Mittelpunki AI: Mesenteric blood vessels: Advances in surgery and physiology. *Arch Surg* 88:1021, 1964.
45. Bounous G, Sutherland NG, McArdle AH, et al: The prophylactic use of an "elemental" diet in experimental hemorrhagic shock and intestinal ischemia. *Ann Surg* 166:312, 1969.
46. Marston A: Causes of death in mesenteric arterial occlusion. II Observations on revascularization of ischemic bowel. *Ann Surg* 158:960, 1963.
47. Bounous G, McArdle AH: Release of intestinal enzymes in acute mesenteric ischemia. *J Surg Res* 9:339, 1969.
48. Resnick RH, Gray SJ: Distribution of serotonin (5-hydroxytryptamine) in the human gastrointestinal tract. *Gastroenterology* 57:599, 1969.
49. Mustala O, Alfthan O, Peltokallio D: 5-hydroxytryptamine

(serotonin) in acute hypotensive shock. *Am J Physiol* 207:215, 1964.
50. Swank RL, Hissen D, Bergentz SE: 5-hydroxytryptamine and aggregation of blood elements after trauma. *Surg Gynecol Obstet* 119:779, 1964.
51. Dardik H, Serdenberg B, Parker J, et al: Intestinal angina with malabsorption treated by elective revascularization. *JAMA* 205:64, 1968.
52. Hildebrand HD, Zierker RE: Mesenteric vascular disease. *Am J Surg* 139:188, 1980.
53. Tomchik FS, Wittenberg J, Ottinger LW: The roentgenographic spectrum of bowel infarction. *Radiology* 96:249, 1970.
54. Boley SJ, Brandt LJ, Veith FJ: Ischemic disorders of the intestines. *Curr Probl Surg* 15(4):1, 1978.
55. Recek C, Kren V, Fixa B, et al: Selective mesenterioradiography as a guide to diagnosis and treatment of acute superior mesenteric artery occlusion. *J Cardiovasc Surg* 9:184, 1968.
56. Bosnick MA, Williams LF, Hastios CA, et al: In vivo arteriography of the bowel wall. *Am J Surg* 114:359, 1967.
57. Rosenman LD, Gruyper AN: Small intestine stenosis caused by infarction: An unusual sequel of mesenteric artery embolism. *Ann Surg* 141:254, 1955.
58. Serjeant JCB: Mesenteric embolus treated with low molecular weight Dextran. *Lancet* 1:139, 1965.
59. Franjndlich D, Taylor RL: Infarction of the small bowel. *JAMA* 189:327, 1965.
60. Vellar ID, Vellar DJ, Goldwasser M, Munk J: Superior mesenteric artery embolism. *Med J Aust* 1:801, 1973.
61. Laufman H: *Significance of Vasospasm in Vascular Occlusion.* Thesis. Northwestern University Medical School, Chicago, 1948.
62. Boley SJ, Regan JA, Tunick PA, et al.: Persistent vasoconstriction; a major factor in nonocclusive mesenteric ischemia. *Surgery* 82:848, 1977.
63. Jackson BB, Lykins R: Serial epidural analysis in mesenteric arterial failure. *Arch Surg* 90:177, 1965.
64. Britt LG, Check RC: Nonocclusive mesenteric vascular disease. *Ann Surg* 169:704, 1969.

65. Rob C: Surgical diseases of the celiac and mesenteric arteries. *Arch Surg* 93:21, 1966.
66. Bussemaker JB, Lindeman J: Comparison of methods to determine viability of small intestine. *Ann Surg* 176:97, 1972.
67. Zarins CK, Skinner DB, James AE Jr: Prediction of the viability of revascularized intestine with radioactive minospheres. *Surg Gynecol Obstet* 138:576, 1974.
68. Cooperman M, Martin EW Jr, Carey LC: Evaluation of ischemic intestine by Doppler ultrasound. *Am J Surg* 139:73, 1980.
69. Buckley AB, Zuidema GD, Hamilton SR, O'Mara CS, Klossmann PG: Intraoperative determination of small intestinal viability following ischemic injury. *Ann Surg* 193:628, 1981.
70. Van Weel MW: Acute mesenteric arterial occlusion. Successful treatment by embolectomy and limited intestinal resection. *Acta Chir Ther* 8:147, 1956.
71. Zuidema GD, Reed D, Turcotte JC, Fry WJ: Superior mesenteric artery embolectomy. *Ann Surg* 159:548, 1964.
72. Zuidema GD: Surgical management of superior mesenteric arterial emboli. *Arch Surg* 82:267, 1961.
73. Krensz MM, Manny J: Acute superior mesenteric arterial occlusion: A plea for early diagnosis. *Surgery* 83:482, 1978.
74. Bergan JJ, Yao JST: Acute intestinal ischemia. In *Vascular Surgery*. Rutherford RR (Ed.). WB Saunders, Philadelphia 1977. p 825.
75. Swan KG, Jacobson ED: Hemodynamics of endotoxin shock in the conscious animal. *Surg Gynecol Obstet* 125:1041, 1967.

11

Mesenteric Venous Occlusive Disease

William L. Smead, M.D.
Patrick S. Vaccaro, M.D.

Introduction

Mesenteric venous thrombosis has been recognized as a clinico-pathologic syndrome distinct from that of arterial occlusion since the landmark descriptions of Warren and Eberhard,[1] Donaldson and Stout[2] in 1935. By 1940, Brown was able to review 104 collected cases of mesenteric venous infarction and further clarify its clinical presentation and pathologic features.[3] In 1949, a postmortem examination of 99 cases documented a wide variety of predisposing clinical disorders as well as a population with no associated etiologic factors.[4] The following year Berry and Bougas[5] reported 13 cases of "agnogenic" mesenteric venous thrombosis in which no predisposing factors could be identified. Jenson and Smith[6] found that the majority of venous occlusions were of this "primary" type and emphasized a significantly improved prognosis in mesenteric venous infarction over that in arterial infarction.

A review of 43 cases in 1965 by Naitove and Weismann[7] established primary or idiopathic mesenteric venous infarction as a distinct entity and stressed the need for early and definitive surgical resective therapy and postoperative anticoagulation. Subsequently, superior mesenteric venous thrombectomy has been described and may limit the length of resection or even obviate the need for resection altogether.[8,9,10,11] Further developments aiding in the early recognition and diagnosis of this clinical syndrome and in the intraoperative assessment of intestinal viability can be expected to improve both survival and the quality of life in patients with this challenging problem.

Incidence

There are few reliable figures on which to base an accurate estimate of the incidence of mesenteric venous occlusive disease. The wide variation in the reported incidence is related to the relative rarity of the syndrome, reflected by the limited number of reports, and the difficulties in establishing the precise etiology of late intestinal infarction. Incidence has been estimated to range between 15 and 55.5% of mesenteric vascular occlusive events.[6,12,13] Approximately 25–55% of patients with mesenteric venous thrombosis have no identifiable etiologic factors and fall into the primary or idiopathic category.[5,6]

Mesenteric venous thrombosis has been reported in a wide age range from 11 months to 89 years with the highest frequency between 30 and 60 years.[15] No uniform difference in sex distribution can be identified.

Clinical Manifestations

The clinical course of mesenteric venous thrombosis has many features that permit the astute clinician to differentiate venous thrombosis from arterial occlusion. The initial manifestations are frequently vague and nonspecific in contrast to the acute, catastrophic onset of superior mesenteric arterial thrombosis or embolism. Early in the course of illness, there are no pathognomonic features or diagnostic studies that establish the diagnosis. Prodromata of ill-defined abdominal discomfort, anorexia, and changes in bowel habits ranging from diarrhea to constipation are characteristically described from 3–21 days prior to the development of severe symptoms.[14] With progression of the disease, colicky midabdominal pain gives way to diffuse abdominal pain with signs of peritoneal irritation. Abdominal distention associated with vomiting is characteristic; hematemesis and melena are not commonly reported. Fever, when present, is generally low grade. Signs of mild-to-moderate dehydration are typical. Examination of the abdomen most frequently shows distention and generalized tenderness, ranging from mild to severe depending on the stage of the disease. Rebound tenderness and associated peritoneal signs are elicited only in far advanced cases with transmural infarction. A discrepancy between signs and symptoms is present in these patients with venous thrombosis, as it is in those with arterial occlusion. Bowel sounds are typically hypoactive or absent, although they may be hyperactive during the early course. Guaiac-positive stool documents profound ischemia with mucosal to transmural infarction.

The nonspecific nature of these signs and symptoms often leads to delay in recognition and, therefore, appropriate therapy prior to the catastrophic consequences of transmural infarction. High morbidity and mortality rates will be improved only by early and specific diagnosis.

Diagnostic Tests

Despite the many diagnostic studies available in the modern hospital, laboratory and roentgenographic tests have been disappointingly nonspecific in patients with mesenteric venous thrombosis. Leukocytosis, generally in the 20,000 range, is characteristic, with a preponderance of polymorphonuclear leukocytes. Hemoconcentration generally reflects the degree of dehydration. Hyperamylasemia and metabolic acidosis are noted only in patients in clinical shock with advanced infarction. The finding of free serosanguinous peritoneal fluid in the majority of these patients (78%) has prompted some authors to recommend paracentesis as a valuable diagnostic test.[6,13,16] Peritonoscopy has also been advocated as "the best and quickest route to the diagnosis of ischemic intestine."[16]

The majority of clinical papers on mesenteric venous thrombosis suggest that radiologic studies seldom assist in the diagnosis,[5–7,11,14,16] but some characteristic findings can confirm the diagnosis if they are carefully evaluated.[17–19] Flat-plate abdominal films show evidence of bowel obstruction in approximately one-half of cases but are otherwise nonspecific. Findings specific to mesenteric venous thrombosis were described by Welson and Eggleston[17] and confirm a specific diagnosis. The affected bowel is identified on sequential films as rigid and thick-walled, with small collections of gas remaining fixed in a straight or curvilinear lumen. As the disease progresses, the bowel wall becomes markedly edematous with narrowing of the lumen and extension of the transition zone. "Thumbprinting" or pseudotumor may be seen in advanced cases.

Barium small bowel studies demonstrate the characteristic radiographic changes associated with severe congestion and edema. The transition zone between involved and uninvolved intestine is characteristically long with progressive thickening of the valvulae to the point of obliteration and progressive narrowing of the lumen due to thickening of the bowel wall.[18] Thickening of the mesentery causes separation of bowel loops. These findings contrast sharply with those of arterial occlusion in which the transition zone is abrupt and extreme edema is uncommon. Ulceration, perforation, and late stricture, characteristics of arterial occlusion, are distinctly uncommon in venous occlusive disease.

Selective superior mesenteric arteriography may demonstrate specific evidence peculiar to venous thrombosis and promote early precise diagnosis. In the arterial phase there is intense spasm in the superior mesenteric artery and its major branches with visualization of few small peripheral branches. Blood flow is remarkably slow or absent, manifested by prolongation of the arterial phase for 20–40 seconds. Contrast staining of the thickened involved bowel wall in the transition zone is intense and prolonged but absent in more severely compromised intestine. In the venous phase there is no opacification of the mesenteric venous system.[18–20] Experimentally produced mesenteric venous lesions reproduced identical arteriographic findings.

Pathophysiology

The gross pathologic changes in intestine involved with mesenteric venous occlusive disease range from mild edema to transmural hemorrhagic infarction. In the typical case, the bowel wall is congested and cyanotic, thickened by edema and intramural hemorrhage. The bowel lumen contains dark bloody fluid and the peritoneal cavity a serosanguinous ascites, reflecting the hemorrhagic infarction. The mesentery is remarkably edematous and hemorrhagic particularly along the affected bowel wall. At resection arterial pulsations are present and cut arteries bleed freely. Thrombus extrudes prominently from the mesenteric veins. Careful examination may reveal different stages of thrombosis, fresh and organized, in a single specimen[14] suggesting that the disease may be intermittent or gradually progressive. Thrombosis may be noted to involve veins in the mesentery of adjacent normal appearing bowel[7] if sufficient collateral venous outflow is maintained.

Review of postmortem and surgical specimens[4,7,21] in

cases of primary mesenteric venous thrombosis suggests that thrombus originates in the mesenteric venous arcades and propagates proximally and/or distally to occlude collateral venous drainage. Hemorrhagic infarction occurs when arcuate, vasa recta, and intramural veins become occluded. Involvement of the superior mesenteric or more proximal veins is varied and not necessary for infarction to occur. The location and rate of spread of thrombosis may be varied and unpredictable. The time interval between initial thrombosis and frank infarction depends on the site of the original lesion and the rapidity of progression, explaining the wide range of clinical presentations. Inferior mesenteric vein thrombosis leading to infarction is distinctly rare and is reported in fewer than 5% of cases in all series reviewed.[7] Late in the course of disease, transmural infarction occurs, and it becomes impossible to differentiate this lesion from that of arterial occlusion.

Microscopic examination of involved intestine demonstrates remarkable edema, hemorrhage, and varying degrees of infarction. Mesenteric veins are filled with red thrombus, usually in the absence of associated inflammatory, allergic, or degenerative processes.[7] Adjacent arteries are widely patent and normal in appearance.

Experimental mesenteric venous occlusion has reproduced identical pathologic lesions.[18] Uniform physiologic changes are tachycardia, hypotension, hemoconcentration, leukocytosis, acidosis, hypovolemia, and decreased mesenteric blood flow.[22]

Etiology

In 50–75% of all reported cases of mesenteric venous thrombosis, a predisposing clinical disorder can be clearly identified. In the large postmortem study reported from the Mayo Clinic,[4] intraperitoneal sepsis was identified as the most frequent etiologic factor, most commonly pyelophlebitis complicating acute appendicitis. Neoplasms can produce vascular occlusion by direct extrinsic compression or invasion as well as thrombosis from hypercoagulability states.[43] Portal hypertension, pre- or postsinusoidal in nature, has been associated with mesenteric venous occlusion, particularly in patients with markedly elevated pressures and hepatofugal flow.[44] Trauma to the mesenteric vessels has been reported as a causative factor in all large series. Injury may result from blunt or penetrating trauma, or surgical misadventure.[21] Of a rather diverse miscellaneous category, one of the most interesting clinical entities associated with venous infarction is Cogan's syndrome.[35] This disease is characterized by nonsyphilitic keratitis, vestibuloauditory dysfunction, aortitis, and systemic vasculitis involving muscular arteries and veins.

A large number of coagulation disorders have been implicated in a small series of patients with venous thrombosis. Hypercoagulability states including polycythemia rubro vera, primary and secondary thrombocytosis, are well represented in case reports. More obscure and specific coagulation defects such as increased factor VIII and IV activity[31] and decreased fibrinolytic activity[10] have been convincingly documented. An association with oral contraceptives has been clearly established;[27–30] by 1977, seventeen cases had been reported with careful documentation. Inherited antithrombin III deficiency is recognized with increasing frequency as diagnostic tests become more widely available.[23–26] In vitro assay of antithrombin III activity is typically less than 50% of normal. Prophylactic and therapeutic anticoagulation with coumadin is an important adjunctive therapy in this population of patients. Sickle cell anemia has been recognized as a predisposing factor; intravascular sludging and hypercoagulability promote venous thrombosis. Multiple reports of postsplenectomy mesenteric venous occlusion and infarction resulting from thrombocytosis are available for review.[32–34] Antiplatelet therapy with aspirin, dypyrimadole, or sulfapyrozone are indicated when platelet counts exceed $1 \times 10^6/cm^3$ as an effort to avoid thrombotic complications.

Treatment

Nonoperative therapy of mesenteric venous thrombosis is associated with a mortality rate of 100%.[6,7] Laparotomy must be undertaken urgently once the diagnosis is suspected and the patient's condition permits if a favorable outcome is to be achieved.

Preoperative preparation must include vigorous fluid resuscitation to correct the moderate-to-severe hypovolemia characteristic of this syndrome. Broad-spectrum antibiotics are indicated in an effort to control the bacteremia and endotoxemia resulting from profoundly ischemic or infarcted intestine. The use of steroids, advocated by some, has not been supported by controlled clinical trials.

Standard surgical treatment consists of resection of all intestine found to be profoundly ischemic or infarcted with end-to-end anastomosis. Naitove and Weismann[7] emphasize the importance of including in the resection areas of adjacent mesentery harboring residual venous thrombosis to avoid subsequent propagation and "recurrent" infarction. Careful judgment is necessary to provide adequate resection but avoid excessive shortening of the small bowel. Recent advances in the assessment of intestinal viability have greatly enhanced the surgeon's accuracy with these difficult decisions.[36,37] Both the Doppler ultrasound and fluorescein techniques have proved highly predictive in the assessment of viability in patients with proved mesenteric venous infarction. In the presence of significant edema of viable remaining intestine, some surgeons have recommended that the ends of the intestine be exteriorized as an enterostomy and that anastomosis be performed following resolution of the acute illness.[16]

The role of superior mesenteric venous thrombectomy is

controversial. In 1967, Mergenthalen and Harris[8] reported the first successful thrombectomy for this disease. Thrombosis complicated pancreaticoduodenectomy; thrombectomy restored circulation and preserved bowel viability. Others[9–11] have reported similar success and suggest that thrombectomy can minimize the extent of resection to include only frankly infarcted bowel and even obviate resection altogether in cases where diagnosis is made early. In the experimental model of venous thrombosis designed by Polk,[22] venous thrombectomy afforded the only survivors but only if performed within two hours of the induced thrombosis.

Routine second-look laparotomy is advocated by some authors[15] 24 hours after the initial procedure, a policy based on the high incidence of recurrent infarction. In a large literature review reported by Jona et al.,[38] the incidence of recurrent thrombosis was 29% with a high mortality of 37%. The majority of recurrences occurred during the early postoperative period, 60% at the site of anastomosis. On the basis of these data, a stance supporting a second-look approach seemed justified. But, with the development of more accurate techniques for the assessment of bowel viability intraoperatively, perhaps the necessity for systematic second-look procedures will diminish. Certainly the threshold for reexploration for suspected recurrent venous thrombosis should be low.

The value of postoperative anticoagulation has been debated as experience has accumulated. Jenson and Smith[6] found no beneficial effect of anticoagulation therapy. Campbell and Mears[39] noted that the additional risks of anticoagulation were not balanced by improvement in survival. While this attitude may be justified in cases of secondary mesenteric venous thrombosis, improved survival with anticoagulation in patients with primary venous occlusion has been documented by several authors. Naitove and Weismann,[7] reviewing 33 cases in which a critical analysis was possible, noted no mortality in patients given anticoagulation therapy, in sharp contrast to a 50% mortality in the group not treated. In Jona's review[38] of 17 cases of recurrent thrombosis, only one patient developed recurrent infarction while adequately anticoagulated. Multiple additional series document this approach[5,13,40,41] and recommend long-term anticoagulation. The currently recommended therapy should include early postoperative heparin anticoagulation by continuous intravenous infusion followed by coumadin oral anticoagulation to be continued for at least three months or longer, depending on associated hematologic disease.

Reported mortality rates of surgical therapy range from 11.1% to 68.2% with recent studies demonstrating progressive improvement that reflects advances in surgical technique and perioperative care. Mesenteric venous occlusive disease clearly carries a better prognosis than that of arterial occlusion, which has a mortality rate of 85%,[42] and that is probably related to a lower incidence of multiple system disease. A high index of suspicion and early, precise treatment can be expected to further improve survival.

References

1. Warren S, Eberhard TP: Mesenteric venous thrombosis. *Surg Gynecol Obstet* 61:102, 1935.
2. Donaldson JK, Stout BF: Mesenteric thrombosis. *Am J Surg* 29:208, 1935.
3. Brown MJ: Mesenteric venous occlusion: a clinical entity. *Am J Surg* 49:242, 1940.
4. Johnson CC, Boggenstoss AH: Mesenteric vascular occlusion. *Proc Mayo Clin* 24:629, 1949.
5. Berry FB, Bougas JA: Agnogenic venous mesenteric thrombosis. *Ann Surg* 132:459, 1950.
6. Jenson CB, Smith GA: Clinical study of 51 cases of mesenteric infarction. *Surgery* 40:930, 1956.
7. Naitove A, Weismann RE: Primary mesenteric venous thrombosis. *Arch Surg* 161:516, 1965.

8. Mergenthalen FW, Harris MN: Superior mesenteric vein thrombosis complicating pancreatoduodenectomy: Successful treatment by thrombectomy. *Ann Surg* 167:106, 1968.
9. Fontaine R, Pietri J, Masson JC, et al: Intestinal mesenteric infarction of venous origin: The place of thrombectomy in the treatment. *J Circ* 97:145, 1969.
10. Bergentz SE: Thrombosis in the superior mesenteric and portal veins: Report of a case treated with thrombectomy. *Surgery* 76:286, 1974.
11. Inahara T: Acute superior mesenteric venous thrombosis: Treatment by thrombectomy. *Ann Surg* 174:956, 1971.
12. Dunson RD, Ferrell TE, Hansbro GL: Acute mesenteric venous thrombosis. *Am J Surg* 83:205, 1952.
13. Mersheimer WL, Winfield JM, Fankhauser RL: Mesenteric vascular occlusion. *Arch Surg* 66:752, 1953.
14. North JP, Wollenman OJ: Venous mesenteric occlusion in the course of migrating thrombophlebitis. *Surg Gynecol Obstet* 95:665, 1952.
15. Khodadadi J, Togencwajg J, Nocasch N, et al: Mesenteric vein thrombosis: The importance of a second look operation. *Arch Surg* 115:315, 1980.
16. Anane-Sifah JC, Blair E, Reckler S: Primary mesenteric venous occlusive disease. *Surg Gynecol Obstet* 141:740, 1975.
17. Welson SW, Eggleston W: Findings on plain roentgenograms of the abdomen associated with mesenteric vascular occlusion with a possible new sign of mesenteric venous thrombosis. *Am J Roentgenol* 83:886, 1960.
18. Clement AR, Chang J: The radiologic diagnosis of spontaneous mesenteric venous thrombosis. *Am J Gastroenterol* 63:211, 1975.
19. Fey PH, Sproyregan S, Ahmed A, et al: Mesenteric vein thrombosis: Angiography in two cases. *Am J Roentgenol* 136:809, 1981.
20. Friendenberg MJ, Polk HC Jr, McAlister WH, et al: Superior mesenteric arteriography in experimental mesenteric venous thrombosis. *Radiology* 85:38, 1965.
21. McCune WS, Keshishian JM, Blades BB: Mesenteric thrombosis following blunt abdominal trauma. *Ann Surg* 135:606, 1952.
22. Polk HC: Experimental mesenteric venous occlusion. *Ann Surg* 163:432, 1956.

23. Gruenberg JC, Smallridge RC, Rosenberg RD: Inherited antithrombin III deficiency causing mesenteric venous infarction. *Ann Surg* 181:791, 1975.
24. Peters TG, Lewis JD, Filip DJ, et al: Antithrombin III deficiency causing postsplenectomy mesenteric venous thrombosis coincident with thrombocytopenia. *Ann Surg* 185:229, 1977.
25. Collins GJ Jr, Zack TF, Zajtchuk R, et al: Hypercoagulability in mesenteric venous occlusion. *Am J Surg* 132:390, 1976.
26. Arko FR, Jewell CT, Dainer P, et al: Primary mesenteric vein thrombosis associated with antithrombin III deficiency. *JAMA* 242:2324, 1979.
27. Civetta JM, Kalodny M: Mesenteric venous thrombosis associated with oral contraceptives. *Gastroenterology* 58:713, 1970.
28. Milne PY, Thomas RJS: Mesenteric venous thrombosis associated with oral contraceptives: A case report. *Aust N Z J Surg* 46:134, 1976.
29. Nesbit RJ Jr, DeWeese JA: Mesenteric venous thrombosis and oral contraceptives. *San M J* 70:360, 1977.
30. Lescher TJ, Bombeck CT: Mesenteric vascular occlusion associated with oral contraceptive use. *Arch Surg* 112:1231, 1977.
31. Hassein MIR, Sepose M, Wilde RC: Mesenteric venous thrombosis in members of the same family: Possible etiologic factor. *Am Surg* 37:418, 1971.
32. Bull S: Mesenteric venous thrombosis following splenectomy: Report of two cases. *Ann Surg* 162:938, 1965.
33. Balz J, Minton JP: Mesenteric thrombosis following splenectomy. *Ann Surg* 181:126, 1975.
34. Nagasue N, Inokuchi K, Kobagashi M, et al: Mesenteric venous thrombosis occurring late after splenectomy. *Br J Surg* 64:781, 1977.
35. LaRoja RD: Cogan syndrome associated with mesenteric vascular insufficiency. *Arch Surg* 111:1028, 1976.
36. Cooperman M, Martin EW, Carey LC: Evaluation of ischemic intestine by Doppler ultrasound. *Am J Surg* 139:73, 1980.
37. Bulkley GB, Zuidema GD, Hamilton SR, et al: Intraoperative determination of small bowel viability following ischemic injury. *Ann Surg* 193:628, 1981.

38. Jona J, Cummins GM, Head HB, et al: Recurrent primary mesenteric venous thrombosis. *JAMA* 227:1033, 1974.
39. Campbell SJ, Mears TW: Mesenteric thrombosis. *Am Surg* 23:543, 1957.
40. Robberson G: Mesenteric venous occlusion. *J Ark Med Soc* 64:143, 1967.
41. Trinkle JK, Bash BF, Fullmer MA, Bryant LR, Rams J: The operative management of idiopathic mesenteric venous thrombosis with intestinal infarction. *Am Surg* 39:338, 1969.
42. Ottinger LW: The surgical management of acute occlusion of the superior mesenteric artery. *Ann Surg* 188:721, 1978.

12

Intestinal Angina

James H. Caldwell, M.D.

Sixty years ago, Klein wrote prophetically, "While mesenteric infarct can by no means be called—as far as we know—an everyday occurrence, there can be no doubt . . . that owing to the difficulty of the diagnosis and to beliefs in its rarity many cases remain unrecognized [and] if these statements hold true for the acute type of the disease, they hold with far greater verity for the chronic."[1] His review of the literature and cases with which he had experience give convincing evidence that a chronic syndrome due to intestinal vascular disease could, on occasion, be recognized prior to the dramatic occurrence of an acute vascular event, and that the outcomes of these lesions depended on the rate and extent of development of an effective collateral circulation. This review also established that the majority of both acute and chronic cases occurred in the presence of coexisting cardiac or peripheral vascular disease. Fifteen years later, Dunphy described the essential characteristics of the pain associated with chronic intestinal vascular disease, finding that seven of 12 patients dying of acute mesenteric thrombosis had experienced abdominal pain for weeks to years before the acute terminal event.[2] The occurrence of severe poorly localized abdominal pain, postprandial at its onset and later becoming constant and sometimes radiating to the back, had in each case been attributed to coexisting coronary artery disease. The description is consistent with our present understanding of the symptoms of mesenteric vascular insufficiency. Since corrective vascular surgery was not available at the time, Dunphy predicted that the importance of recognizing the vascular origin of this type of chronic abdominal pain was that it preceded intestinal infarction. The recognition of nonthrombotic etiologies of intestinal infarction has diminished to some extent the prescience of this prediction, but the observation is still valid for some cases of mesenteric vascular disease. For example, the report of an early case diagnosed preoperatively and electively corrected by endarterectomy includes mention of five similar cases seen in a relatively brief period, all of whom progressed to frank infarction before elective correction could be performed.[3] This paper, which did much to popularize the term "intestinal angina" also led to the expectation that many such cases were awaiting recognition and surgical correction. One of the goals of this chapter is to reexamine this expectation in an effort to place the syndrome of chronic intestinal vascular insufficiency in perspective.

Incidence

There are few reliable figures on which to base an accurate estimate of the incidence of intestinal angina. Only about 200 cases of surgically corrected intestinal angina had been reported in the two decades since the report of the first successful operation.[4] A worldwide incidence of 10 cases per year may have been on the mind of the anonymous editorialist who wrote, "chronic intestinal ischemia does not rate all the attention it has received."[5] A survey of five series comprising 133 patients reported more recently suggests that intestinal angina is uncommon but not vanishingly rare.[6–10] This series from five large centers reflects the combined experience of 11 to 17 years (mean 15 years) and yields a calculated average of approximately two patients per year (range, 1–3) in major referral hospitals with active vascular surgery services.

Hildebrand and Zierler found six patients with intestinal angina among 75 patients with acute intestinal infarction.[11] Similarly, a medical record audit at The Ohio State University Hospitals disclosed 2 cases of intestinal angina among 23 patients with acute gut ischemia of all causes, while total annual admissions were 24,300.[12] These figures are consistent with reported rates of acute mesenteric infarction of 1:1,000 admissions[13–17] and suggest that intestinal angina occurs in about 1:12,000 admissions. Since there are an estimated 35,000,000 hospital admissions per year in the United States, nearly 3,000 cases might be anticipated per year. Thus, intestinal angina occurs infrequently enough that many physicians might not encounter it in a lifetime. On the other hand, the consultant in a referral center seeing many patients with abdominal pain will encounter this disease and should be familiar with the principal clinical features and diagnostic approaches.

Clinical Features

The hallmark of intestinal angina is postprandial abdominal pain, and Dunphy's early description[2] has not been changed by time. Mavor expanded the clinical features of the syndrome to include altered bowel habit, occult blood in the stool, weight loss, and, on occasion, evidence of malabsorption.[18] Bowel changes are variable, with both diarrhea and constipation recorded with varying frequency. On the other hand, weight loss is almost unvarying, owing largely to the association of pain with eating and the adoption of a diet of small meals. The combination of pain and weight loss is present in over 90% of patients and atypical presentations are distinctly uncommon. Many patients are thought to harbor an occult neoplasm before consideration is given to intestinal vascular disease.

In contrast to the virtually stereotyped history, there are no specific physical findings of chronic intestinal vascular disease. Nearly all patients evidence weight loss in excess of 10% of body weight, and evidence of ischemic cardiac disease, peripheral vascular disease, or abdominal aortic aneurysm will be present in the majority. In the series cited previously[6–10] 65% of patients had abdominal bruits. The significance of this finding will be further discussed.

Age and sex data are surprising, for in contrast to the expectations for patients with multiple sites of vascular disease, women predominate. Although female to male ratios vary from 1:1 to 4:1 in different series, the ratio was 88:45 in the series previously cited.[6–10] The average age in most series is the fifties. In one series, the average age of women was 51, while that of men was 63.[10] It is apparent that the typical patient with intestinal angina is likely to be a middle-aged woman.

Diagnosis

Although many patients with intestinal angina have abdominal bruits, the significance of this physical finding has been questioned because of its nonspecificity. It is widely recognized that many normal persons have audible abdominal vascular sounds with a reported frequency of 6.5%[19] to 29%.[20] It is less well known that the quality of the bruit and the age of the person influence the interpretation of this finding. Rivin[21] found that 18% of 500 normal subjects had bruits. The incidence was 44% in those under 25 years of age, and only 4% in those 51 years or older. Thus, an abdominal bruit as a normal finding becomes less common with age, and therefore more significant. In addition, the detection of a diastolic component may have special significance. Watson et al. reported that five of six patients with extrinsic compression of the celiac artery had a diastolic sound detectable by phonoangiography not found in normal persons.[20] Sarr et al. recently used this technique in two patients not previously suspected of having intestinal angina and reported that the discovery of a diastolic component in the bruit prompted angiography and led to the correct diagnosis, subsequently confirmed at operation.[22] Additional experience is necessary to confirm these findings, but there is a real possibility that further attention to this aspect of the syndrome will result in more precise diagnosis.

The incidence of malabsorption in patients with intestinal angina is unknown, but it was recognized and reported in the first cases diagnosed preoperatively and undergoing elective surgical correction.[23] Correction of steatorrhea and D-xylose malabsorption by revascularization of the intestine is good evidence that ischemia impairs absorptive mucosal function.[24] Unfortunately, clearcut evidence of malabsorption is present in a minority of patients, so absorptive function studies are of little diagnostic assistance in most. Nonetheless, it is important to be aware of intestinal ischemia in the differential diagnosis of steatorrhea, especially since an exceptional patient will have barium contrast X-ray studies suggestive of malabsorption. Although most patients with intestinal angina have normal gastrointestinal roentgenograms, stasis, dilatation, and disordered jejunal peristalsis have been described.[25] These findings would ordinarily suggest one of the mucosal diseases such as gluten enteropathy.

Angiographic visualization of the mesenteric vessels is essential. Lateral views during aortic injection are critical to evaluate the root of each vessel, for atherosclerosis usually affects the first few centimeters of each artery. A-P views serve principally to demonstrate the presence or absence of collateral circulation between the celiac and superior mesenteric distribution, or from branches of the inferior mesenteric artery to the superior mesenteric through the arc of Riolan. The usual findings in intestinal angina are high-grade stenosis or complete occlusion of two or three mesenteric vessels, with involvement of the celiac and superior mesenteric artery most common (Figure 1A). The finding of a large, meandering inferior mesenteric artery (Figure 1B) supplying flow through the left colic branch to the superior mesenteric artery via its middle colic branch is evidence of significant impairment of flow from

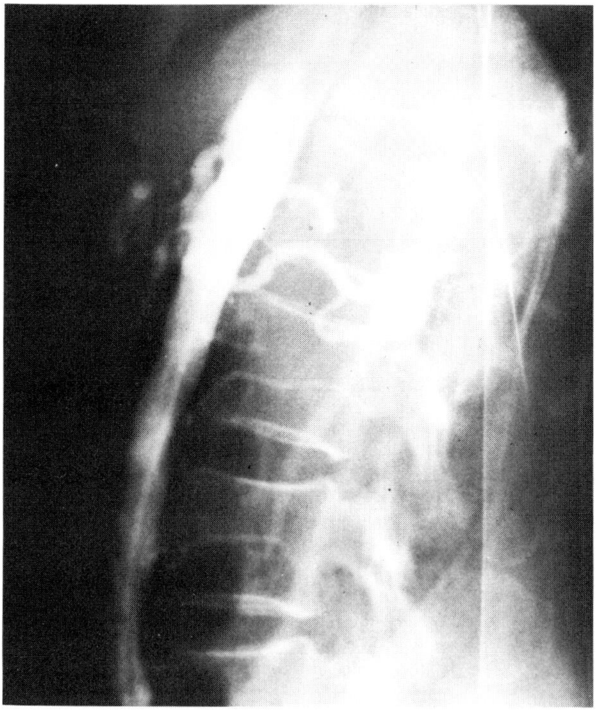

Figure 1A. Lateral view of aortogram showing high grade stenosis of origins of celiac artery and superior mesenteric artery.

the proximal arteries.[16] It is likely that flow through the inferior mesenteric artery is sufficient to maintain intestinal nutrition at rest but incapable of increasing sufficiently in response to a meal, producing the characteristic clinical picture.[26] Unfortunately, although collaterals accompanying severe disease in two of the three principal visceral branches are the usual angiographic finding in intestinal angina, angiography produces only qualitative results that may be consistent with but not diagnostic of intestinal angina. Mesenteric vascular disease is found in the majority of individuals over 45[16] and one-third of patients

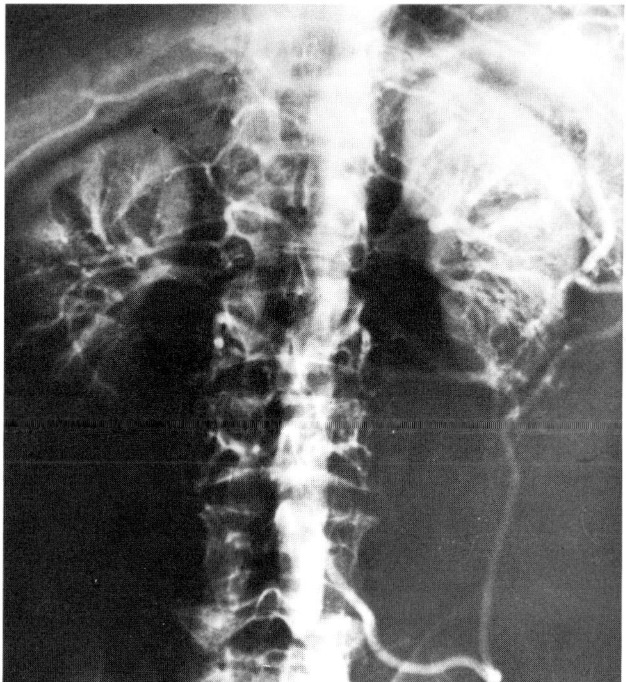

Figure 1B. Anterior view of aortogram showing prominent inferior mesenteric artery with proximal collateral (meandering mesenteric artery).

having aortography for any reason have been found to have asymptomatic celiac axis obstruction.[7] Since intestinal angina is uncommon even in the face of significant angiographic abnormalities, most of the asymptomatic patients must have well developed collateral circulations.

An attempt to find quantitative diagnostic angiographic changes in intestinal angina was reported by Dick et al. in 1967.[27] Estimated cross-sectional areas of the celiac, SMA, and IMA from patients with intestinal angina were compared with those from patients having aortography for claudication, aneurysm, suspected renal artery stenosis and other indications. The mean cross-sectional area in patients with angina was significantly less than that of other patients, but there was overlap between the two groups. Since only area and not flow can be measured by angiography, numerical estimates of reduced vessel diameter often are not accurately correlated with the presence or absence of symptoms.

Hansen and co-workers provided valuable data on splanchnic blood flow in these patients and contributed to an understanding of the pathophysiology as well as diagnosis.[28] Using a dye method for measuring total hepatic blood flow (which is equivalent to splanchnic blood flow), they measured fasting and postprandial flow before and after revascularization in patients with intestinal angina. These results were compared with flow before and after meals in controls and in patients suspected of abdominal angina with less severe angiographic findings than those operated upon. They found no difference in fasting blood flow in patients with intestinal angina compared with that in the other groups. Postprandial flow increased 40% above fasting flow in controls and those with minimal vascular disease, but not in patients with angina. Following revascularization, fasting flow was increased above preoperative levels and further increased postprandially to normal values. The authors proposed that absence of a postprandial increase in splanchnic blood flow favors the diagnosis of abdominal angina, while an appropriate increase after the test meal is evidence against the diagnosis.

Measurement of splanchnic blood flow is not a commonly performed diagnostic test. Nonetheless, it can be performed in any facility equipped for angiography and cardiac catheterization, procedures likely to be performed in a center prepared to do vascular surgery. Further experience with blood flow measurements in patients with intestinal angina provide additional information about the feasibility, utility, and precision of this technique.

Treatment

Surgical correction of intestinal vascular disease is indicated when a confident diagnosis is established, for there is no effective medical therapy. In contrast to the forbidding mortality of acute intestinal infarction, more than 90% of patients with intestinal angina undergoing elective operation survive. In spite of the frequently coexisting vascular disease in other organs, five-year survival of 83% and ten-year survival of 62% has been reported.[29] In most series, nearly all survivors are completely relieved of symptoms. Although no controlled study has been performed to demonstrate whether elective surgical treatment prevents progression to acute infarction, the long-term survival results and the infrequency of acute ischemia following successful elective treatment suggest that this is an additional benefit of therapy.

The type of correction varies with the experience of the surgeon, the location of the lesions, the severity of coexisting aortic disease, and the need for simultaneous correction of other lesions, such as aneurysm, renal artery lesions, or iliofemoral disease. The first successful operation reported was endarterectomy,[23] but the availability of suitable graft materials and wide experience with bypass grafts in other locations has resulted in bypass as the preferred procedure in most cases.[7,10,29] Most authors favor synthetic prosthetic grafts over vein grafts. Arguments in favor of synthetic grafts include: less tendency to kink when positioned near the mesenteric root;[6] ready availability and technically easier attachment to the aorta in the presence of aortic disease or the need for aortic replacement;[7] a higher rate of stricture or occlusion of vein grafts;[8] and less tendency to deform with posture changes.[10] Reimplantation is infrequently recommended because of coexisting aortic disease, but is applicable to the hypertrophied inferior mesenteric artery if an aortic graft is required. Most surgeons will also revascularize the celiac or superior mesenteric artery in this situation. Although some advocate single-vessel repair regardless of the number of vessels involved, Hollier et al.[30] have presented experience suggesting that late recurrence is lower when all affected vessels are revascularized. Their data also indicate that correction of all diseased vessels is more important than the choice of graft material.

One of the reasons bypass operations have been favored over endarterectomy is that it is difficult to expose the origin of the celiac and SMA by an anterior abdominal approach. Stoney et al.[8] advocate transaortic endarterectomy by a thoracoretroperitoneal approach to overcome these difficulties, especially if endarterectomy of the renal arteries is to be undertaken simultaneously. For patients with a patent IMA and disease confined to the celiac and SMA, they advocate aortoceliac bypass alone as their results suggest residual SMA disease alone does not influence outcome. Another report of extensive experience with endarterectomy comes from Russia.[31] These authors also favor endarterectomy for multiple vessel disease, but favor resection and replacement rather than bypass grafts if there is extensive disease. Their results are difficult to evaluate, since only about 40% of their patients had symptoms of chronic intestinal ischemia and half of these had isolated extravascular compression of the celiac artery. The rest had a prophylactic intestinal vascular operation performed in the course of aortic or renal artery procedures.

Summary

The syndrome of chronic intestinal angina due to atherosclerosis of the mesenteric vessels produces a readily recognized clinical picture of postprandial abdominal pain and weight loss. Exclusion of the principal differential diagnoses of complicated peptic ulcer disease, biliary or pancreatic disease, inflammatory bowel disease or other structural intestinal lesions, and digestive tract neoplasm can be readily accomplished with modern diagnostic techniques. In the absence of other diagnoses, abdominal angiography is indicated and yields information about the anatomy, and to some extent, the functional state of the mesenteric circulation. Further experience with measurement of the postprandial splanchnic blood flow response can make diagnosis quantitatively precise and predict the outcome of surgical treatment. Several standard surgical approaches are available and the postoperative results are excellent. The proportion of the population at risk is increasing, and advances in vascular surgery will prolong the lives of many patients at special risk.

References

1. Klein E: Embolism and thrombosis of the superior mesenteric artery. *Surg Gynecol Obstet* 33:385, 1921.
2. Dunphy JE: Abdominal pains of vascular origin. *Am J Med Sci* 192:109, 1936.
3. Mikkelsen WP, Zaro JA: Intestinal angina: Report of a case with preoperative diagnosis and surgical relief. *N Engl J Med* 260:912, 1959.
4. Eklof B, Hoevels J, Ihase I: The surgical treatment of chronic intestinal ischemia. *Ann Surg* 187:318, 1978.
5. Chronic intestinal ischemia. Editorial, *Lancet* 2:1332, 1977.
6. Hertzer NR, Beven EG, Humphries AW: Chronic intestinal ischemia. *Surg Gynecol Obstet* 145:321, 1977.
7. Crawford ES, Morris GC, Myhre HO, et al: Celiac axis, su-

perior mesenteric artery, and inferior mesenteric artery occlusion: surgical considerations. *Surgery* 82:856, 1977.

8. Stoney RJ, Ehrenfeld WK, Wylie EJ: Revascularization methods in chronic visceral ischemia caused by atherosclerosis. *Ann Surg* 186:468, 1977.
9. Robb HJ, Ketonen P, Ketonen L, et al: Clinical experience with surgical treatment of chronic intestinal ischemia. *Ann Chirurg Gynecol* 67:70, 1978.
10. Zelenock GB, Graham LM, Whitehouse WM, et al: Splanchnic arteriosclerotic disease and intestinal angina. *Arch Surg* 115:497, 1980.
11. Hildebrand HD, Zierler RE: Mesenteric vascular disease. *Am J Surg* 139:188, 1980.
12. Cooperman M, Martin EW, Carey LC: Evaluation of ischemic intestine by Doppler ultrasound. *Am J Surg* 139:73, 1980.
13. Wilson GSM, Block J: Mesenteric vascular occlusion. *Arch Surg* 73:330, 1956.
14. Ottinger LW, Austen WG: A study of 136 patients with mesenteric infarction. *Surg Gynecol Obstet* 124:251, 1967.
15. Kairaluoma MI, Karkola P, Heikkinen E, et al: Mesenteric infarction. *Am J Surg* 133:188, 1977.
16. Boley SJ, Brandt LJ, Veith FJ: Ischemic disorders of the intestines. *Curr Probl Surg* 15:1, 1978.
17. Marston A: Acute mesenteric vascular occlusions. In *Vascular Disorders of the Intestine.* Boley SJ, Schwartz SS, Williams LF (Eds.) Appleton-Century-Crofts, New York 1971. p 509.
18. Mavor GE, Lyall AD, Chrystal KMR, et al: Mesenteric infarction as a vascular emergency. *Br J Surg* 50:219, 1962.
19. Edwards AJ, Hamilton JD, Nichol WD, et al: Experience with coeliac axis compression syndrome. *Br Med J* 1:342, 1970.
20. Watson WC, Williams PB, Duffy G: Epigastric bruits in patients with and without celiac axis compression. *Ann Intern Med* 79:211, 1973.
21. Rivin AU: Abdominal vascular sounds. *JAMA* 221:688, 1972.
22. Sarr MG, Dickson ER, Newcomer AD: Diastolic bruit in chronic intestinal ischemia: Recognition by abdominal phonoangiography. *Dig Dis Sci* 25:761, 1980.
23. Shaw RS, Maynard EP: Acute and chronic thrombosis of

mesenteric arteries associated with malabsorption: A report of two cases successfully treated by thromboendarterectomy. *N Engl J Med* 258:874, 1958.

24. Dardik H, Seidenberg B, Parker JG, et al: Intestinal angina with malabsorption treated by elective revascularization. *JAMA* 194:148, 1965.
25. Meyers MA, Kaplowitz N, Bloom AA: Malabsorption secondary to mesenteric ischemia. *Am J Roentgenol* 119:352, 1973.
26. Saegesser F: Acute abdomen arising from vascular disorders in the elderly. In *Clinics in Gastroenterology*: Vol 10. Forsali A (Ed.) WB Saunders Co, London 1981. pp 145–176.
27. Dick AP, Graff R, Gregg DM, et al: An arteriographic study of mesenteric arterial disease. *Gut* 8:206, 1967.
28. Hansen HJB, Engell HC, Ring-Larsen H, et al: Splanchnic blood flow in patients with abdominal angina before and after arterial reconstruction. *Ann Surg* 186:216, 1977.
29. McCollum CH, Graham JM, DeBakey ME: Chronic mesenteric arterial insufficiency: Results of revascularization in 33 cases. *South Med J* 69:1266, 1976.
30. Hollier LH, Bernatz PE, Pairolero PC, et al: Surgical management of chronic intestinal ischemia: A reappraisal. *Surgery* 90:940, 1981.
31. Pokrovsky AV, Kasantchjan PO: Surgical treatment of chronic occlusive disease of the enteric visceral branches of the abdominal aorta. *Ann Surg* 191:51, 1980.

13

Spontaneous Ischemic Colitis

John J. Ferrara, M.D.

Spontaneous ischemic colitis (SIC) has only recently been identified as an entity distinct from all other inflammatory diseases of the colon. Recognition of this fact has led to earlier, more accurate diagnosis, and hence to improvement in the treatment of patients with this disease. Knowledge concerning SIC has been derived from both animal experimentation and human clinical observations.

History

Until the 1960s, patients who would now be recognized to have SIC were believed to have symptoms and signs suggestive of inflammatory bowel disease. However, in 1963 Boley et al.[1] reported five patients with similar symptoms, crampy abdominal pain followed closely by bloody diarrhea and abdominal tenderness. Barium enema examination in each demonstrated nodular filling defects arising from the colon wall, some of which could later be visualized and biopsied on sigmoidoscopy. The described "thumbprinting" of the colon (Figure 1) represented areas of submucosal hemorrhage. Since Boley was able to recreate the findings by ligating the vascular supply to the

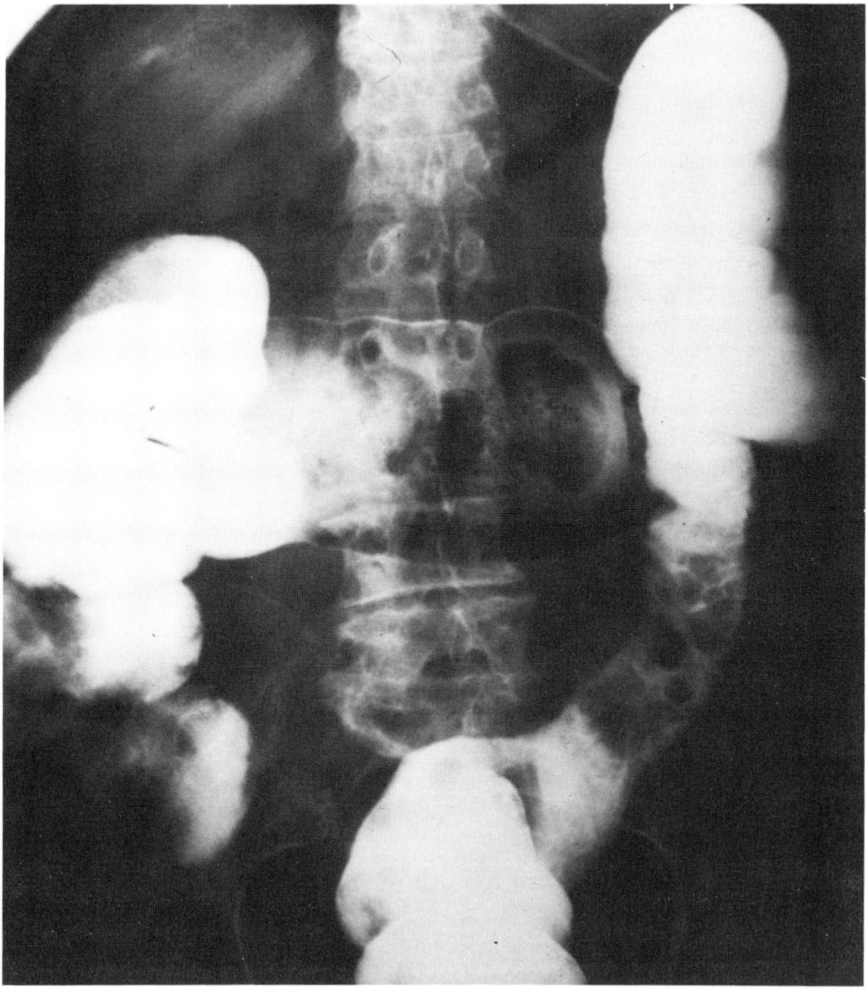

Figure 1. Barium contrast examination of the colon in a patient with SIC. Note the extensive *thumbprinting* of the sigmoid colon.

descending colon in mongrel dogs, he called this disease *vascular occlusion of the colon.* Through close follow-up of his patients, he determined that the disease was essentially self-limited and resolved with simple supportive measures. He therefore added the term *reversible* to the newly described clinical entity.

Marston et al.[2] continued to develop clinicopathologic criteria for the disease, which they called *ischemic colitis.* Detailed clinical analysis of 16 patients led to further categorization into three distinct groups of patients based upon the outcome of the ischemic insult. The first group demonstrated severe ischemic injury leading to transmural colonic infarction that required emergency surgical intervention. An intermediate state of ischemia led to a less fulminant course that could be managed nonoperatively by aggressive medical support. However, the involved colon segments healed by forming strictures that often required resection at a time well distant from the original insult. The final group consisted of patients who, like those in Boley's series, had transient, mild ischemia characterized by a benign clinical course with colon segments that healed rapidly without significant damage.

While Marston's classification has thus far stood the test of time, others have been proposed. Williams et al.[3] have questioned whether it is necessary to categorize patients into separate groups based on clinical outcome. They suggest two categories determined by the necessity for surgical intervention. Patients in the first group require surgery for either fulminant progression or prolongation of disease (dense fibrotic strictures). In the second group are patients whose disease is either completely reversible or in whom mild strictures occur and who can be managed without surgical intervention.

Regardless of the classification used, work by these original investigators has led to numerous clinical reports confirming that SIC exists as a disease entity with a readily identifiable set of symptoms and signs.

Pathogenesis

Following Boley's experimental data[1] that suggested the etiology of SIC to be vascular occlusion, numerous investigators have attempted to further relate the clinical findings to the pathophysiology of the disease. Several points are to be made from these studies. There appear to be two well defined populations who develop SIC.[4] Patients in the first group are generally at least 50 years of age. Diseased colon segments, while not confined to a specific area, are located distal to the midtransverse colon in the majority of instances. Occurrence of SIC is postulated to be secondary to occlusive atheromatous vascular disease of involved colon segments.

In contrast to this larger group, there is a more recently defined smaller group whose age at onset is usually under 50 years. Again, while diseased segments may occur throughout the colon, most are found in the right side. Finally, the pathogenesis of SIC in these patients is only rarely atheromatous in nature. Rather, any of a number of predisposing factors have been postulated, including collagen vascular disease,[5] drug abuse,[6] and hormone therapy.[7] While the presumed common factor in these patients is a period of prolonged hypotension leading to ischemia, quite often no cause can be found.[8,9]

Regardless of the classification of patients, the opinion that SIC is a result of vascular occlusion or nonocclusive colon hypoperfusion is nearly universal. This theory has remained essentially unchanged since the experimental work of Boley,[1] though several refinements have been made. For instance, it was noted that most cases of SIC in the elderly involve the left colon, particularly at the splenic flexure. Griffith[10] identified what he considered a critical anastomotic series between branches of the ascending left colic artery and the marginal artery of Drummond at the point where the former vessel joins the left branch of the middle colic artery (Figure 2). A poor communication in

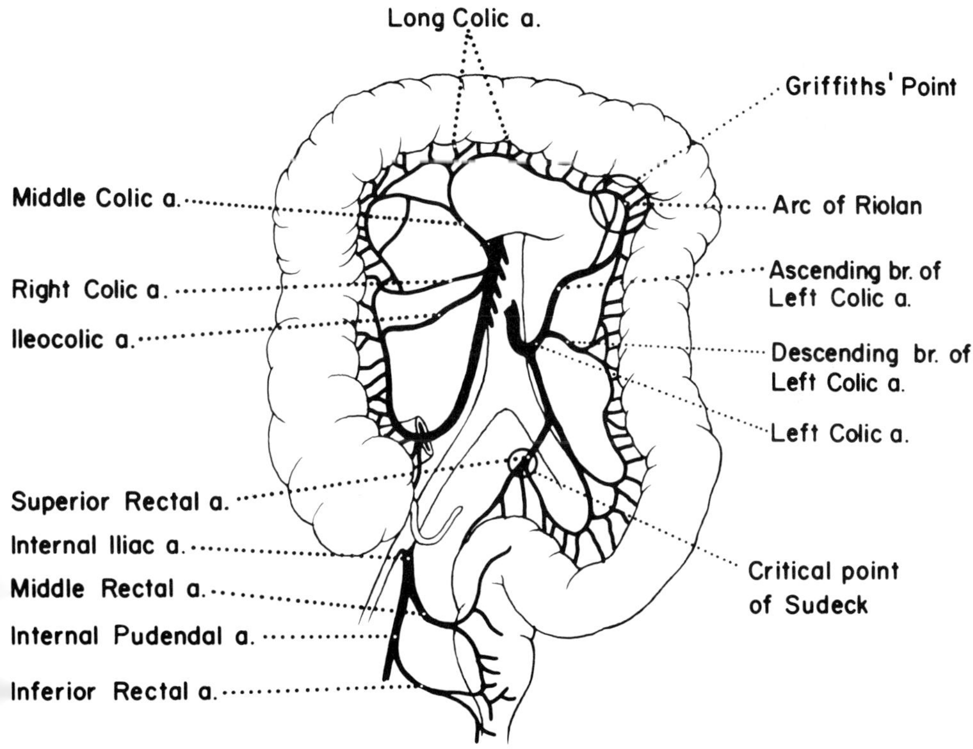

Figure 2. Schematic representation of the arterial supply to the colon.

this area results in a watershed effect corresponding to the descending portion of the splenic flexure, with no dominant arterial supply. Meyers[11] performed selective angiography on 58 human necropsy specimens and found a tenuous arterial communication at Griffith's point in over one-half of the cases. Presumably, in an older patient with generalized atherosclerotic vessels, this area would be vulnerable to diminished perfusion, thereby leading to the high incidence of left-sided SIC. While Binns and Isaacson[12] were unable to confirm a consistent absence of anastomoses at Griffith's point, they did demonstrate a significant increase in tortuosity of the long colic arteries with age. The resultant increased resistance to forward flow to the colon acts as a contributing factor to mucosal ischemia in the elderly.

In an extensive review of patients who presented with SIC at the Institut de Pathologie CHUV, Saegesser et al.[13] identified four factors that they believed contributed to the development of colon ischemia. The foremost was a lack of adequate vascular anastomosis not only at Griffith's point, but also at the point of Sudek. (See Figure 2.) This latter watershed area lies at the sigmoid colon where superior and middle hemorrhoidal arteries form anastomotic arcades. The second factor involves an insult that causes a reduction of splanchnic flow. This results in colonic arteriolar vasoconstriction and localized ischemia, particularly at the aforementioned critical anastomotic points. A third factor requires development of increasing intramural pressure secondary to distal colonic obstruction and a competent ileocecal valve. While this generally results in cecal disease (secondary to the well known law of Laplace), there will also be increased pressure distributed throughout the colon. In already compromised points of the left colon, distention results in further mural ischemia. Finally, the presence of colonic microflora in areas of vascular compromise would augment colonic damage. These four factors then, alone or in combination, contribute to development of SIC in the presence of either occlusive or nonocclusive colon hypoperfusion.

Pathology

Both gross and histologic findings in patients with SIC depend upon the stage of the disease process. As described initially by Boley,[1] the acute ischemic phase is characterized by areas of submucosal hemorrhage and intramural bleeding through mucosal breaks. The microscopic appearance of acute colon ischemia is well delineated by Whitehead[14] and Allen.[15] There is dilation of superficial capillaries with necrosis of mucosal structures and infiltration of underlying tissue with polymorphonuclear leukocytes. Should the ischemic insult persist, progression to gangrene will follow, with full-thickness necrosis, tissue sloughing, and perforation following formation of mural microabscesses.

In most instances, however, the period of ischemia is shortlived, and recovery is possible. There is a gradual resolution of submucosal hemorrhages fostering the formation of ulcers where mucosal breaks occur.

Morson[16] aptly described the microscopic appearance as one of full-thickness mucosal loss with ulceration covered by granulation tissue. Epithelialization occurs from the edges of the ulcers. Submucosal layers are thickened with dilated capillaries and hemosiderin-laden macrophages, which characterize the healing phase of SIC.[4] Under propitious conditions, healing is complete, with total restoration of normal anatomy. At times, however, the ischemic period is too severe for total resolution of disease, and strictures form. Marston[2] notes that ischemic strictures are generally short areas with patchy mucosal ulceration and thickened submucosa filled with white granulation. Attempts at epithelial regeneration are present along the borders of the lesion. Again, hemosiderin-filled macrophages are scattered in the submucosa. Inflammation may carry through the muscularis propria to pericolic tissues, resulting in fibrosis.

Clinical Manifestations

Little can be added to Boley's[1] initial description of the patient with SIC. The triad of abdominal pain, lower abdominal tenderness, and bloody diarrhea still serves as the best guide to diagnosis. The abdominal pain is usually sudden in onset and is characterized as mild, though crampy.

Within 24 hours of the onset of pain, diarrhea ensues, often bloody. Lower quadrant tenderness is present by then, confined at least initially to the affected side of the colon. Wittenberg et al.[17] found that nearly three-fourths of patients had crampy abdominal pain and tenderness, while two-thirds developed bloody diarrhea. In a review of their experience, Hagihara et al.[18] found that the extent of disease could be fairly well characterized by the symptoms. Those with mild to moderate disease developed only minimal early abdominal pain with little to no tenderness. Diarrhea followed almost immediately after the onset of pain. It consisted of large amounts of mucus mixed with blood. In contrast, those with moderate to severe disease had a dramatic onset of severe crampy pain, and often, localized rebound tenderness. Onset of diarrhea, while at times immediate, might be delayed by a rapidly developing ileus. Finally, patients with gangrene presented in a state of shock, unable to give a clear history or submit to physical examination.

Most, but not all, patients with SIC have fever and leukocytosis, reflecting the inflammatory nature of the disease. The major benefit of serial determination of both values lies in evaluating the success of therapy.

Differential Diagnosis

In order to establish the diagnosis of SIC, several more common diseases should be disproved. This is, at times, a most difficult task. Abdominal pain in patients with SIC may be so mild as to make it difficcult to differentiate this disease from the generally asymptomatic hemorrhage from colon diverticulae or angiodysplasia. In such cases, barium enema and colonoscopy may fail to yield a definite diagnosis. Angiography is helpful in identifying the source of hemorrhage if the patient is bleeding at a rate of 1–2 cc/min. Usually, however, the bleeding is slow and one must rely on careful clinical evaluation and prolonged follow-up to confirm the diagnosis of SIC. Repeated episodes of hemorrhage are more common in diverticular disease or angiodysplasia; recurrent bleeding is rarely reported in SIC.

It is often more difficult to differentiate the symptoms and radiographic signs of SIC from those of other inflammatory forms of colitis. The initial presentation and even the pathologic findings may be identical to those of either granulomatous or ulcerative colitis. Follow-up is of considerable assistance, since patients with SIC have localized segmental involvement that remains unchanged in site; furthermore, there is usually little response to steroid therapy.

Examination of stool specimens for ova, parasites, white cells, and *Clostridia* species is essential to rule out an infectious etiology. Antibiotic-induced bacterial overgrowth leading to pseudomembraneous colitis is to be disproved as well.

One might, at times, have a difficult time differentiating SIC from acute small bowel ischemia. In the latter disease, pain is usually periumbilical but may be located in the lower quadrants of the abdomen. Symptoms are described as severe, though findings on abdominal examination are at first quite benign. Bloody diarrhea is a later manifestation in small bowel disease, and is accompanied by increasing tenderness to palpation secondary to diffuse peritonitis. If the distinction between large and small bowel ischemia remains uncertain, selective angiography is indicated before barium contrast studies are performed. The complications of superior mesenteric artery occlusion are so devastating that this problem must be dealt with immediately.

Diagnostic Evaluation

Once the diagnosis of SIC is considered on clinical grounds, several diagnostic tests have been recommended. Since, in most patients the disease is confined to the left colon, sigmoidoscopy or fiberoptic colonoscopy may be used both as a diagnostic procedure and as a means of following the progression of the disease. Hagihara et al.[18] performed colonoscopy as soon as the diagnosis of SIC was suspected. In patients with mild SIC, the involved segments of colon demonstrated mild edema and submucosal hemorrhage. The mucosal surface, while intact, was easily traumatized into bleeding. In more advanced disease, there was severe blunting of mucosal folds and ballooning of the mucosa into the colon lumen. Patients with severe SIC showed fibrous coating of the mucosa with areas of denuded submucosa in a still edematous bowel wall. Great care is to be taken in the examination of these patients because of the extreme fragility of the bowel wall. Should disease progress even further, thick pseudomembrane covers the inside of the colon. Bleeding will be encountered only when healthy mucosa is identified. The edema has given way to a thinned-out bowel wall quite susceptible to perforation.

Hagihara performed serial examinations in several patients to establish the course of the disease. This technique was considered quite helpful in determining whether or not surgical intervention was necessary. He also performed histologic examination by colonoscopic biopsy. The biopsies only confirmed what could be viewed endoscopically and were, in general, not thought to be of significant diagnostic value.

Radiographic examination of the colon is thought by most authors to be an essential part of the diagnostic evaluation. Plain abdominal films may demonstrate only an adynamic ileus. In more severe cases with progression to bowel infarction, there may be haustral thickening and dilation of the colon proximal to diseased segments. Free air under a hemidiaphragm is, of course, an ominous sign of frank gangrene with perforation. All of these radiographic changes are, however, quite nonspecific. Therefore, a barium contrast enema examination should be performed. In films made within 72 hours of onset of symptoms, the pathognomonic features of "thumbprinting" or "sawtooth" irregularity of the involved colonic segments are present. (See Figure 1.) These intraluminal defects, or pseudotumors, are the result of protruding submucosal hemorrhages. Radiographic changes such as intramural extravasation of barium and loss of the mucosal pattern seen on a postevacuation film will parallel the clinical progression of the disease. While a carefully performed barium enema has been accompanied by no apparent morbidity in these patients, there is little enthusiasm for performing this study in more than moderately ill patients for fear of perforation by barium injected under even a small amount of pressure.

Follow-up examinations are an essential feature in the care of patients with SIC. In those who have recovered from mild disease, a barium enema performed 10 to 21 days following onset of the illness will be normal. This stresses the importance of an early barium enema to confirm the diagnosis. When symptoms of intermittent diarrhea and a change in bowel habits persist following apparent recovery from SIC, a repeat barium examination is essential. Quite often the previously involved segment of colon will have formed a fibrous stricture that may require resection if symptoms are debilitating.

With the general belief that the etiology of SIC involves the arterial supply of the colon, one would expect angiography to be of diagnostic value. However, the results of selective mesenteric injection have been inconclusive, for several reasons. Mesenteric angiography performed for reasons other than to confirm SIC demonstrates occlusive disease of the superior and inferior mesenteric vessels along with their collaterals in a high percentage of cases. Therefore, the failure to identify collateral circulation in patients with SIC thought to be secondary to occlusive disease would not be diagnostic. Reuter et al.[19] were able to demonstrate a hyperemic state in involved segments of colon in two patients who underwent mesenteric angiography several days following onset of symptoms. They do state that these changes are indicative only of inflammation from any of a variety of sources and are not specific for SIC.

Angiography has been performed on young patients thought to have SIC on a nonocclusive basis. The studies have generally been normal, confirming the nonocclusive nature of the disease in this group.

It would therefore appear that, at present, angiography plays a limited role in the diagnosis of SIC since the findings, when present, are nonspecific. The examination is invasive, with documented morbidity, including a report of colitis secondary to the performance of mesenteric angiography. The test should be used only when necessary to exclude other disease, such as superior mesenteric occlusion.

Treatment

Any patient suspected to have SIC should be hospitalized for diagnostic evaluation and therapy. As noted previously, the course of the disease is so unpredictable that all patients should receive in-hospital care. It is important to point out that treatment regimens are based upon previous experience rather than upon data from prospective trials; this disease is so uncommon as to preclude such studies.

Administration of intravenous fluids is essential to replenish volume deficit, maintain urine output, and correct electrolyte and metabolic abnormalities. Nasogastric suction is important to diminish gaseous distension from an evolving ileus or mechanical bowel obstruction. Rectal tube insertion, although beneficial in decompressing distal colon segments, is attended by an increased risk of perforation and pressure necrosis where it lies against the colon mucosa, and should not be performed.

Saegesser et al.[13] recommend the avoidance of any drugs that could have a vasospastic effect upon the splanchnic circulation, including digitalis. Patients who cannot tolerate a reduction in such medications should have concomitant treatment with intravenous papaverine. In addition, they feel that vigorous attempts should be made to maintain an adequate cardiac output and, thereby, splanchnic flow. These measures should include correction of cardiac arrhythmias when feasible.

Since the ischemic segments of colon act as a culture medium for existing bacterial flora, high-dose intravenous broad-spectrum antibiotics are indicated. One must be careful not to superimpose a pseudomembraneous enterocolitis secondary to drugs such as clindamycin. Frequent sigmoidoscopic examinations, then, are essential, should the patient develop a pattern of worsening diarrhea or other signs indicating progression of the disease. Steroids, once thought to be helpful in diminishing the inflammatory stages of disease, are now thought to be contraindicated since they increase the probability of superinfection.

While it is helpful to evaluate serial leukocyte counts, electrolytes, blood gases, and amylase levels, continuing assessment of the patient's vital signs and general well-being, and repeated abdominal examinations are the mainstay in following the results of therapy. It appears that, regardless of the initial impression of the extent of disease, the described therapy can result in complete reversal of disease, even if there is total involvement of the colon.

Treated according to this protocol, about one-half the patients with mild SIC will demonstrate symptomatic improvement over five to seven days. A barium enema performed two to four weeks thereafter will yield normal findings. Almost one-third will follow a more prolonged hospital course before recovery. Unfortunately, a high percentage of these will form strictures in previously diseased segments. While some can be managed nonoperatively, the remainder will require resection due to (1) symptoms of intermittent obstruction, (2) bloody diarrhea from exposed granulation tissue in the strictured area, or (3) difficulty in differentiation of stricture from a colon malignancy.

The remainder of patients are either admitted with or rapidly progress to severe SIC in fulminant septic shock and rapidly progressive multiple organ systems failure.

These patients require immediate and aggressive resuscitation before operation is undertaken. At exploration, all diseased segments of colon must be removed. While transmural gangrene is easy to identify, it is important to remember that normal-appearing serosa may conceal frankly necrotic colon mucosa. This has led some authors to suggest resection of obviously gangrenous bowel followed by operative endoscopy of remaining segments. This will help to determine whether the lines of resection are adequate, since the mucosal surface can be carefully inspected. However, this maneuver adds considerable time to the operative procedure and may be of little benefit. A more practical approach is to perform a generous resection of gangrenous segments of colon based upon either abscence of arterial pulsations by Doppler ultrasound or nonfluorescence of necrotic segments following an intravenous injection of fluorescien. End-colostomy with mucous fistula should follow, rather than a primary anastomosis. Immediate colocolostomy in these patients is associated with a high incidence of anastomotic leak and should not be done. Furthermore, the exteriorization will permit the monitoring of the viability of the colon by direct visualization.

It is essential, however, to resect all grossly necrotic bowel rather than to perform a simple decompressive or diverting colostomy. There was initial enthusiasm for the latter procedures because of a short anesthesia time, but additional experience has shown that these alternative procedures did little to alter the course of the disease and were accompanied by excessive mortality. Thus, resection with exteriorization is the present procedure of choice in these seriously ill patients. Despite optimum resection, the mortality rate in this group remains at least 50%.

Summary

Spontaneous ischemic colitis has only recently been recognized as an entity distinct from all other forms of colitis.

It appears to result from either acute colonic hypoperfusion secondary to hypotension or occlusive atheromatous arterial disease of the colon. Initial pathologic changes are submucosal hemorrhages which either resolve completely or progress to full-thickness necrosis with gangrene and perforation. The clinical triad of abdominal pain, lower abdominal tenderness, and bloody diarrhea should direct suspicion to this disease. Barium enema in the acute stages will demonstrate "thumbprinting" of the colon lumen secondary to the submucosal hemorrhages; this examination remains the cornerstone of both initial diagnosis and follow-up.

Patients may follow one of three clinical courses. In most cases, the disease is self-limited, and the colon regains normal anatomic configuration within one month after the appearance of symptoms. A smaller group of patients will have a more protracted, indolent course, but will recover without requiring surgical intervention in the acute stages of disease. However, a high percentage will develop fibrotic strictures representing failure of colonic repair, and most of these will mandate resection and primary anastomosis. In both groups, initial management consists of nasogastric decompression, correction of metabolic imbalances, broad spectrum intravenous antibiotics, and nutritional support. Steroids are contraindicated in this form of colitis.

The remainder of patients will present in septic shock from rapidly progressive disease. Resuscitation followed by emergency surgery is indicated. Generous resection of the involved segments with colostomy and mucous fistula is the treatment of choice. Mortality in this group approaches 70% despite aggressive care.

References

1. Boley SJ, Schwartz S, Lash J, Sternhill V: Reversible vascular occlusion of the colon. *Surg Gynecol Obstet* 116:53–60, 1963.
2. Marston A, Pheils MT, Thomas ML, Morson BC: Ischaemic colitis. *Gut* 7:3–15, 1966.

3. Williams LF, Wittenberg J: Ischemic colitis: an useful clinical diagnosis, but is it ischemic? *Ann Surg* 182:439–446, 1975.
4. Byrne JJ, Wittenberg J, Grimes ET, Williams LF: Ischemic diseases of the bowel. II. Ischemic colitis. *Dis Colon Rectum* 13:283–289, 1970.
5. Kiston MM, Kaplan MM, Harrington JT: Diffuse ischemic colitis associated with systemic lupus erythematosus. Response to subtotal colectomy. *Gastroenterology* 75:1147–1151, 1978.
6. Turnbull AR, Isaacson PJ: Ischaemic colitis and drug abuse. *Br Med J* 2:1000, 1977.
7. Barcewicz PA, Nulch JP: Ischemic colitis in young adults. *Dis Colon Rectum* 23:109–114, 1980.
8. Clark AW, Lloyd-Mostyn RH, Sadler MRdeC: "Ischaemic" colitis in young adults. *Br Med J* 4:70–72, 1972.
9. Duffy TJ: Reversible ischaemic colitis in young adults. *Br J Surg* 68:34–37, 1981.
10. Griffith JD: Blood supply of the colon. *Proc Roy Soc Med* 881–882, 1966.
11. Meyers MA: Griffiths' point: Critical anastomosis at the splenic flexure. Significance in ischemia of the colon. *Am J Roentgenol* 126:77–94, 1976.
12. Binns JC, Isaacson P: Age-related changes in the colonic blood supply: their relevance to ischaemic colitis. *Gut* 19: 384–390, 1978.
13. Saegesser F, Loosli H, Robinson JWL, Roenspies U: Ischemic diseases of the large intestine. *Int Surg* 66:103–117, 1981.
14. Whitehead R: The pathology of ischemia of the intestines. In *Pathology Annual*. Sommers SC (Ed.) 1976.
15. Allen AC: Unified concept of the vascular pathogenesis of enterocolitis of varied etiology. A pathophysiologic analysis. *Am J Gastroenterol* 55:347–378, 1971.
16. Morson BC: Pathology of ischaemic colitis. In *Inflammation in Gut*. Karger, New York 1970. pp 134–136.
17. Wittenberg J, Athanasoulis CA, Williams LF et al: Ischemic colitis. Radiology and Pathophysiology. *Am J Roentgenol* 123:287–295, 1975.
18. Hagihara PF, Parker JC, Griffen WO: Spontaneous ischemic colitis. *Dis Colon Rectum* 20:236–251, 1977.
19. Reuter SR, Kanter IE, Redman H: Angiography in reversible colonic ischemia. *Radiology* 97:371–375, 1970.

14

Intestinal Ischemia and Gangrene in Obstruction

E. Christopher Ellison, M.D.

Intestinal obstruction is one of the most common surgical problems. Mortality of simple, uncomplicated intestinal obstruction has remained constant at 3 to 7% for the last twenty years since the recognition of the need for adequate preoperative volume restoration. In contrast, when obstruction is associated with strangulation, mortality rises from 20 to 70%. Silen[1] has stated that strangulation accounted for more than 50% of deaths from intestinal obstruction. In fact, only two series reported in the last twenty years show mortality rates lower than 10% when gangrenous bowel complicated intestinal obstruction. Zollinger[2] relates this excessive mortality directly to four factors: (1) delay in diagnosis; (2) uncertain management after the diagnosis is made; (3) insufficient preoperative preparation; and (4) technical errors. With these factors in mind, this chapter addresses the pathophysiology of intestinal ischemia and gangrene in obstruction and outlines principles of diagnosis and treatment that may diminish operative mortality and morbidity.

Pathophysiology

Alterations of blood flow to intestine during the obstructed state may result from two mechanisms (Table I). Strangulation and gangrene result when blood flow to the intestine is impaired. This may be the consequence of mechanical obstruction, a closed loop obstruction or external hernia. Impairment of intestinal blood flow may also occur in simple distention.

Strangulation

Obstructed bowel becomes distended initially with air and intestinal secretions that are no longer absorbed. Intestinal secretions may amount to 8 to 10 liters daily, up to three times the total plasma volume. Secretion of water and electrolytes in addition to failure of reabsorption exacerbates the situation. Progressive distention leads to ve-

Table I

Pathophysiology of Intestinal Ischemia in Bowel Obstruction

INTESTINAL OBSTRUCTION

↙ ↘

Distention Strangulation

↘ ↙

Venous Congestion

↓

Hypovolemia ⇐⇒ ↓BLOOD FLOW ← Vascular Disease

↓ C.O.
Shock
↑ Viscosity

Shunting of blood to serosa
Capillary thrombosis and rupture
Hemorrhagic infarction
Transmural necrosis and gangrene
Perforation

Vascular Disease
Digoxin

nous congestion. As intraluminal pressure exceeds venous pressure within the obstructed segment of bowel, there is venous engorgement and an increase in venous pressure with increasing interstitial pressure that leads to capillary rupture and hemorrhagic infiltration of the submucosa-mucosa and eventually all layers of the bowel. Thrombosis of the intramural and eventually the mesenteric veins secondary to stasis hastens the congestion and results in localized ischemia. Necrosis eventually occurs, and the necrotic segment eventually perforates.

The time course of the natural history of strangulation varies and probably depends on many interrelated factors that affect blood flow to the areas of the bowel involved. These are decreased cardiac output, changes in vascular resistance, effects of local and systemic vasoconstrictors, influence of hypovolemia, hemoconcentration with increased viscosity, effects of bacterial toxins that enter the ischemic wall and may lead to further thrombosis, and the effects of medical intervention such as the use of vasopressors to maintain blood pressure in a hypotensive patient. All of these factors must be considered in the progression of potentially reversible ischemia to strangulation and gangrene. It is pertinent that following the relief of obstruction and the return of normal blood flow, there may be propagation of the intramural thrombus which may produce delayed infarction, so that perforation may occur hours or days later. In addition, a strangulated loop of bowel that is released before actual perforation has taken place may subsequently fibrose, resulting in stricture and bowel obstruction.

Altered Blood Flow in Simple Distention

Even in the absence of strangulation, ischemic changes may progress to full-thickness ischemia and perforation as a result of the pressure necrosis and vascular disturbances secondary to distention alone. Pressure necrosis may occur at any site where a tight band crosses the bowel, such as an incarcerated inguinal hernia or a foreign body or impacted feces producing mucosal ulceration. In these instances, the pressure necrosis and injury to the bowel seem to be a local phenomenon. However, it has been demonstrated by numerous experiences in the laboratory and by clinical observations that progressive vascular disturbances occur throughout the distended bowel. As long ago as 1907, Van Zwalenburg[3] observed interruption of capillary flow and complete circulatory standstill in distended bowel wall. This was confirmed later by Van Buren,[4] who noted the susceptibility of the mesenteric border of the bowel wall, and later, in the 1940s, by Oppenheimer.[5] Noer and colleagues[6] noted progressive circulatory disturbances brought about by increasing distention and demonstrated that irreversible intravascular agglutination occurs under high pressure distention.

Sperling and colleagues[7] studied the degree of pressure elevation in small bowel obstruction, noting that pressure in the small bowel ranged from 4 to 18 cm H_2O in the obstructed state and rose to 20 to 30 cm H_2O during peristalsis. In the colon, pressures range from 12 to 52 cm H_2O. In both small and large bowel, Boley et al.[8] noted increases over 30 mm Hg in intraluminal pressure resulted in stepwise decreases in total intestinal blood flow until an irreducible level of 20 to 25% was reached. This level of intestinal blood flow was maintained even at pressures as high as 210 mm Hg.

It was further noted that arteriovenous shunting occurred during intestinal obstruction.[8] This was evidenced by decreased oxygen extraction with decreasing blood flow. The authors hypothesized that blood is shunted away from the mucosa and muscularis propria with preferential filling of the submucosal and serosal arteries. This shunting of highly oxygenated blood from the inner bowel layers to the serosa is reflected in the frequent clinical observation of normal external appearance of bowel masking extensive mucosal infarction. Also, this supports the clinical impression of the unreliability of bowel appearance in determining intestinal viability that is discussed in other chapters of this textbook.

In later work, Tunick along with Boley[4] demonstrated that intermittent increases in intraluminal pressure significantly reduce blood flow not only to the local distended segment, but to the entire small bowel, and this diminution in flow persisted for hours after the relief of the obstruction or distention.

In summary, then, intestinal ischemia during obstruction can result in infarcted bowel just from simple distention alone. Its effect is observed not only in areas near the point of obstruction where one would expect the maximum amount of intraluminal pressure, but also in distant areas. Therefore, ischemia, gangrene, and perforation of intestine can occur at sites distant to the point of obstruction. Strangulation develops when the circulation to the obstructed bowel becomes impaired. A special case is the closed loop obstruction that occurs when a segment of bowel is affected at two points along its length.

Clinical Prediction of Intestinal Viability During Obstruction

Regardless of the etiology of obstruction, the suspicion of nonviable bowel mandates surgical intervention. Many investigators have discussed the clinical signs of strangulation and have emphasized features that suggest its diagnosis.[10–13] These are shown in Table II. It should be noted that there is general agreement about the lack of correlation between the presence of any one of these "classic" features and the presence of strangulated bowel. Silen[1] noted that strangulation is easily recognized in the presence of severe pain, tachycardia, fever, tenderness, rigidity, pal-

Table II

Clinical Indicators of Gangrenous Intestine in Obstruction

Abdominal tenderness	Guarding
Tachycardia	Palpable mass (incarcerated hernia)
Leukocytosis	Shock
Severe constant pain (replaces cramps)	Hypothermia
	Bloody diarrhea
Fever	

pable mass, and leukocytosis. However, only a few patients will have all or a majority of these pathognomonic signs. In addition, many patients with simple nonstrangulated obstruction may manifest one or more of these pathognomonic signs as well. The differentiation between simple and strangulating obstruction is often difficult and sometimes impossible. In Silen's series,[1] 37% of patients with strangulated obstruction were judged to have some condition other than intestinal obstruction. This is in contrast to the opinion of Stewardson and colleagues,[14] who noted that in the absence of all classic signs, no patient had gangrenous bowel. They felt that a delayed operation was reasonably safe in patients who showed neither leukocytosis, fever, tachycardia, or localized tenderness. The weight of information in the literature supports early operative intervention in all patients with intestinal obstruction after reasonable delay for fluid resuscitation.

X-ray criteria for obstruction with gangrene include air within the bowel wall, edema and thickening of the valvulae convinentes, and excessive peritoneal fluid. These findings are rarely present in all or even the majority of patients with strangulated obstruction, and if they are present may be quite subtle and perceived only in retrospect. One of the most serious errors in the diagnosis of strangulating obstruction is the not infrequent occurrence of normal or nondiagnostic X-ray of the abdomen. The abdominal X-ray is often normal in the course of strangulation.[15] In closed loop obstruction air-fluid levels are seldom seen, since the bowel loop fills with blood and fluid. The presence of an isolated short and dilated loop may be the only finding. A normal roentgenogram of the abdomen in the presence of symptoms suggestive of obstruction should always raise the question of strangulation.

In summary, X-rays of the abdomen are of little help in making the diagnosis of strangulated obstruction. Most important is recognition that the absence of radiographic evidence of strangulated bowel must not delay surgical intervention.

Laboratory Studies of Intestinal Ischemia

Because of the difficulties in making the diagnosis of intestinal obstruction with strangulation on the basis of clinical findings and X-ray evidence, various other tests are used to aid the physician preoperatively.

Peritoneal tap, using a fine-gauge needle, may be valuable in perplexing cases.[16] Intestinal infarction is suggested by finding of fluid that is reddish brown, has a fetid odor, has gram-negative rods on gram stain, or shows an increased amylase level, usually over 1000 units. In patients with distended bowel, this is a risky procedure and should be used with discretion in order to avoid iatrogenic bowel perforation and peritoneal contamination.

Various serum and laboratory tests to predict intestinal viability have been suggested. Amylase elevation has been suggested to indicate intestinal necrosis. This finding is nonspecific. Hyperamylasemia may occur from a variety of causes and in particular may result from simple obstruction alone. A large base deficit and lactic acidosis with a fall in serum bicarbonate concentration may be observed in cases of intestinal ischemia. In work by Brooks and

Carey,[17] this was clearly demonstrated in superior mesenteric artery occlusion. This has been observed occasionally on a clinical basis in patients with strangulated obstruction; however, no experimental data have been generated to support these anecdotal cases. In addition, a rise in the small intestine alkaline phosphatase has been observed after acute mesenteric infarction, but whether or not this occurs with a localized intestinal obstruction such as a closed loop or strangulated obstruction has not been well documented.[18]

Most recently, Jamieson and co-workers[18,19] studied the value of serum, urine, and peritoneal phosphate levels in the diagnosis of intestinal infarction. They found that inorganic phosphate levels were significantly elevated in animals with ligated superior mesenteric arteries. In a review of seven patients with massive intestinal infarction who had phosphate determinations, the phosphate levels were uniformly elevated above normal values. Jamieson also found elevated peritoneal fluid phosphate levels in experimental animals. He, however, noted that with venous ligation, the degree of hyperphosphatemia was less. Lores and colleagues[21] demonstrated that serum phosphate levels were reliable indicators of *irreversible* massive intestinal ischemia after four hours. Therefore, measurement of serum phosphate does not seem to aid in the early recognition of strangulation or of intestinal necrosis, but rather may reflect irreversible ischemic damage.

The use of serum phosphate and peritoneal phosphate measurements in the diagnosis of intestinal ischemia in the presence of bowel obstruction has not been tested clinically or experimentally. Jamieson noted, however, that if only a small area of intestine is necrotic, the peripheral vein phosphate levels did not rise. Therefore, it can be surmised that serum phosphate levels may not rise in strangulated obstruction, as short segments of bowel are usually involved and as there is usually venous obstruction.

In summation, although the clinical signs, radiographic

findings, and biochemical indicators of strangulation must be sought, there is no infallible method of detecting intestinal gangrene preoperatively.

Operative Management of Strangulated Intestinal Obstruction

Initial management should consist of fluid and electrolyte replacement with central venous pressure monitoring, establishment of adequate urine output (1 cc/kg/hour), intestinal decompression with the use of a nasogastric tube preferably of the sump type, restoration of blood volume, and administration of parenteral antibiotics. Parenteral antibiotics are given as prophylaxis against contamination of the peritoneal cavity and are not to be considered a substitute for resection of gangrenous intestine. Although this point seems self-evident, it should be emphasized that symptoms and findings usually improve with the use of these measures, even in the patient with gangrenous intestine.

The timing of operation depends on three factors: (1) the duration of obstruction which affects the severity of fluid and electrolyte and acid-base abnormalities and hence dictates the time needed for fluid resuscitation: (2) the cardiovascular stability and concomitant medical problems of the patient; and (3) consideration of the risk of strangulation. As previously stated, since there is no reliable way to predict intestinal gangrene preoperatively, operation should be performed as soon as reasonable in patients with complete bowel obstruction.

Operative Management

Endotracheal anesthesia should be used in all patients with intestinal obstruction in order to prevent massive tracheobronchial aspiration of feculent vomitus, regardless of the competence of the anesthesiologist and surgeon. In the absence of external hernia, exploration is carried out through a midline incision. The obstructive point is identified and the obstruction relieved.

Once the obstruction is released, it is often difficult to determine intestinal viability. Although the ability of the ischemic, traumatized bowel to resume its normal appearance and characteristics is indeed remarkable, this may take a considerable length of time. Inordinately long periods of examination and evaluation should be avoided in deciding whether a segment of bowel should be resected. After relieving the obstruction, warm, moist packs should be applied to the bowel and after 10 minutes, viability should be assessed. Clinical indicators of viability include return to a pink color, return of mesenteric pulsations, a bright, glistening surface, intact serosal surface without damage, and active peristalsis. Bowel of questionable status may be further improved by the injection of lidocaine into the root of the mesentery. This theoretically produces a transient local sympathectomy and increased blood flow.

Clinical indicators of intestinal viability in the operating room have been shown to be unreliable. This has led to the development of various noninvasive methods for determining the adequacy of blood flow to the intestine. Wright et al.[22] and Cooperman et al.[23] have demonstrated the accuracy of determining intestinal viability with Doppler ultrasound. Others have demonstrated the superiority of fluorescent indicators over standard clinical criteria in determining intestinal viability.[24–26] This technique involves illumination of questionable bowel with a high intensity ultraviolet lamp (360 to 400 angstrom units) after the intravenous injection of a nontoxic dose of fluorescein (15 mg/kg). These two techniques are roughly comparable in assessing intestinal blood flow. It has been our experience that fluorescence of the bowel and the segment in question may appear before Doppler pulsations come back, but both techniques are accurate.

These techniques do require the availability of special equipment in the operating room, and in some hospitals this may not be possible. However, only limited experience is required to become adept at either approach.

If either of the above methods demonstrate nonviable bowel, it should be resected and an end-to-end anastomosis performed if the small bowel is involved, and standard principles of colon surgery applied if the large colon is affected. If there is reasonable doubt of the bowel's viability without the application of either test, it should be resected in order to avoid the possibility of leaving nonviable intestine within the abdomen.

Management of Strangulated External Hernia

General Considerations

A subtype of strangulated intestinal obstruction is the hernia with gangrenous contents. Strangulation occurs when the blood supply of the hernia contents is impaired at the neck of the sac. The mortality of strangulated hernia ranges from 14 to 15% for inguinal and femoral hernias to 42% for umbilical hernias. Hernia may be classified as extraabdominal and intraabdominal as shown in Table III.

Vascular impairment of the hernia contents should be suspected in the presence of a tense, tender mass at the hernia site, or the development of intestinal obstruction. These signs may vary with the trapped viscus.

Differential Diagnosis

The two most common errors leading to misdiagnosis and delayed operation in the patient who does have necrotic hernia contents are (1) assuming that such a hernia is not strangulated because symptoms are not acute, and (2) over-

Table III

Classification of Hernias Causing Strangulation

Extraabdominal
Inguinal
Femoral
Umbilical
Incisional
Diaphragmatic
Special hernias (Obturator, Richter's, Littre's)
Intraabdominal
Congenital
Acquired
Operative defects
Pelvic floor

looking a small hernia deeply imbedded in the abdominal fat.

A strangulated inguinal hernia must be differentiated from an incarcerated inguinal hernia, enlarged inguinal lymph nodes, hydrocele of the cord, torsion of the testis, and thrombosis of the pampiniform plexus. A strangulated femoral hernia may be confused with inflamed inguinal nodes, thrombosis of a saphenous varicosity, a localized neoplasm, or a psoas abscess pointing inferior to the inguinal ligament. Acute incarceration and subsequent strangulation occur most frequently with femoral hernia.

A strangulated obturator hernia should be suspected in a patient with signs and symptoms of intestinal obstruction complaining of pain on the medial aspect of the thigh, corresponding to the sensory distribution of the obturator nerve (Howship-Romberg sign). In the female, the diagnosis may be confirmed by a vaginal examination demonstrating a firm mass high in the lateral wall of the pelvis. In the male, no mass is accessible to the examining finger. In each type of hernia the major decision affecting therapy is the differentiation between an incarcerated hernia and one that is strangulated and contains gangrenous bowel.

Treatment

In the surgical community there is disagreement about the initial management of incarcerated and possibly strangulated inguinal hernia. There are two points of view. First, some contend that all patients with incarcerated hernias should undergo emergency operation because of the uncertain viability of the bowel. Others, however, believe that an attempt should be made to reduce the incarcerated hernia by taxis.

Reasons for not attempting nonoperative hernia reduction in the adult have been summarized by Kauffman[27]: (1) difficulty in detecting a strangulated hernia, (2) reduction of gangrenous bowel with an attendant increased morbidity and mortality, (3) reduction en masse, and (4) trauma to the intestine during taxis. Although each is a valid argument against nonoperative reduction, each can be contested.

Several authors have noted that strangulated intestine can usually be differentiated from simple hernia incarceration. In fact, in Kauffman's series of strangulated hernias, all were diagnosed correctly preoperatively and all errors in diagnosis were made in the opposite direction, that is, diagnosis of strangulated bowel was made in a patient with an uncomplicated incarceration. However, as in the case of intestinal obstruction, the clinical and laboratory studies suggesting gangrenous bowel are not uniformly reliable.

Although a rare occurrence, reduction of gangrenous bowel would be expected to lead to increased mortality. This is supported in the literature. The mortality of reducing nonviable bowel ranges from 0 to 4%. Interestingly, the mortality of emergency surgery in a patient with viable bowel with an incarcerated hernia ranges from 8 to 11%.

Deaths were attributed to emergency operations in poorly prepared patients with uncorrected and severe cardiac and pulmonary problems. The greater operative mortality in patients with viable bowel than in those with nonviable bowel reflects the risk of operating upon all patients with incarcerated hernia without an attempt at nonoperative reduction.

Reduction en masse of groin hernia is defined as displacement of the hernia sac and contents to the properitoneal position without relief of the incarceration or strangulation.[28] The incidence is 1 in 13,000 groin hernias; 95% of cases result from attempts at reduction. In 5% of cases, the reduction is spontaneous. Reduction en masse is suspected when symptoms of intestinal obstruction and intestinal necrosis continue after a hernia is apparently reduced. It is certainly a rare occurrence and must be considered when manipulating a hernia; however, it should not be a major reason to avoid nonoperative hernia reduction.

The final objection to hernia reduction is potential injury to the bowel. There are no supporting data regarding intestinal rupture as a complication of inguinal hernia reduction.

Attempts at hernia reduction should be made when the contents of the hernia are thought to be viable.[29] Approximately one quarter of hernias can be reduced without the use of relaxants. The use of barbiturates, narcotics, and/or muscle relaxants doubles the number of successful reductions. Hernia reduction permits delayed and elective surgery which is particularly important in the poor-risk patient. If the hernia cannot be reduced or if gangrenous intestine is suspected, emergency operative intervention is indicated.

If strangulated obstruction is suspected, several principles should be respected. First, the incision is made directly over the hernia sac and should be ample, affording easy access to the hernia and its contents. The sac should be opened, and its contents grasped by the assistant to avoid their retraction into the abdomen. The constricting band should then be divided. If at this point, the contents are lost into the peritoneal cavity or if adequate exposure is not possible, an incision in the midline is necessary. If the bowel has been inadvertently reduced to the peritoneal cavity, the hernia should be repaired before making a second incision.

Bowel viability may be determined by the method described previously. However, the presence of gangrenous bowel is usually made obvious by the dark, odoriferous, hemorrhagic fluid within the sac. Bowel of questionable viability should be resected. A closed anastomosis is preferable. A Cooper's ligament repair should be done in inguinal and femoral hernias.

The resection of gangrenous bowel must be adequate.[30] The bowel distal and proximal to the area of strangulation must be examined carefully. Although it is rare, gangrene has occurred in a segment of bowel within the abdomen. This has been termed retrograde strangulation and may occur as the result of two mechanisms. Extension of a thrombotic process from clotted vessels within the herniated mesentery may lead to necrosis of a proximal or distal segment of intestine. Alternatively, proximal and distal segments of a hernia may become infolded, forming a "W" with infarction of the infolded portion. This is termed a "W" or Maydl's hernia.

Contamination of the peritoneal cavity and subcutaneous tissues should be prevented. Dennis and Varco[30] suggested a method of excising strangulated femoral hernia that reduces spillage of fluid. The technique involves en bloc removal of the sac and contents, so that the fibrous neck at the ring is removed intact and not divided, and the involved loops of bowel and hernia sac are clamped and removed without opening the sac.

In cases of a suspected reduction en masse[28] and in strangulated obturator hernias,[31] the abdominal approach is the preferred method of treatment.

Summary

The morbidity and mortality of strangulation occurring either in the course of intestinal obstruction from adhesions or from external herniation greatly exceed that of simple obstruction without vascular compromise of the intestine or hernial contents. For this reason, early diagnosis of strangulation is imperative. Unfortunately, the reliability of clinical signs, physical examination, radiologic signs, and biochemical indicators of intestinal viability in these situations is poor. Therefore, operative intervention should be undertaken as soon as feasible in all patients with suspected complete bowel obstruction and in those with tender, irreducible, and incarcerated external hernias. At the time of operation, clinical indicators of intestinal viability are often not accurate. Doppler ultrasound and fluorescence of the bowel after an injection of intravenous fluorescein have been used to facilitate the determination of intestinal blood flow. It should be pointed out that excessive time spent trying to assess intestinal viability may be deleterious to the patient, and therefore any segments of questionable viability should be resected without undue delay.

References

1. Silen WK, Hein MF, Goldman L: Strangulation obstruction of the small intestine. *Arch Surg* 85:137, 1962.
2. Zollinger RM, Kinsey DC: Diagnosis and management of intestinal obstruction. *Am Surg* 30:1, 1964.
3. Van Zwalenburg C: Strangulation resulting from distention of hollow viscus. *Ann Surg* 46:780, 1907.
4. Van Buren FT: The mechanism of intestinal perforation due to distention. *Ann Surg* 83:69, 1926.
5. Oppenheimer MJ, Mann FC: Intestinal capillary circulation during distention. *Surgery* 13:548, 1943.
6. Noer RJ, Derr JW: Effect of distention on intestinal revascularization. *Arch Surg* 63:520, 1951.

7. Sperling L, Paine JR, Wangensteen OH: Intra-enteric pressure in experimental and clinical intestinal obstruction. *Proc Soc Exp Biol Med* 32:1504, 1935.
8. Boley SJ, Agrawal GP, Warren AR, et al.: Pathophysiologic effects of bowel distention on intestinal blood flow. *Am J Surg* 117:228, 1969.
9. Tunick PA, Treiber WF, Frank M, Veith FJ, Glierdeman ML, Boley SJ: Pathophysiologic effects of bowel distention on intestinal blood flow II. *Curr Topics Surg Res* 2:59, 1970.
10. Davis SS, Sperling L: Obstruction of the small intestine. *Arch Surg* 99:424, 1969.
11. Greene WW: Bowel obstruction in the aged patient. *Am J Surg* 118:541, 1969.
12. Leffall LD, Syphox B: Clinical aids in strangulated intestinal obstruction. *Am J Surg* 120:756, 1970.
13. Snyder EN, McCranie D: Closed loop obstruction of the small bowel. *Am J Surg* 111:398, 1966.
14. Stewardson RH, Bombeck CT, Nyhus LM: Critical operative management of small bowel obstruction. *Ann Surg* 187:189, 1978.
15. Gough IR: Strangulating adhesive small bowel obstruction with normal radiographs. *Br J Surg* 65:431, 1978.
16. Gray EB Jr, Amador LS: Acute mesenteric venous thrombosis simulating acute pancreatitis. Value of peritoneal fluid analysis. *JAMA* 167:1734, 1958.
17. Brooks DH, Carey LC: Base deficit in superior mesenteric artery occlusion as an aid to early diagnosis. *Amer Surg* 177:352, 1973.
18. Caldwell JH: Small intestinal choline phosphatase after acute mesenteric infarction. (Abstr) *Gastroenterology* 66:670, 1974.
19. Jamieson WE, Waul WJ, Durand D: Changes in serum phosphate levels associated with intestinal infarction and necrosis. *Surg Gynecol Obstet* 140:19, 1975.
20. Sarver B, Jamieson WG, Durand D: The significance of elevated peritoneal fluid phosphate level in intestinal infarction. *Surg Gynecol Obstet* 146:43, 1978.
21. Lores ME, Canizares O, Rosselle PJ: The significance of elevated serum phosphate levels in experimental intestinal ischemia. *Surg Gynecol Obstet* 152:593, 1980.

22. Wright CB, Hobson RW: Prediction of intestinal viability during Doppler ultrasound technics. *Am J Surg* 129:642, 1975.
23. Cooperman M, Pace WG, Martin EW Jr et al.: Determination of viability of ischemic intestine by Doppler ultrasound. *Surgery* 83:705, 1978.
24. Bulkley GB, Weaton CB, Strandberg JD, Zuidema GD: Assessment of small intestine recovery from ischemic injury after segmental arterial, venous, and arteriovenous occlusion. *Surg Forum* 30:210, 1979.
25. Bulkley GB, Zuidema GD, Hamilton SR et al.: Intraoperative determination of small intestine viability following ischemic injury: A prospective, controlled trial of two adjuvant methods, Doppler and fluorescein, compared to standard clinical judgement. *Ann Surg* 193:628, 1981.
26. Marfuggi RA, Greenspan M: Reliable intraoperative prediction of intestinal viability using a fluorescent indicator. *Surg Gynecol Obstet* 152:33, 1981.
27. Kauffman HM, O'Brien DP: Selective reduction of incarcerated inguinal hernia. *Am J Surg* 119:660, 1970.
28. Minges H, Olson JD: Reduction "en masse" of groin hernia. *Arch Surg* 90:764, 1965.
29. Rogers FA: Strangulated femoral hernia. A review of 170 cases. *Ann Surg* 149:9, 1959.
30. Dennis C, Varco RL: Femoral hernia with gangrenous bowel. *Surgery* 22:312, 1947.
31. Gray SW, Skondalakis JE, Soria RE, Rowe JS: Strangulated obturator hernia. *Surgery* 75:20, 1974.

15

Intestinal Volvulus

Marc Cooperman, M.D.

Volvulus is a torsion of the intestine and its mesentery that results in intestinal obstruction. A rotation of the bowel around its mesenteric axis of at least 180 degrees is required to produce a volvulus, although the degree of twisting is often much more severe.

Volvulus of the colon occurs most commonly, with volvulus of the small intestine being much less common, and volvulus of the stomach quite rare. Colonic volvulus involves the sigmoid colon most often, followed by the cecum and transverse colon. Volvulus of the colon has been reported to account for 3–5% of cases of intestinal obstruction in the United States and 10–13% of acute large bowel obstructions.[1] Colonic volvulus is more common in Scandinavia and Eastern Europe, where it causes 30–50% of intestinal obstructions,[2] and small bowel volvulus is encountered most commonly in Africa, Asia, and the Middle East.[3]

In order for a volvulus to occur, the bowel must be mobile and have a fixed point about which to twist. Other factors implicated in the development of chronic volvulus include colonic distension by feces, pregnancy, adhesions from previous operations, and congenital abnormalities.[4]

The clinical picture is initially dominated by signs and symptoms of intestinal obstruction until gangrene develops, with resultant peritonitis and sepsis. Plain radiographs of the abdomen are often helpful, but frequently barium enema examination is required to confirm the diagnosis.

Successful management depends on prompt diagnosis and treatment before intestinal infarction occurs. Mortality from colonic volvulus increases dramatically once gangrene has developed. In a recent series of 81 cases of colonic volvulus, Kerry reported 13 deaths, accounting for 16% mortality; however, mortality was 75% in those with gangrene.[5] In a collected series of volvulus of the sigmoid colon, Webster reports an average mortality rate of 12.5% if the bowel is viable, compared to a 49.2% mortality with nonviable bowel.[1]

Cecal Volvulus

Initially described by Rokitansky in 1837,[6] cecal volvulus has become a well recognized clinical entity. It is responsible for 25–40% of colonic volvulus and 1% of intestinal obstructions.[7] In a sense, the term, cecal volvulus, is a misnomer as the terminal ileum and ascending colon are also involved in the torsion. For reasons that are not understood, this condition is encountered more commonly in Eastern Europe and Scandinavia than in the United States.[8] The diagnosis must be made rapidly to avoid infarction with perforation and peritonitis.

Etiology

In order for cecal volvulus to occur, abnormal mobility of the cecum must be present. This results from failure of fusion of the ascending colon and cecum with the posterior parietal peritoneum. Autopsy studies have shown sufficient mobility of the cecum for volvulus to occur in 11.2% of adults.[9] There must also be a fixed point around which the bowel may twist. Frequently, adhesions from prior surgery serve as the fulcrum for the torsion. In cecal volvulus, the twist is usually clockwise in direction. Less common than the axial twist is the cecal bascule, in which the cecum folds anteriorly on to the ascending colon, producing obstruction at the transverse fold. Cecal bascules may account for 10% of cases of cecal volvulus.[10]

Certain conditions have been clearly associated with the development of cecal volvulus. These include previous abdominal operations, pregnancy, distal colonic obstruction, and increased peristalsis. Previous operations have been reported in up to 83% of patients developing cecal volvulus.[11] Pregnancy may precipitate cecal volvulus by displacing the abnormally mobile cecum from its normal position in the right lower quadrant. The incidence of distal obstructing lesions of the colon in patients with cecal volvulus varies from 0–50% in reported series.[8,12–14] Ritvo et al. report significant colonic lesions distal to the volvulus in 6 of 12 cases,[13] and Kippaehne et al. found distal obstructing lesions in 8 of 22 patients.[14] The incidence of distal lesions is high enough to warrant radiologic examination of the distal colon in all patients with cecal volvulus.

Clinical Presentation

The majority of patients exhibit signs and symptoms of small bowel obstruction. Cramping abdominal pain is invariably the primary complaint. Abdominal distension and nausea and vomiting will be present in approximately 50% of patients. The abdomen is frequently mildly distended and tender. Bowel sounds are often hyperactive.

The clinical presentation is more fulminant if gangrene is present. The picture is dominated by sepsis, and shock may be present. Abdominal examination discloses the findings of peritonitis with rigidity, rebound, and absent bowel sounds. The incidence of gangrene reported varies from 8–65%, but approximates 30% in most series.[8,12,14–16]

Uncommonly, cecal volvulus may be a chronic recurrent problem. Patients have intermittent abdominal distension and cramping abdominal pain that resolves spontaneously. Such patients represent only a small minority of those with cecal volvulus. Grover et al. report only one patient with chronic recurrent volvulus among 13 patients with cecal volvulus treated over a five-year period,[17] and O'Mara et al. report chronic recurrent symptoms in 9 of 50 patients.[10]

Diagnosis

Physical examination is generally not diagnostic, and findings are usually those of small intestinal obstruction. Diffuse moderate abdominal tenderness is the most common finding, followed by abdominal distension and either hyperactive or absent bowel sounds. An abdominal mass may be palpable in approximately 20% of patients.[10]

Plain radiographs of the abdomen are abnormal in almost all patients, but rarely are diagnostic. O'Mara et al. report abnormal abdominal radiographs in 38 of 40 patients with acute cecal volvulus.[10] However, the diagnosis of cecal volvulus was made in only 2 patients. Abnormal findings included small bowel dilatation in 12, proximal colon dilatation in 11, and dilatation of both small bowel and proximal colon in 15.

The finding of a greatly dilated cecum containing an air-fluid level which is located in the epigastrium or left upper quadrant should strongly suggest the diagnosis of cecal volvulus.[18] The other classical findings of distended small bowel loops with air-fluid levels and absence of colonic gas are nonspecific and may be found in cases of small bowel obstruction from a variety of causes.

Barium enema should be performed in all patients in

whom the diagnosis of cecal volvulus is suspected. Classically, the barium column will stop in a tapered, beaklike fashion, at the site of the torsion. A small amount of barium may pass through the twist and enter the markedly dilated cecum.[18] O'Mara reports that barium enema was diagnostic in 69% of the patients who underwent the procedure (Figures 1 and 2).[10]

Treatment

The treatment for cecal volvulus is prompt operation to avoid the sequelae of gangrene and perforation. If the bowel has suffered irreversible ischemia, all nonviable bowel must be resected. In the majority of cases, primary reanastomosis will be safe. However, if perforation has occurred and frank peritonitis is present, then the safer course is to perform an ileostomy and mucous fistula, which may be closed at a later date. As discussed in Chapter VII, techniques to objectively determine bowel viability are available, and they should be employed rather than relying on clinical judgment alone.

In the absence of irreversibly ischemic bowel, the operative management of cecal volvulus is controversial. Advocated treatment ranges from simple detorsion to resection.

Resection of the right colon with iliocolostomy was first advocated by Melchior in 1949 to reduce the incidence of recurrent volvulus after two recurrences shortly following cecopexy.[19] Others have also reported recurrences after cecopexy and endorsed the use of resection to avoid this problem.[20–24] However, hemicolectomy on an emergency basis in the patient with unprepared bowel is a major operative procedure associated with significant morbidity. O'Mara reports postoperative complications in 43% of those treated by resection.[10] In the absence of a high recurrence rate following fixation procedures alone, it is difficult to justify hemicolectomy in the absence of nonviable bowel.

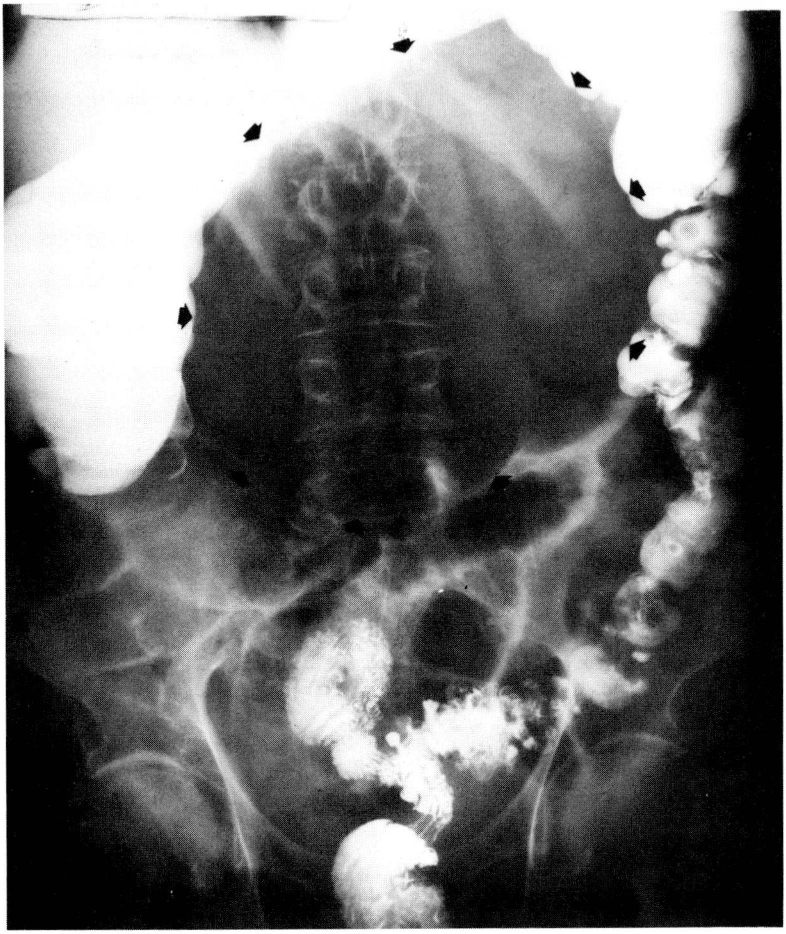

Figure 1. Barium enema in a patient with cecal volvulus. Barium does not enter the hugely dilated cecum located in the left upper quadrant. The cecum is outlined by arrows.

In the absence of gangrenous bowel, cecopexy is the treatment of choice for cecal volvulus. After the bowel is untwisted, the abnormally mobile cecum and right colon are sutured to the lateral peritoneum with interrupted nonabsorbable sutures. The use of a lateral peritoneal flap to ensure adequate fixation has been advocated,[25] but this

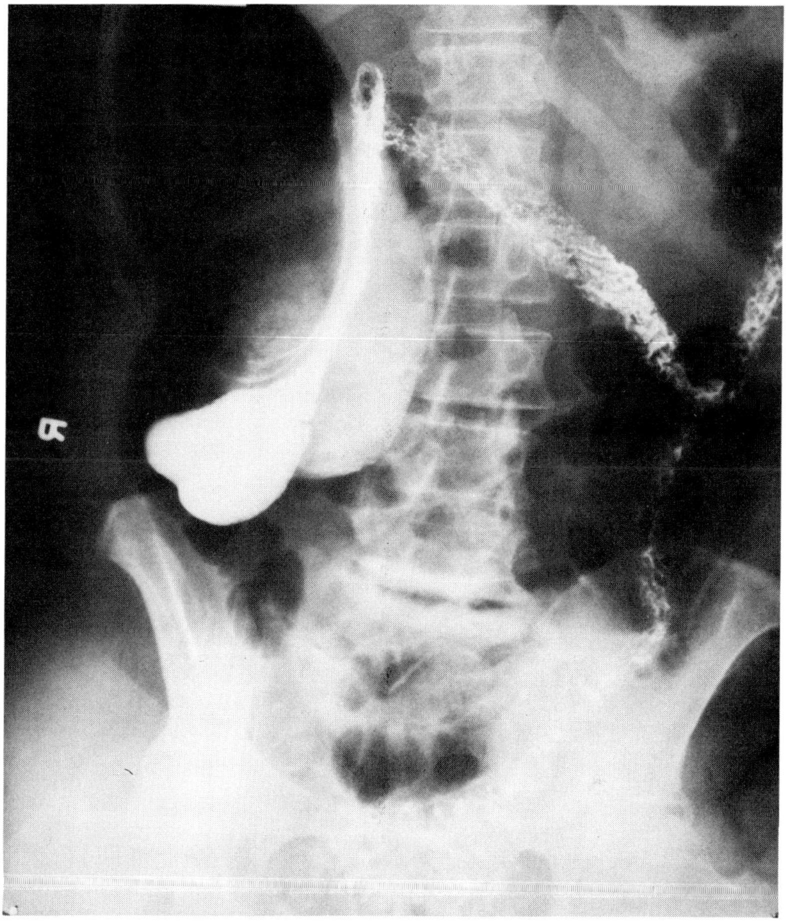

Figure 2. Barium enema in a patient with cecal bascule. The cecum is folded into the right upper quadrant and does not fill with barium.

technique has not been widely employed. Most surgeons report good results with cecopexy. In a collected series, Anderson et al. report a recurrence rate of less than 5%.[8]

Tube cecostomy has also been advocated as a means of assuring adequate fixation of the cecum. Todd reports no recurrences with the use of this technique.[26] However, cecostomy has the inherent disadvantage of opening the bowel with the attendant increased risk of complications. An increased incidence of wound infection as well as abdominal wall sepsis and persistent fecal fistula have been reported after cecostomy.[10]

Results

The mortality of cecal volvulus depends largely on whether or not gangrenous bowel is present. O'Mara et al. report a mortality rate of 33% if nonviable bowel is present, compared to 7% in the absence of gangrenous bowel.[10] In a collected series of 151 patients, Todd reports an overall mortality of 22.5%.[26] The mortality was 41.4% in those with gangrene and 14.5% in those without gangrene.

Volvulus of the Transverse Colon

Volvulus of the transverse colon is extremely rare, with fewer than 70 cases having been reported in the English literature.[27] Volvulus of the transverse colon accounts for less than 4% of cases of colonic volvulus[28] and occurs more commonly in women by a two to one margin. The mean age of patients is slightly less than 50 years.[27]

Etiology

The rarity of this entity is due to the normal anatomy of the transverse colon. The mesentery is quite short and the colon is relatively fixed at the hepatic and splenic flexures. In patients with volvulus of the transverse colon, the following anatomic defects have been reported: an abnormally long transverse mesocolon; absence of the mesentery with abnormally mobile bowel; and close approximation of the points of fixation at the flexures, allowing torsion to occur.[28] The most common precipitating cause of transverse colon volvulus is distal colon obstruction.[29] Hirschsprung's disease, strictures, carcinoma of the colon, and adhesions have been reported as causes of the distal obstruction. Chronic constipation, mental retardation, and laxative abuse have also been implicated.[28]

Clinical Presentation

The signs and symptoms of volvulus of the transverse colon are those of acute intestinal obstruction. Cramping abdominal pain is usually severe and sudden in onset. Abdominal distension and vomiting are often present. Bowel sounds may be hyperactive and obstructive in character, or decreased. Signs of peritonitis may be present if gangrene or perforation has occurred.

Diagnosis

Plain abdominal x-rays may suggest the diagnosis by demonstrating a double closed loop. Air-fluid levels will be present in the twisted transverse colon, as well as the ascending colon if the ileocecal valve is competent. Air-fluid levels in the small intestine may be present as well. Gas is usually absent in the colon distal to the volvulus. Barium enema will demonstrate obstruction at the site of the volvulus and will occasionally show breaking at the site of the twist.

Treatment

The treatment of volvulus of the transverse colon is prompt surgical exploration. If gangrenous bowel is present it must be resected and either a primary anastomosis or colostomy and mucous fistula performed. The former has the advantage of requiring only one operative procedure but exposes the patient to the risks attendant to the anastomosis of unprepared colon. On the other hand, if a colostomy and mucous fistula is performed, a second operative procedure will be required to reestablish intestinal continuity. The safer course in the presence of gangrenous bowel is to avoid an anastomosis and perform a temporary colostomy and mucous fistula.

If the bowel is viable after the torsion has been corrected, resection is still the preferred method of treatment. Colopexy for volvulus of the transverse colon is followed by a high recurrence rate and therefore is inadvisable. Anderson et al. report recurrence in 3 of 4 patients in whom the volvulus was not resected.[27] Successful detorsion of a volvulus of the transverse colon using the colonoscope has been reported.[30] However, this technique should be reserved for only patients with medical illnesses that make the risk of laparotomy prohibitive.

Results

Mortality of 15% was reported by Zinkin et al. in a collected series of 34 patients.[29] Recurrence is rare in patients treated by resection, but will be frequent if colopexy rather than resection is performed.

Sigmoid Volvulus

The sigmoid is the most common site of colonic volvulus. Sigmoid volvulus is the third most common cause of large bowel obstruction, exceeded only by carcinoma and diverticular disease. It has been reported to account for 3–5% of intestinal obstructions in the United States. Elsewhere, particularly in the Middle East, the incidence is even higher. In Edinburgh, Anderson identified 134 patients with sigmoid volvulus among 3387 patients admitted with acute intestinal obstruction. Sigmoid volvulus was present in 4% of cases of intestinal obstruction and in 69.4% of patients with colonic volvulus.[32]

Etiology

In contrast to cecal volvulus and volvulus of the transverse colon, which tend to occur in younger patients and twice as often in women, sigmoid volvulus is typically a disease of the elderly and shows no sexual predilection. In a study of 99 patients reported by Arnold and Nance, 54 patients were men and 45 women. The highest incidence occurred in the eighth decade; 53% were over 70 years of age.[33] Not surprisingly, other serious medical illnesses are often present in these elderly patients. Arnold and Nance reported a 70.4% incidence of serious cardiovascular and respiratory problems, with cardiovascular disease being most common.[33]

The occurrence of sigmoid volvulus in patients with psychiatric disorders has been well documented. String and DeCosse report that psychiatric disease was present in 48% of patients,[34] and the incidence has been cited as being as high as 75% by others.[33] It is thought that chronic constipation is an important factor in the development of sigmoid volvulus, explaining the high frequency in psychiatric and nursing home patients.

Anatomically, the sigmoid colon and mesocolon are markedly elongated. The base of the mesentery is narrowed, with two closely spaced points of fixation, making it easy for twisting to occur. Scarring at the base of the mesentery from previous episodes of torsion, which serves to further narrow this area, may be present. The volvulus may occur with either clockwise or counterclockwise rotation of at least 180 degrees. If the ileocecal valve is competent, this will produce a second closed loop obstruction of the proximal colon as well.

Clinical Presentation

Delay from the onset of symptoms to diagnosis is common. Arnold reported an average duration of symptoms prior to admission of 5.2 days.[33] Significant delay on the part of the physician in instituting definitive treatment may occur also. In fact, String and DeCosse reported that patients admitted through the emergency room were more promptly and successfully treated than those who developed sigmoid volvulus during a hospital stay under physician observation for another problem.[34]

Cramping abdominal pain and abdominal distension are the two most common symptoms.[32] These are followed in frequency by constipation, nausea and vomiting, and diarrhea.

Abdominal distension is an almost uniform finding. Bowel sounds are abnormal in most patients and usually are hyperactive and obstructive in character. Absence of bowel sounds is the most reliable indicator of the presence of gangrenous bowel. Of 15 patients with absent bowel sounds in one series, gangrenous colon was present in 13.[32]

Diagnosis

Plain roentgenograms of the abdomen will suggest the diagnosis in the majority of patients (Figure 3). The diagnosis of sigmoid volvulus was made roentgenographically in 35% of patients in one series, with colonic obstruction being diagnosed in an additional 60%. In a review of 45 patients with sigmoid volvulus, Hines et al.[35] reported that the correct diagnosis could have been made from plain films alone in 42 patients. Typically, the sigmoid is hugely dilated, with the ends located in the left lower quadrant. Terms such as "bent inner tube," "ace of spades," and "bird beak" have been used to describe the appearance.

Barium enema will demonstrate the point of torsion (Figures 4 and 5). Barium may pass into the obstructed loop demonstrating the spiral where the twist occurs.

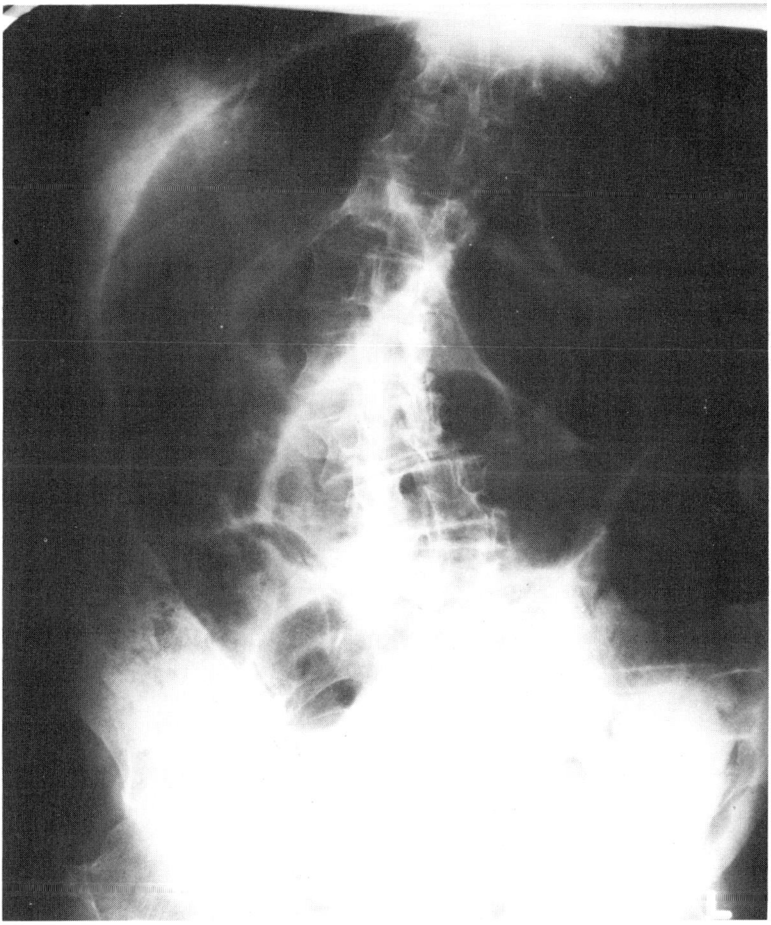

Figure 3. Sigmoid volvulus, plain film.

Treatment

Unless there is strong suspicion that gangrenous bowel is present or perforation has occurred, initial treatment should be directed at nonoperative decompression of the volvulus. Sigmoidoscopic decompression of sigmoid volvulus was first advocated by Bruusgard in 1947.[36] Numerous reports since then have documented the efficacy and safety

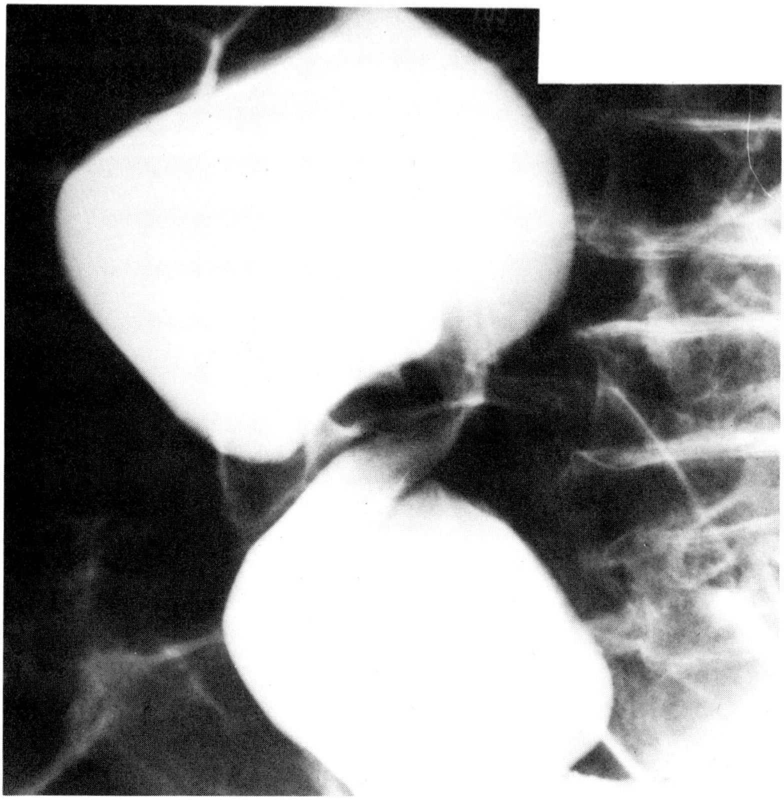

Figure 4. Sigmoid volvulus, barium enema demonstrating twist.

of this technique. For example, Arnold reported the success rate of sigmoidoscopic decompression to be 77% with only one perforation in 118 procedures.[33]

If nonoperative detorsion is unsuccessful, urgent operation is essential. Although the optimum operative procedure is controversial, there is general agreement that simple detorsion alone is insufficient due to the high rate of recurrence. The incidence of recurrent volvulus after operative detorsion has reported to range from 27–89%.[33,37,38] Resection of the volvulus with colostomy and mucous fistula with subsequent colostomy closure is the treatment of

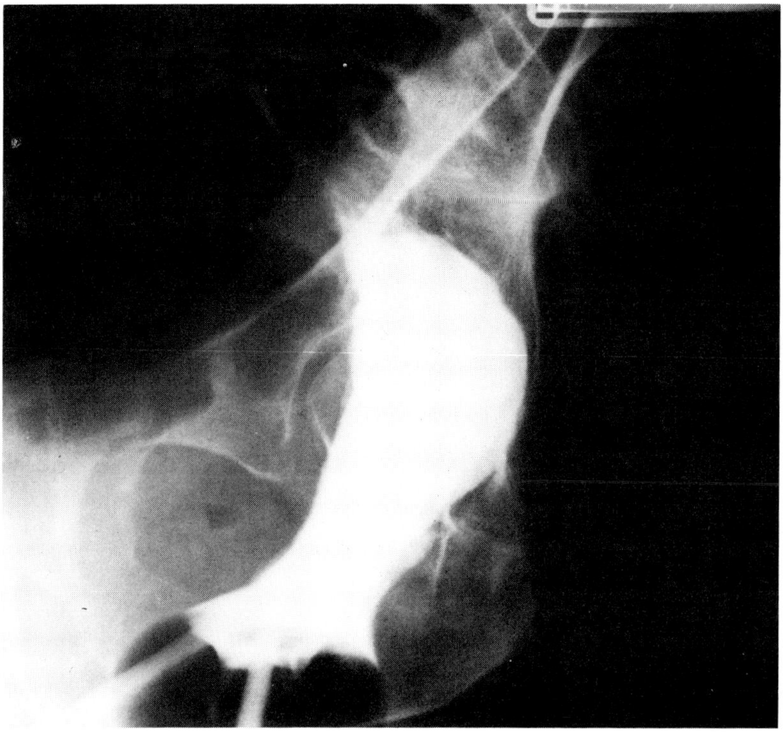

Figure 5. Sigmoid volvulus, barium enema demonstrating typical "bird's beak" appearance.

choice and is followed by a low recurrence rate and is safer than a one-stage procedure. Resection is always indicated in the presence of gangrenous bowel. Again, a two-stage procedure with creation of a temporary colostomy is the procedure of choice.

The management of the patient who has undergone unsuccessful nonoperative detorsion is controversial. In good risk patients, elective resection is advisable, as nonoperative detorsion has been shown to be followed by a high rate of recurrence. The mortality of the second episode has also been reported to be higher than that of the first. String and DeCosse report a recurrence rate of 28%, with a mortality rate in these patients of 43%.[34] Hines reported a mortality of 40% in patients with recurrent volvulus, compared to 22% in those with the first episode.[35]

However, the risk of recurrence must be weighed against the risk of elective resection. Arnold reports 15% mortality following elective resection.[33] In this series, although recurrent volvulus occurred in 55% of patients following detorsion, the mortality in those treated by detorsion alone was only 9.3%, less than the risk of elective resection. Clearly, the further treatment of patients in whom nonoperative detorsion is successful needs to be individualized. Elective resection may be prohibitively dangerous in the patient with significant associated medical diseases. However, younger good-risk patients should be strongly considered for elective resection.

Results

Gangrene occurs in approximately 10% of patients with sigmoid volvulus[32] and is associated with a high mortality. Sharpton reports a mortality of 50% in 10 patients with gangrenous colon treated by resection and colostomy.[39] Anderson reports 10 deaths in 13 patients with nonviable bowel.[32]

The mortality is less if gangrenous bowel is not present. Anderson reports 18 deaths in 121 patients with viable bowel for a mortality rate of 15%. String and DeCosse report an overall mortality rate of 28% in 25 patients. Factors associated with mortality were inordinate delay to diagnosis and treatment, severe associated medical diseases, and inappropriate treatment.[34]

Volvulus of the Small Intestine

The incidence of small bowel volvulus varies dramatically, depending upon whether the diagnosis is restricted to primary small bowel volvulus occurring in the absence of previous operations or one includes small bowel torsion secondary to adhesions from prior operations. If volvulus secondary to adhesions is included, then the small bowel is the most common site at which volvulus occurs. On the other hand, primary small bowel volvulus is extremely rare, particularly in the United States. (Strangulated intestinal obstruction is discussed in detail in Chapter XIV and small bowel volvulus in infancy is covered in Chapter VIII.) The following section is confined to primary small bowel volvulus in the adult.

Etiology

Primary volvulus of the small intestine is extremely rare in the United States and Western Europe and occurs most commonly in Africa, Asia, and the Middle East. Patients with this disease have been shown to consume a high-fiber, high-bulk diet and have elongated small bowel mesenteries facilitating torsion.[40] Sudden entrance of a large bulky meal into the jejunum is thought to drag the mobile jejunum into the left lower quadrant, initiating torsion.

Clinical Presentation

Small bowel volvulus should be suspected in the patient with signs and symptoms of acute small bowel obstruction who has not undergone previous operations. Cramping abdominal pain usually precedes the nausea, vomiting, and abdominal distension that are almost always present. Abdominal examination demonstrates moderate tenderness, distension, and abnormal bowel sounds. Bowel sounds are usually hyperactive and obstructive in character. The absence of bowel sounds should raise the suspicion that intestinal infarction has occurred.

If infarction or perforation has taken place in the twisted segment of bowel, physical examination may demonstrate the findings of peritonitis with diffuse tenderness, guarding, and rebound. The absence of peritoneal signs, however, does not disprove the presence of gangrenous bowel.

Diagnosis

Abdominal x-rays will demonstrate the presence of small bowel obstruction. Distended loops of small bowel with air-fluid levels will be present. A long air-fluid level may be seen in the twisted segment. Little or no gas will be present distal to the volvulus. Angiography performed in these patients when the diagnosis of superior mesenteric artery embolus or thrombosis is suspected may give the correct diagnosis by demonstrating the "barber pole" sign, with spiraling of the branches of the twisted superior mesenteric artery.[41]

Treatment

After rapid correction of fluid and electrolyte imbalances, prompt operation is mandatory. Often the diagnosis of volvulus is not made preoperatively and the patient is operated on with a preoperative diagnosis of either small bowel obstruction or intestinal infarction. The operative management depends on whether the involved bowel is judged to be viable after detorsion of the volvulus. Because long segments of small bowel are involved, it is important to preserve all viable intestine, and Doppler ultrasound or fluorescein dye injection may be used to confirm viability. If the bowel is viable, detorsion of the volvulus suffices. Nonviable bowel must be resected; remaining viable bowel may be reanastomosed primarily.

Results

The mortality of primary small bowel volvulus has been reported to range from 10–67%. In a series of 26 patients with primary small bowel volvulus reported by Duke and Yar,[40] 3 patients died, establishing the mortality rate at 11.6%. A low mortality rate in this series from an Afghanistanian hospital is due in part to a high preoperative index of suspicion of the diagnosis, leading to rapid resuscitation and surgical exploration. In Western countries, where the entity is much less common, an increased delay in diagnosis and operation may be expected to result in a higher incidence of intestinal infarction and increased morbidity and mortality.

Gastric Volvulus

Gastric volvulus is extremely rare and fewer than 300 cases have been reported.[44] Two types of gastric volvulus may occur. The more common is termed organo-axial, in which the twist occurs around the long axis of the stomach. The mesenterioaxial volvulus in which rotation occurs from right to left around the sagittal plane is less common. Either part or all of the stomach may be involved, and the volvulus may be chronic and intermittent in nature or acute. Even a rotation of 180 degrees is sufficient to produce gastric gangrene.

Etiology

Usually a predisposing cause for gastric volvulus can be identified. Abnormal laxity and elongation of the ligamentous attachments of the stomach at the pylorus and esophagus are often present. However, one of the following may be present as well: paraesophageal hiatal hernia; diaphragmatic hernia; eventration of the left hemidiaphragm; or pyloric or duodenal obstruction resulting in gastric distension. A heavy meal may be the precipitating event.[45]

Symptoms

Gastric volvulus may be a chronic intermittent phenomenon with symptoms suggestive of peptic ulcer disease. Dysphagia may result from distortion of the esophagogastric junction. Bloating during meals is common. Some patients have epigastric pain and vomiting after eating.

The clinical presentation of acute gastric volvulus is much more consistent and should allow for a prompt, correct diagnosis. As pointed out by Maingot,[44] the three typical findings are early vomiting followed by retching with inability to vomit, severe epigastric pain, and progressive epigastric distension and inability to pass a nasogastric tube into the stomach.

Treatment

The treatment of acute gastric volvulus is immediate surgical exploration to prevent the development of gangrene. If gangrene is present, a near-total or total gastrectomy will be required. In the absence of gangrene, the surgeon's goal must be to prevent future recurrence of the volvulus. Underlying causes such as paraesophageal or other types of diaphragmatic hernias must be repaired. The duodenum and pylorus should be carefully inspected for evidence of obstruction, which, if present, must be corrected.

Gastropexy to fix the stomach to the anterior abdominal wall should be performed, but this by itself may not be enough to prevent recurrent volvulus. Tanner has advocated a "colonic displacement" operation in which the gastrocolic omentum is completely divided, freeing the stomach from the colon.[45] The transverse colon is then free to rise into the subdiaphragmatic space without exerting traction on the greater curvature of the stomach. Tanner reported successful results in 12 of 14 patients treated by this procedure.

Results

The mortality of acute gastric volvulus has been cited by Maingot as 30–40%.[44]

References

1. Wertkin MG, Aufses AH, Jr: Management of volvulus of the colon. *Dis Col and Rect* 21:40, 1978.
2. Bruusgard C: Volvulus of the sigmoid colon and its treatment. *Surgery* 22:466, 1947.
3. Fink W, Cohen A, Greenstein AJ: Small bowel volvulus in association with recurrent Crohn's disease. *Am J Gastroenterol* 74:337, 1980.
4. Nemer FD, Hagihara PF, Mays ET, Griffen WO Jr: Volvulus of the colon—a continuing surgical problem. *Dis Col and Rect* 19:321, 1976.
5. Kerry RL, Ranson HK: Volvulus of the colon. *Arch Surg* 99:215, 1969.
6. Rokitansky C: Intestinal strangulation. *Arch Gen Med* 14:202, 1837.
7. O'Mara CS, Wilson TH Jr, Stonesifer GL, Cameron JL: Cecal volvulus: analysis of 50 patients with long-term follow-up. *Curr Surg* 37:132, 1980.
8. Andersson A, Bergdahl L, Ven Der Linden W: Volvulus of the cecum. *Ann Surg* 181:876, 1975.
9. Wolfer JA, Beaton LE, Anson BJ: Volvulus of the cecum. Anatomical factors in its etiology. Report of a case. *Surg Gynecol Obstet* 74:882, 1942.
10. O'Mara CS, Wilson TH, Stonesifer GL, Cameron JL: Cecal

volvulus, analysis of 50 patients with long-term follow-up. *Ann Surg* 189:724, 1979.
11. Dixon CV, Meyer AC: Volvulus of the cecum. *Surg Clin North Am* 28:953, 1948.
12. Smith WR, Goodwin JN: Cecal volvulus. *Am J Surg* 126:215, 1973.
13. Ritvo M, Farrell GE, Shauffer IA: The association of volvulus of the cecum and ascending colon with other obstructive colonic lesions. *Am J Roentgenol* 78:587, 1957.
14. Kippaehne WK, Vetto RM, Jenkins CC: Volvulus of the ascending colon: a report of 22 cases. *Am J Surg* 114:323, 1967.
15. Peterson HI: Volvulus of the cecum. *Ann Surg* 116:296, 1967.
16. Hinshaw DB, Carter R, Joergenson EJ: Volvulus of the cecum or right colon. *Am J Surg* 98:175, 1959.
17. Grover NK, Gulati SM, Tagore NK, Taneja OP: Volvulus of the cecum and ascending colon. *Am J Surg* 125:672, 1973.
18. Haskin PH, Teplick SK, Teplick JG, Haskin ME: Volvulus of the cecum and right colon. *JAMA* 245:2433, 1981.
19. Melchior E: Volvulus of the cecum: an appeal for primary resection with report of six cases. *Surgery* 25:251, 1949.
20. Meyers JR, Heifetz CJ, Baue AE: Cecal volvulus: a lesion requiring resection. *Arch Surg* 104:594, 1972.
21. Sawyer RB, Sawyer KC Jr, Sawyer KC: Volvulus of the colon. *Am J Surg* 104:468, 1962.
22. Saint JH: Acute volvulus of the cecum. *Am J Surg* 95:798, 1958.
23. Speer CS, Bacon HE: Volvulus of the cecum: report of a case. *Dis Col and Rect* 5:306, 1982.
24. Thomas CV: Volvulus of the cecum and ascending colon. *Aust New Zeal J Surg* 35:77, 1965.
25. Smith WR, Goodwin JN: Cecal volvulus. *Am J Surg* 126:215, 1973.
26. Todd GJ, Forde KA: Volvulus of the cecum: choice of operation. *Am J Surg* 138:632, 1979.
27. Anderson JR, Lee D, Taylor TV, McLean Ross AH: Volvulus of the transverse colon. *Br J Surg* 68:179, 1981.
28. Budd DC, Nidlinger EL, Sturts DL, Fouty WJ Jr: Transverse colon volvulus associated with scleroderma. *Am J Surg* 133:370, 1977.
29. Zinkin LD, Kratz LD, Rosin JD: Volvulus of the transverse

colon: report of a case and review of the literature. *Dis Col and Rect* 22:492, 1979.
30. Cuderman BS, Roback SA, Weintraub WH, Leonard AS: Volvulus of the transverse colon. *Surgery* 69:797, 1971.
31. Joergensen K, Kronborg O: The colonoscope in volvulus of the transverse colon. *Dis Col and Rect* 23:357, 1980.
32. Anderson JR, Lee D. The management of acute sigmoid volvulus. *Br J Surg* 68:117, 1981.
33. Arnold GJ, Nance FC: Volvulus of the sigmoid colon. *Ann Surg* 177:527, 1973.
34. String ST, DeCosse JJ: Sigmoid volvulus: An examination of the mortality. *Am J Surg* 121:293, 1971.
35. Hines JR, Gearkink RE, Bass RT: Recurrence and mortality rates in sigmoid volvulus. *Surg Gynecol Obstet* 124:567, 1967.
36. Bruusgard C: Volvulus of the sigmoid colon and its treatment. *Surgery* 122:466, 1947.
37. Shepard JJ: Treatment of volvulus of the sigmoid colon: a review of 425 cases. *Br Med J* 2:280, 1968.
38. Sutcliffe MML: Volvulus of the sigmoid colon. *Br J Surg* 55:903, 1968.
39. Sharpton B, Cheek RC: Volvulus of the sigmoid colon. *Am Surg* 436, 1976.
40. Duke JH Jr, Yar MS: Primary small bowel volvulus: cause and management. *Arch Surg* 112:685, 1977.
41. Burnanasiri SI, Baum S, Nusbarum M, et al: The angiographic diagnosis of midgut malrotation with volvulus in adults. *Radiology* 109:555, 1973.
42. Juler GL, Stemmer EA, Connolly JE: Preoperative diagnosis of small bowel volvulus in adults. *Am J Gastroenterol* 36:235, 1972.
43. Gulati SM, Grover NK, Tagore NK, et al: Volvulus of the small bowel in India. *Am J Surg* 126:661, 1973.
44. Maingot R: Duodenal ileus and gastric volvulus. In *Abdominal Operations*. Maingot R (Ed), Appleton-Century-Crofts, New York 1980. p 469.
45. Tanner NC: Chronic and recurrent volvulus of the stomach. *Am J Surg* 115:505, 1968.

16

Intestinal Ischemia Following Aortic Reconstructions

Patrick S. Vaccaro, M.D.
William L. Smead, M.D.

Introduction

Improvements in operative technique, anesthesia, and physiologic monitoring have resulted in decreased morbidity and mortality associated with abdominal aortic reconstructions. However, the incidence of intestinal ischemia following such procedures remains unchanged, and the occurrence of complications and death remains significant. Prompt recognition and treatment of potentially lethal episodes of intestinal ischemia are necessary if the results are to be improved, yet maximal improvement will be obtained only when preventative measures that reduce the actual incidence of intestinal ischemia are observed. Intestinal ischemia following abdominal aortic reconstructive procedures is reviewed, and the principles of diagnosis, treatment, and prevention are discussed.

Historical Perspective

The first report of intestinal ischemia following abdominal aortic reconstruction was that by Moore in 1954.[38] Following abdominal aortic aneurysmectomy in which the inferior mesenteric and both hypogastric arteries were ligated, the patient developed a rectal stricture. The following year Movius reported ten cases of aneurysmectomy with a 90% incidence of diarrhea and two cases of rectal stricture.[41] Subsequent reports by Cannon, Barnes and associates, and McKain and Schumacher described infarction of the left colon following aneurysmectomy.[1,9,37] In 1958 Gwathmey and associates reported necrosis of the left colon following operation for aortoiliac occlusive disease, and shortly thereafter, Bernatz, and Smith and Szilagyi reported similar findings.[2,23,47] All reports emphasized the appearance of diarrhea, left colon gangrene, and the need for immediate operative intervention. In 1963 Young and associates, from the Cleveland Clinic, in a review of the literature that included 8 cases of their own reported 42 cases of intestinal ischemia following aortic reconstruction, the majority having only colon involvement.[55] However, in 1965 Kountz, Laub, and Connolly described a controversial new entity, aortoiliac steal, which resulted in ischemia and necrosis of the small intestine following aortic reconstruction for aortoiliac occlusive disease in patients with concomitant occlusive disease of the celiac and superior mesenteric arteries.[30] Since that time reports of intestinal ischemia following aortic reconstruction have continued to appear.

Incidence and Classification

Colon ischemia following aortic reconstructive procedures is generally stated to occur in 1 to 2% of cases.[2,5,20,24,25,28,32,42,44] An isolated retrospective report of 120 cases by

Smith and Szilagyi set the incidence as high as 10%. However, in a prospective study by Hagihara, Ernst, and Griffin in which colonoscopy was performed within 2.8 days of aortic reconstruction on 75% of 180 patients, the incidence of colon ischemia was 6.7% following repair for occlusive disease to 6.8% after elective or urgent aneurysmectomy.[24] In patients operated upon for ruptured abdominal aortic aneurysms, the incidence was 60%. However, the incidence of small bowel ischemia following abdominal aortic reconstruction is 0.15%.[28]

In most centers mortality following abdominal aortic reconstructions is approximately 5% or less for elective procedures and 50% for ruptured aortic aneurysms, although recent reports for ruptured abdominal aortic aneurysms show a survival in excess of 70%.[11,16,33,36,50] Although the incidence of ischemic complications following reconstruction appears relatively low, it is significant because mortality associated with colon ischemia varies from 40 to 65%, approaching 100% in association with aortic aneurysm rupture, and in small intestinal ischemia it approaches 90%.[28,42,44]

Although intestinal ischemia may follow bypass grafting or endarterectomy of the occluded aortoiliac segment, it occurs most often following graft replacement of abdominal aortic aneurysms. Boley and associates classified colon ischemia into three clinical types: (1) reversible transient ischemic colitis, (2) ischemic colonic stricture, and (3) ischemic colonic gangrene.[6] Each can be identified histopathologically. The mucosa, which has the highest metabolic rate of the intestinal wall, is the most sensitive to ischemic insult. Mild ischemia may cause submucosal ischemia and hemorrhage leading to increased submucosal friability. Loss of mucosal integrity heralds the development of inflammation and bacterial invasion from the lumen which may lead to actual mucosal sloughing with ulceration. Gross bleeding into the lumen may follow, but generally complete healing ensues. Moderate ischemia results in similar mucosal and submucosal changes, but in addition produces alterations in the cells of the muscularis propria. Healing occurs by fibrosis resulting in scarring of the gut wall and stricture formation. With severe ischemia, a full-thickness injury occurs to the gut wall, resulting in gangrene and disruption in the intestinal integrity. Such an irreparable injury leads to peritonitis and is the condition most often cited in reports of intestinal ischemia following aortic reconstructions, since it is the most obvious clinically. The prototypic model of colon ischemia following aortic reconstruction would occur in the patient undergoing aneurysmectomy with ligation of the inferior mesenteric artery and resultant development of sigmoid colon ischemia.

Anatomy

Appreciation of the events involved in the development of intestinal ischemia following aortic operations requires a basic understanding of arterial anatomy. The three major arterial circuits supplying blood to the intestines are the superior mesenteric, inferior mesenteric, and hypogastric arteries. The superior mesenteric artery (SMA) primarily supplies the small intestine through the jejunal and ileal branches, and the right and transverse colon through the right and middle colic arteries. The inferior mesenteric artery (IMA) supplies the colon from the splenic flexure to the proximal rectum via the left colic, sigmoid, and superior rectal arteries. The distal two-thirds of the rectum are supplied by the middle and inferior rectal branches of the hypogastric arteries.

Important collateral vessels maintain a continuity of flow between these three circuits. Of utmost importance is the marginal artery of Drummond supplying an important connection between the SMA and IMA circuits. Coursing in the periphery of the colonic mesentary in close approximation to the colonic wall, this vessel remains most constant in the region of the transverse and descending colons. Early studies on the blood supply to the colon have shown this continuity to be absent in the ascending colon in 5% of individuals, 20% in the sigmoid region, and more frequently at the junction of the rectosigmoid especially in association with progressive arteriosclerotic disease.[49] An area of particular importance located in the region of the splenic flexure is known as Griffith's point.[22] At this point the continuity of the marginal artery of Drummond is established by the anastomosis between the middle colic artery of the SMA and the left colic branch of the IMA. The precarious nature of anastomoses in this area is well known. The major collateral channels in the region of the distal colon and rectum are between the middle and inferior rectal branches of the hypogastric and superior rectal branch of the IMA. The dense network of the anastomoses between these two systems makes this area well vascularized.

One can see that each circuit is not a separate entity, but that all are dynamically intercommunicating. An example of the importance of these communications can be seen in the event that the middle colic artery is congenitally absent. Although Sonneland found this vessel to be congenitally absent in 3.6% in a large series of autopsies, others have reported the incidence to be as high as 20–22%.[3,22,48] Should such a patient undergo aortic reconstruction in which the IMA was ligated, the communication between the hypogastric and IMA circuits and the contribution of the right colic artery would assume protean importance.

Several other collateral systems may also assume importance in the vascular supply to the intestines, especially in the presence of advanced arteriosclerotic disease. The meandering mesenteric artery, also called the central anastomotic artery, marginal artery, mesomesenteric artery, middle colic-left colic collateral, artery of Drummond, arc of Treves, or the arc of Riolan, is the result of a communication between the left branch of the middle colic artery and the ascending branch of the left colic artery, and is said to be present in up to two-thirds of normal individuals.[18,40] Enlargement of this vessel has been described as being indicative of IMA and/or SMA stenosis.[12,18,28] In patients with SMA stenosis, flow is upward from the left colic artery through the meandering mesenteric artery to the superior mesenteric artery to supply the small intestine and right colon. In 27% of the patients with aortic aneurysmal disease and in 35% of patients with aortic occlusive disease, an enlarged meandering artery may be seen angiographically with the flow from the superior mesenteric system coursing downward to opacify the inferior mesenteric system.[20] In the presence of occlusion of the superior mesenteric artery, not only the meandering mesenteric artery but also the pancreaticoduodenal branches of the celiac artery may form important collaterals. A further communication to supply the left colon may be established through the ileolumbar artery, the circumflex iliac artery, the inferior epigastric artery, and the circumflex femoral artery.

The gradual development of occlusive disease is a strong stimulus for the development of collaterals. On the other hand, aneurysmal disease is not always associated with occlusive processes and may not stimulate development of collaterals to the same extent. This may partially explain why the occurrence of intestinal ischemia is higher after aortic reconstruction for aneurysmal disease when the IMA is sacrified.

Pathophysiology and Clinical Manifestations

While most patients undergoing ligation of the inferior mesenteric artery during aortic reconstruction will tolerate this maneuver well, a few will develop intestinal ischemia. In fact, in most reports concerning intestinal ischemia following aortic reconstruction, ligation of the IMA is the most common event.[2,3,19,20,28,35,42,45] Ernst and associates have recently shown that the inferior mesenteric artery may be seen in preoperative angiograms in only 40% of patients with aneurysmal disease and 52% with occlusive disease.[20] Others have reported the incidence of preoperative occlusion of the IMA in association with aneurysmal disease to be as high as 80%.[46] Since most cases of postoperative intestinal ischemia follow the repair of abdominal aortic aneurysms and since the IMA is occluded preoperatively in most such cases, it is reasonable to assume that factors other than ligation of the IMA may also contribute to the occurrence of intestinal ischemia. Other factors cited are improper ligation of the IMA, failure to resume hypogastric flow, congenital absence or injury to collaterals, operative trauma to the colon secondary to excessive retraction, low perfusion and hypotension, loss of collateral supply secondary to cholesterol emboli, aneurysmal rupture with mesenteric compression, and compromise of the inferior mesenteric vein. Whatever the cause, however, the response to the ischemic event is determined by the duration of ischemia and the adequacy of collaterals. The most likely reason for the lower incidence of intestinal ischemia following operations for occlusive disease is related to the gradual development of collateral systems which may be less advanced in the case of aneurysmal disease.

The existence and pathophysiology of the aortoiliac steal syndrome remains more controversial.[12,13,21,25,30,31,54] The syndrome is said to occur in patients undergoing arterial reconstruction for aortoiliac occlusive disease with concomitant severe occlusive disease of the celiac and superior mesenteric arteries. Kountz and associates in 1965 postulated that shunting of blood by bypass or endarterectomy into previously blocked leg vessels steals blood from the stenotic or occluded mesenteric circulation and leads to ischemia and gangrene of the small intestine.[30] Such a borrowing–lending phenomenon between vascular systems was first proposed by DeBakey et al in 1947.[17] In an attempt to validate their proposal, Kountz and associates performed hemodynamic studies in dogs showing that after sympathectomy and lower aortic occlusion followed by release of the occlusion the mesenteric flow decreased from 42 to 72% below preoperative levels.[30] These early and subsequent reports of aortoiliac steal noted an enlarged meandering mesenteric artery. Early ischemia is believed secondary to hemometakinesia, the borrowing–lending phenomenon, while late ischemia, occurring months to years later, appears to be due to superimposed thrombosis of stenotic mesenteric vessels, progression of underlying disease, or a combination of both. In the presence of visceral vessel stenosis, prophylactic revascularization has been recommended.[12] Opponents of the steal phenomenon stress that other events may be responsible for the ensuing ischemia.[51] Stoney stresses that the phenomenon reported by Kountz et al may more likely be secondary to (1) vasomotor responses to operative shock altering collateral flow, (2) low cardiac output resulting in nonocclusive intestinal infarction, or (3) operative damage to a vital portion of the mesenteric blood supply, such as damage to the orifice of or embolization into the inferior mesenteric artery resulting in decreased upward flow through the meandering mesenteric artery to the superior mesenteric artery, or to direct operative interruption of the meandering artery.

The signs and symptoms of intestinal ischemia vary with the degree of involvement. With mild ischemia, increased motility and decreased absorptive capacity of the gut may produce diarrhea that is self-limiting. With moderate ischemia, the diarrhea may be more persistent and severe, and occasionally bloody. Depending upon the extent of stricture formation, intestinal obstruction may ensue. The manifestations of severe ischemia are generally more dramatic, and may initially occur in the first 24 to 48 hours following operation. In 50 to 68% of patients the diarrhea may become bloody.[4,42] Pain may be moderate to severe, and is usually out of proportion to that expected following an uneventful aortic operation. The pain, usually crampy but occasionally constant, and tenderness are located in the lower abdomen, most frequently in the left lower quadrant. Generalized abdominal distension may become prominent, and with perforation, signs of peritonitis are apparent. Nonspecific systemic manifestations of sepsis including marked leucocytosis, fever, metabolic acidosis, progressive hypotension, and hypovolemia manifested by unusually massive crystalloid requirements may also be present.

Diagnosis

The incidence of death following transmural colonic ischemia has been reported to be 70 to 90%.[28,35] Such alarming mortality rates will continue unless earlier diagnoses are made. Ottinger and associates showed that in five of 13 patients with transmural ischemic colitis, diagnosis was delayed from six to 20 days when the diagnosis was based on the signs and symptoms of perforation.[42] Clearly, early diagnosis is of utmost importance and is enhanced by the surgeon's heightened suspicion in patients at highest risk of intestinal ischemia.

Of all the signs and symptoms of postoperative intestinal ischemia, the early onset of diarrhea should alert the surgeon to the diagnosis. Suspicion should also be aroused by marked leucocytosis and refractory metabolic acidosis. The appearance of free air under the diaphragm on abdominal radiography confirms the presence of perforation.

Sigmoidoscopy, more specifically fiberoptic colonoscopy, remains the most helpful procedure for establishing the early diagnosis of colon ischemia. In mild cases, hemorrhage and edema may be seen, while in more advanced cases erosions, ulcers, and pseudomembranes are present. In the most severe episodes when the colonic segment is frankly gangrenous, a yellowish green, necrotic noncontractile surface is seen. Ernst and associates showed the efficacy of endoscopy in a prospective trial in 1976.[20] All patients who underwent aortic reconstruction had colonoscopy within four days of operation. They noted a 6% incidence of ischemic changes, and also observed that ischemic changes may be visible before the onset of diarrhea. In the presence of aortic rupture, the incidence rose sharply.

Several other points also warrant emphasis. First, serial examinations are necessary to observe progression or resolution of the ischemic process. Only with such attention can surgical intervention be appropriately timed. Second, once the involved segment is visualized, one should resist the urge to advance the instrument beyond this area, thus lessening the chance of perforation. Since it is rare for the ischemic process to occur without involvement of the left colon, it is rarely necessary to pass the colonoscope beyond 40 centimeters.

Although barium enema may be useful in diagnosing stenotic lesions resulting from ischemia, it is rarely necessary for diagnosis of the acute process, and may lead to perforation. Similarly, angiography is of limited assistance. Although ultrasonography and computerized axial tomography are helpful in diagnosing aneurysmal disease, they are of no assistance in the diagnosis of intestinal ischemia.

Treatment

Occasionally ischemic injury to the colon is noted intraoperatively at the time of initial aortic reconstruction. Under these circumstances there are two courses of action. The first alternative would be to attempt mesenteric revascularization either by reimplantation of the IMA if it has been sacrificed, or by bypass to the IMA or SMA. There has been a report of bypass grafting directly from the aortic prosthesis to the meandering mesenteric artery under such circumstances.[21] When such procedures result in an improved appearance of the bowel, the operation is terminated. If bypassing fails to improve the appearance of the intestine or when it is impossible, all compromised intestine should be removed and an end colostomy with Hartmann's pouch or mucus fistula performed. Primary anastomosis should be avoided. Intestinal resection should be performed only after all prosthetic material has been suitably reperitonealized.

When intestinal ischemia occurs in the postoperative period, the surgeon is faced with the decision as to necessity of reoperation. On the basis of serial examinations, including colonoscopy, one must decide whether the condition is progressing or improving. When improvement in clinical signs, laboratory parameters, and appearance of the colon is apparent on repeated studies, nonoperative management may be continued. Such management consists of placing the gut at rest, fluid and electrolyte correction, and the administration of broad spectrum antibiotics.[45]

If the patient's condition worsens, showing deterioration in clinical signs or progression of the ischemic process on repeated colonoscopy, the patient should be prepared for urgent reoperation. During laparotomy all nonviable intestine should be excised, and end colostomy with Hartmann's pouch or mucus fistula performed. At no time should reanastomosis of the colon be attempted. Whether or not to reanastomose small intestine should be up to the surgeon's discretion. If it can be shown that the margins of resection are unquestionably viable by either the appearance of fluorescein staining or presence of Doppler signals, then an anastomosis should be attempted.[7,14,27,28,34] If the viability after resection remains questionable, then the ends of intestine should be brought through the abdominal wall for reanastomosis at a later time. At all times during intestinal operations, the prosthetic graft should never be exposed to avoid the chance of graft infection.

Progressive rectal ischemia may occur in 0.5% of cases and requires excision of all nonviable intestine with the creation of an end colostomy and insertion of adequate perineal drains.[32]

Prevention

The surgeon must adopt a preventive preoperative attitude to postoperative intestinal ischemia. A systematic evaluation should predict which patients are at highest risk for the development of postoperative ischemia. A history compatible with chronic visceral ischemia places the patient at an increased risk for the development of postoperative ischemia and should alert the surgeon to the need for preoperative angiograms with appropriate views of the visceral vessels. Similarly, the presence of an abdominal aortic aneurysm increases the patient's risk of ischemia.

Precise delineation of the vascular anatomy can be obtained only by careful preoperative angiography. Not only the primary anatomy but also the collateral circulation should be carefully evaluated in both anteroposterior and lateral views. As previously noted, in 60 to 80% of patients with aneurysms and nearly half of patients with aortoiliac occlusion the IMA will fail to opacify on preoperative angiography.[20,46] It is the patient with the patent IMA who has this vessel ligated at the time of aortic reconstruction that runs the greatest risk of postoperative ischemia. Similarly, 13% of patients with aneurysms and 30% with occlusive disease will show concomitant occlusion of the hypogastric arteries.[20] The importance of the communication between the IMA and hypogastric systems has already been stressed, and in patients in whom the IMA is ligated at operation, the maintenance of flow through the hypogastric systems assumes greater importance.

The meandering mesenteric artery may be seen angiographically in 27% of patients with aneurysmal disease and 35% of patients with occlusive disease, signifying concomitant occlusive disease of the SMA or IMA.[12,18,20,28] An attempt should be made to determine the direction of flow through this vessel by serial X-rays. If the flow is from the SMA to IMA, signifying occlusion of the IMA, the patient is at a lower risk for the occurrence of intestinal ischemia than if the direction of flow is reversed. If reversed flow is present, lateral views of the origin of the SMA should be obtained to determine the degree and location of occlusion in this vessel. In such cases concomitant aortosuperior mesenteric artery bypass or reimplantation of the IMA or both may be necessary to avoid the development of postoperative ischemia. In the patient with aortoiliac occlusive disease, an end-to-side rather than end-to-end proximal aorta-to-graft anastomosis may be preferred to preserve antegrade IMA flow.

Several other factors employed preoperatively may also lessen the risk for postoperative ischemia. As suggested by Whittemore et al, the maintenance of optimal cardiac performance determined preoperatively with the aid of a Swan-Ganz catheter will reduce operative mortality.[53] Such a preventive approach may reduce the occurrence of hypotension and diminished intravascular perfusion during operation, lessening the possibility of thrombosis in the smaller, but important, collateral vessels to the intestine. Preoperative mechanical cleansing of the colon will reduce the sheer bulk of this structure and may decrease the incidence of retraction-related injury to the colon and mesocolon during operation. Finally, although controversial, the administration of preoperative antibiotics may diminish the insult to the intestine should postoperative ischemia develop.[3,4,5,32]

Although such thorough preoperative assessment and preparation may aid in the prevention of intestinal ischemia, all advantage is lost if the operation is not adeptly performed. Although most patients appear to tolerate ligation of the IMA, a tolerable situation may be made intolerable by improper ligation technique. It is imperative that ligation be performed as close to the origin of the IMA as possible so that important collateral channels to the colon are not interrupted. The best technique for avoiding improper ligation is to oversew the orifice of the IMA from within the aneurysmal sac once it is open.

As in any operation, gentleness in handling tissue is extremely important. Great care should be exercised in dissection around the aorta to avoid the possible embolization of debris into the vessels of the legs, pelvis, or intestine. Care in handling the colon and mesocolon during retraction and packing for exposure may prevent direct trauma to these structures and their collateral circulation, especially the meandering mesenteric artery. The use of heparin during the operation may prevent thrombosis of the collateral circulation during periods of lower perfusion pressure, whether secondary to hypotension, clamp occlusion, or extrinsic compression. Also of importance is the exposure to the left external iliac artery, best obtained by gently retracting the sigmoid colon superiorly and medially with an incision in the lateral mesocolon giving easy access. To attempt to expose this vessel from the medial side of the sigmoid may necessitate excessive retraction on the colon resulting in injury to both the structure and its collateral circulation.

An attempt should be made to maintain flow into one and preferably both hypogastric arteries, and rarely is there a need for endarterectomy or bypass to these vessels. Flow to these vessels is maintained in an antegrade fashion by placing the distal graft anastomosis to either the terminal aorta if possible, or more commonly, into the common iliac arteries. Should disease in the common iliac vessels preclude such a reconstruction, retrograde perfusion of the hypogastrics may be obtained by end-to-side anastomosis to the external iliac or common femoral arteries, with ligation of the common iliac vessels proximally.

The question of when to reimplant the IMA remains. Obviously the vessel could be reimplanted every time it is found to be patent, but this is time consuming and unnecessary in most cases. Ottinger et al have suggested several ways of dealing with this problem.[42] One approach is to temporarily occlude the IMA with a bulldog clamp prior to its division and observe the appearance of the colon. If ischemia develops, the IMA is reimplanted. Another technique is to divide the IMA just distal to its origin and observe the back bleeding. Should the backflow appear pulsatile, then the circulation is assumed to be adequate and reimplantation is unnecessary. In the presence of poor back bleeding, particularly if the IMA appears enlarged, or the hypogastrics are occluded, reimplantation is suggested. Although these techniques have merit, it is still possible for infarction to occur in a colon that appears normal at the termination of operation.

Since criteria of intestinal viability including color, peristalsis, and arterial pulsations are frequently inadequate, several techniques have been introduced to aid in decision making. In the past, techniques that were difficult in application and time consuming utilized technetium-labeled albumin microspheres, surface temperature and pH determinations, vital dye injections, or electromyography.[8,39,43,52,56] More recently, Doppler ultrasonography, fluorescein staining, and IMA pressure determinations have each been shown to be simple to apply and accurate in assessing intestinal viability.[7,14,19,27,28,34] Several investigators have shown the value of the Doppler ultrasonic flowmeter in the determination of intestinal viability in gastrointestinal surgery. Hobson and colleagues in 1976 and 1979 reported the efficacy of this technique in predicting intestinal viability during aortic reconstruction.[27,28] Before and after temporary occlusion of the IMA, arterial flow signals are recorded over the IMA, the large bowel mesentery, and the serosal surface of the left colon. If arterial flow over the latter two areas remained unchanged with occlusion of the IMA, this structure was ligated if necessary and reimplantation not performed. On the other hand, if signals markedly diminished or disappeared, the IMA was reimplanted or an end-to-side proximal aortic anastomosis performed to maintain flow to the IMA through the native aorta. A total of 155 patients were studied and in 8% the flow through the IMA was preserved, based on the Doppler technique. No cases of clinical intestinal ischemia developed. Opponents of this technique state that audible flow signals may be present even though the actual perfusion pressure may be less than necessary for maintenance flow in the mucosal vessels. The significance of this point remains unclear.

Fluorescein staining has been shown to be effective in the prediction of small intestinal viability and is simple to use, requiring only a Wood's light. Buckley et al have suggested that this technique may be a more accurate predictor than either clinical judgement or Doppler assessment.[7] Supporters of this technique believe that fluorescence indicates adequate perfusion, and that the total area in question may be studied at once rather than by multiple applications of the Doppler probe. Opponents of this technique cite the possible and extremely rare anaphylactoid reaction to fluorescein as a strong deterrent to its use. Advocates of the Doppler technique ascribe the discrepancy in results presented by Buckley et al to improper application of the technique. Although fluorescein studies have dealt mainly with the viability of flaps and small intestine, its use in the determination of colonic viability appears valid.

Ernst and colleagues have shown that the determination of the IMA stump pressure is a reliable index of safety for ligation of the IMA during aortic reconstruction, especially for aneurysmal disease.[19] The distal IMA is cannulated with an 18-gauge Teflon catheter after division of the IMA, or the orifice of the IMA is so cannulated from within the opened aneurysm wall. In the presence of normal systemic arterial pressure, a postreconstruction mean IMA pressure of greater than 40 mm Hg or mean IMA/systemic pressure ratio greater than 0.40, precludes the development of ischemic colitis and the IMA is safely ligated. This is true even in the absence of flow through the hypogastric arteries, and the technique may have its widest application when it is impossible to reconstitute hypogastric flow. Ernst et al are the only investigators to correlate pressure recordings with postoperative colonoscopic examinations, and the only patient who developed ischemic colitis had a postreconstruction pressure and ratio of 30 mm Hg and 0.37, respectively. Overall, it appears that all three techniques are applicable, and the surgeon should use the technique with which he is most familiar.

There are several techniques for reattachment of the IMA and the surgeon should be familiar with all. When feasible, the best method for reattachment of the IMA to the graft is that described by Crawford for reattachment of visceral vessels during thoracoabdominal aortic aneurysm reconstruction.[15] The orifice of the IMA is sewn around an oval opening in the graft leaving the aneurysmal wall intact to allow hemostatic closure of the sac over the prosthetic graft. Other techniques use the patch reattachment popularized by Carrel,[10] application of the spatulated IMA directly to the graft, or interposition of reversed saphenous vein or Dacron tube graft between the aortic graft and distal cut end of IMA.

References

1. Barnes WH, Ellis FH, Kirklin JW, Edwards JE: Experiences with 165 aortic homografts. *Surg Gynecol and Obstet* 106:49, 1958.
2. Bernatz P: Necrosis of the colon following resection for abdominal aortic aneurysms. *Arch Surg* 81:373, 1960.
3. Berstein WC, Bernstein EF: Ischemic ulcerative colitis following inferior mesenteric arterial ligation. *Dis Colon and Rectum* 6:54, 1969.

4. Bicks RO, Bale GF, Howard H, McBurney RF: Acute and delayed colon ischemia after aortic aneurysm surgery. *Arch Intern Med* 122:249, 1968.
5. Birnbaum W, Rudy L, Wylie E: Colonic and rectal ischemia following abdominal aneurysmectomy. *Dis Colon and Rectum* 7:293, 1964.
6. Boley JJ, Brandt LJ, Veith FJ: Ischemic disorders of the intestines. *Curr Probs in Surg* 15:1978.
7. Bulkley GB, Zuidema GD, Hamilton SR, O'Mara CS, Klacsmann PG, Horn SD: Intraoperative determination of intestinal viability following ischemic injury. *Ann Surg* 190:628, 1981.
8. Bussemaker JB, Lindeman J: Comparison of methods to determine viability of small intestine. *Ann Surg* 176:97, 1972.
9. Cannon JA: In discussion of Payne JH et al: *Am J Surg* 90:314, 1955.
10. Carrel A: Technique and remote results of vascular anastomoses: *Surg Gynecol Obstet* 14:246, 1912.
11. Chiariello L, Reul GJ, Wukasch DC, Sandiford FM, Hallman GL, Cooley DA: Ruptured abdominal aortic aneurysm. Treatment and review of eighty-seven patients. *Am J Surg* 128:735, 1974.
12. Connolly JE, Kwaan JH: Prophylactic revascularization of the gut. *Ann Surg* 190:514, 1979.
13. Connolly JE, Stemmer EA: Intestinal gangrene as the result of mesenteric arterial steal. *Am J Surg* 126:197, 1973.
14. Cooperman M, Pace WG, Martin EW et al: Viability of ischemic intestine by Doppler ultrasound. *Surg* 83:705, 1978.
15. Crawford ES: Thoraco-abdominal and abdominal aortic aneurysms involving renal, superior mesenteric and celiac arteries. *Ann Surg* 179:763, 1974.
16. Crawford ES, Saleh SA, Babb JW, Glaeser DH, Vaccaro PS, Silvers A: Infrarenal abdominal aortic aneurysm: factors influencing survival after operation performed over a 25-year period. *Ann Surg* 193:699, 1981.
17. DeBakey ME, Burch G, Ray T, Ochsner A: The "borrowing—lending" hemodynamic phenomenon (hemometakinesia) and its therapeutic application in peripheral vascular disturbances. *Ann Surg* 126:850, 1947.
18. Ernst CB: Colon ischemia following abdominal aortic recon-

struction. In *Complications in Vascular Surgery* by Bernhard VM, Towne JB. Grune and Stratton, New York 1980. p. 379.

19. Ernst CB, Hagihara PF, Daugherty ME, Griffen WO: Inferior mesenteric artery stump pressure: a reliable index for safe IMA ligation during abdominal aortic aneurysmectomy. *Ann Surg* 187:641, 1978.
20. Ernst CB, Hagihara PF, Daugherty ME, Satchatello CR, Griffen WO: Ischemic colitis incidence following abdominal aortic reconstruction: a prospective study. *Surgery* 80:417, 1976.
21. Gonzalez LL, Jaffe MS: Mesenteric arterial insufficiency following abdominal aortic resection. *Arch Surg* 93:10, 1966.
22. Griffiths JD: Surgical anatomy of the blood supply of the distal colon. *Ann Roy Coll Surgeons,* England 19:241, 1956.
23. Gwathmey O, Pierpont HC, Blades B: Clinical experience with the surgical treatment of acquired aortic vascular disease. *Surg Gynecol and Obstet* 107:205, 1958.
24. Hagihara PF, Ernst CB, Griffen WO: Incidence of ischemic colitis following abdominal aortic reconstruction. *Surg Gynecol and Obstet* 149:571, 1979.
25. Hayward RH, Calhoun TR, Korompai FL: Gastrointestinal complications of vascular surgery. *Surg Clin North Am* 59:885, 1979.
26. Hobson RW, Wright CB, O'Donnell JA, Jamil Z, Lamberth WC, Najen Z: Determination of intestinal viability by Doppler ultrasound. *Arch Surg* 114:165, 1979.
27. Hobson RW, Wright CB, Rich NM, Collins GT: Assessment of colonic ischemia during aortic surgery by Doppler ultrasound. *J Surg Research* 20:231, 1976.
28. Johnson WC, Nabseth DC: Visceral infarction following aortic surgery. *Ann Surg* 180:312, 1974.
29. Katz S, Wahab A, Murray W, Williams LE: New parametics of viability in ischemic bowel disease. *Am J Surg* 127:136, 1974.
30. Kountz SL, Laub DR, Connolly JE: "Aortoiliac steal" syndrome. *Arch Surg* 92:490, 1966.
31. Lancaster JR, Payan HM, Jacobs WH, Gerwig WH: Aortoiliac steal syndrome and necrosis of gastrointestinal tract. *Arch Surg* 94:172, 1967.
32. Launer DP, Miscall BG, Beil AR: Colorectal infarction fol-

lowing resection of abdominal aortic aneurysms. *Dis Col and Rectum* 21:613, 1967.

33. Lawrie GM, Crawford ES, Morris GC, Howell JF: Progress in the treatment of ruptured abdominal aortic aneurysm. *World J Surg* 4:653, 1980.
34. Lee BY, Trainor FS, Kavner D, McCann WJ: Intraoperative assessment of intestinal viability with Doppler ultrasound. *Surg Gynecol and Obstet* 149:671, 1979.
35. McBurney RP, Howard H, Bicks RO, Bale F: Ischemic and gangrene of the colon following abdominal aortic resection. *Am Surg* 36:205, 1970.
36. McCabe CJ, Coleman WS, Brewster DC: The advantage of early operation for abdominal aortic aneurysm. *Arch Surg* 116:1025, 1981.
37. McKain J, Shumacher HB: Ischemia of the left colon associated with abdominal aortic aneurysms and their treatment. *Arch Surg* 76:355, 1958.
38. Moore SW: Resection of the abdominal aorta with defect replaced by homologous graft. *Surg Gynecol and Obstet* 99:745, 1954.
39. Moosa AR, Skinner DB, Stark V, Hoffer P: Assessment of bowel viability using ^{99m}technetium tagged albumin microspheres. *J Surg Res* 16:466, 1974.
40. Moskowitz M, Zimmerman H, Felson B: The meandering mesenteric artery of the colon. *Am J Roentgenol* 92:1088, 1964.
41. Movius HJ: Resection of abdominal arteriosclerotic aneurysm. *Am J Surg* 90:298, 1955.
42. Ottinger LW, Darling RC, Nathan MJ, Linton RR: Left colon ischemia complicating aorto-iliac reconstruction. *Arch Surg* 105:841, 1979.
43. Papachristun D, Fortner JG: Prediction of intestinal viability by intra-arterial dye injection; a simple test. *Am J Surg* 132:573, 1976.
44. Papadopoulos CD, Mancini HW, Marino AW: Ischemic necrosis of the colon following aortic aneurysmectomy. *J Cardiovasc Surg* 15:494, 1974.
45. Perdue GD, Lowry K: Arterial insufficiency to the colon following resection of abdominal aortic aneurysms. *Surg Gynecol and Obstet* 115:39, 1962.

46. Rösch J, Keller FS, Porter JM, Baur GM: Value of angiography in the management of abdominal aortic aneurysms. *Cardiovasc Radiol* 1:83, 1978.
47. Smith RF, Szilagyi DE: Ischemia of the colon as a complication in the surgery of the abdominal aorta. *Arch Surg* 80:114, 1960.
48. Sonneland J, Anson BJ, Beaton LE: Surgical anatomy of the arterial supply to the colon for the superior mesenteric artery based upon a study of 600 specimens. *Surg Gynecol Obstet* 106:885, 1958.
49. Steward JA, Rankin FU: Blood supply of large intestine: its surgical considerations. *Arch Surg* 26:843, 1933.
50. Stokes J, Butcher HR: Abdominal aortic aneurysms. Factors influencing operative mortality and criteria of operability. *Arch Surg* 107:297, 1973.
51. Stoney RJ in Discussion of Connolly JE, Stemmer EA: Intestinal gangrene as a result of mesenteric arterial steal. *Am J Surg* 126:202, 1973.
52. Wapnick S, Solowiejczyk M, Grosman E: Detection of intestinal ischemia. II. Temperature difference between mesenteric and antimesenteric margins of bowel as a criterion of intestinal anastomosis viability. *Rev Surg* 33:371, 1977.
53. Whittemore AD, Clowes AW, Hechtman HB, Mannick JA: Aortic aneurysm repair: reduced operative mortality associated with maintenance of optimal cardiac output. *Ann Surg* 192:414, 1980.
54. Williams LF, Kim RM, Tompkins W, Byrne JJ: Aortoiliac steal—a cause of intestinal ischemia. *N Engl J Med* 278:777, 1968.
55. Young JR, Humphries AW, deWolfe VG, Le Fevre FA: Complications of abdominal aortic surgery. *Arch Surg* 86:51–59, 1963.
56. Zarins CK, Skinner DB, Rhodes BA, James AE: Predictions of the viability of revascularized intestine with radioactive microspheres. *Surg Gynecol Obstet* 138:576, 1974.

17

Intestinal Ischemia in Radiation Enteritis

Peter J. Fabri, M.D.

Radiation as a therapeutic modality in cancer treatment has experienced continued and progressive acceptance over the past 75 years. While the complications of radiation have been long recognized, new applications of radiotherapy in the treatment of neoplastic diseases such as Hodgkin's and non-Hodgkin's lymphoma, testicular carcinomas, embryonal tumors, sarcomas, and gynecological and scrotal malignancies continue to emerge with good clinical response. While the position of radiation in the oncologic armamentarium is well established, radiotherapy continues to provide some of the most difficult, long-term management problems in clinical medicine in terms of acute and chronic radiation injury to the bowel. Chronic radiation damage results in obliterative endarteritis and subsequent intestinal ischemia. It is the purpose of this review to summarize our current knowledge of the pathophysiology and management of radiation induced intestinal abnormalities with specific emphasis on the ischemic injury.

Definition of the Problem

It is estimated that 50% of all cancer patients will receive radiotherapy at some stage of their treatment. While many receive palliative treatment to control symptoms of advanced disease, a continued place exists for radiation as primary treatment of many solid neoplasms. Virtually all patients receiving radiation to the abdomen will develop early symptoms of radiation injury to the bowel and 5–20% will be left with long-term sequelae of treatment collectively referred to as radiation enteritis. Fortunately, the early effects are self-limiting and easily controlled. On the other hand, chronic radiation enteritis, while rare, is, for the most part, an incurable disease.

Irradiation of the pelvis for gynecologic malignancies accounts for[1,2,3,4] the majority of cases of symptomatic radiation enteritis and proctitis. Approximately 20% of women undergoing radiation for carcinoma of the cervix will develop annoying gastrointestinal symptoms and 3–8% will develop severe to incapacitating symptoms. The majority of these (75%) will involve radiation damage to the anterior rectal wall, behind the cervix. Women having previous surgery in the pelvis with small bowel adherence are also at risk of developing small bowel involvement.

Patients receiving radiation for carcinoma of the bladder or prostate cannot be protected completely from exposure of the rectosigmoid and therefore, radiation proctitis is virtually certain in the majority.[5] Small bowel involvement is less common unless previous lower abdominal surgery, e.g. appendectomy, has resulted in intestinal fixation.

Virtually all patients receiving radiation to the abdomen will develop acute radiation damage during therapy.[6] While bothersome and occasionally a limiting factor in total radiation dose, acute radiation enteritis is self-limiting and also poorly correlated with chronic damage. Chronic radiation damage, a combination of fibrosis and endarteritis results in irreversible ischemia of segments of bowel.

While this may result in bothersome symptoms, malabsorption, and occasionally hemorrhage, obstruction, or perforation, the major risk of chronic radiation injury appears to exist during subsequent abdominal surgical procedures in which the intestinal ischemia frequently limits the success of otherwise successful procedures because of leaking intestinal anastomoses, perforation, abscess formation, or fistulae.[7]

Occurrence

Radiation enteritis and proctitis occur only after significant doses of therapeutic radiation and then only within the area of the radiation port. Damage due to scatter outside the port is virtually nonexistent. Careful delineation of the therapeutic port clearly defines the area of the abdominal cavity—and its contents—at risk.

Radiation enteritis occurs in three forms: acute, subacute, and chronic. Acute injury occurs during the course of treatment in virtually all patients receiving abdominal radiation and seems to be unrelated to total dose but rather to amount of radiation per unit time. Over 1000 rads per week is very likely to cause symptoms which may be minimized by providing rest periods at regular intervals to allow recovery.

Subacute radiation enteritis is the occurrence months later of recurrent symptoms, primarily bleeding, diarrhea, etc., and may include ulceration of the rectum, free perforation, or fistulization. Subacute problems are fortunately less frequent than acute enteritis and again are most frequent following pelvic irradiation, particularly after surgery.

Chronic radiation damage manifests itself months to years after radiation and may be a crippling or even fatal disease. It occurs in 3–20% depending on the diligence of the search, the indications for radiation, and preradiation pelvic surgery.[8] Intestinal malabsorption,[9] obstruction, and fistulization represent the most common expression of the disease. Carcinoma has also been described as a late manifestation of radiation damage to the colon.[10]

While acute radiation enteritis is most closely correlated with radiation dose per unit time, subacute and chronic radiation damage are related to total dose. The incidence begins to rise after 4000 rads and is most common after doses above 6000 rads. Previous pelvic inflammation (PID, appendicitis, or pelvic surgery) increases the likelihood by fixing the small intestine in the pelvis. Diabetes, hypertension, vascular disease, and chemotherapy[11] seem to be contributing factors, increasing the probability of radiation injury as well as decreasing the total dose likely to cause damage.

While acute enteritis is not uncommon during upper abdominal radiation, chronic problems are seen less often than after pelvic therapy. This has been attributed to mobility of the upper abdominal viscera, limitations of total dose, a more extensive, complex blood supply, and less focused radiation. Therapy which delivers more concentrated radiation, comparable to the colpostat used in intracavitary radiation of the uterine cervix, might be expected to cause similar radiation problems if it were used in the upper abdomen because of the administration of a high dose in a small area.

Pathophysiology

Therapeutic radiation produces complex cellular damage by a variety of mechanisms. While the exact biochemical events leading to cell destruction are unclear, essential factors include formation of active radicals, chromosomal damage, and possibly cellular dehydration. Cellular destruction is not dependent on structure—at a high enough dose any cell can be destroyed by radiation. Radiation sensitive cells, however, are characterized by continued cell turnover, presumably because cells are more susceptible to radiation in the early post-mitotic period.

Stable populations of cells, e.g. brain, are more resistant to radiation while structures with continued cell replacement, e.g. gastrointestinal mucosa, are more sensitive. Vascular endothelium seems susceptible in a more chronic fashion with thrombosis and obliteration commonly seen histologically. These two sequences, destruction of rapid turnover cells and obliteration of blood vessels, combined with an unusual fibroblastic response, seem to comprise the scope of the radiation-induced abnormalities.

Acute radiation enteritis is due to destruction of the rapidly dividing cells at the base of the crypts of the gastrointestinal mucosa. Lack of replacement of the villus epithelium results in secondary blunting which is reversed over 10–14 days by cellular replacement. During the period of mucosal destruction, integrity against bacteria may be lost with transmural migration and subsequent infectious complications. Most of the insult associated with acute radiation injury is related to the loss of absorptive surface, edema, and dysmotility. Vascular changes are a very minor component of this early lesion.

Subacute and chronic radiation damage are characterized by fibrosis and vascular obliteration. The fibrosis consists of bizarre fibroblasts through all layers of the bowel associated with edema and hyaline degeneration. The vascular injury consists primarily of early thrombosis associated with hyaline plugs. Both arterial and venous involvement are prominent leading to endarteritis and endophlebitis. Telangectasia are common gross manifestations and are frequently surrounded by a characteristic marble-like appearance to the bowel wall.

While acute radiation damage is characterized by diarrhea, tenesmus and nausea, chronic damage seems to be most commonly associated with fibrotic narrowing, malabsorption, and occasionally bacterial overgrowth. Ulceration may occur and progress to full-thickness loss with perforation or fistulization. Crampy pain, weight loss, chronic diarrhea, failure to thrive, or bleeding may be the first manifestation of chronic radiation enteritis or proctitis. While histologic changes and endoscopic abnormalities can be identified in virtually everyone who has received pelvic radiation, those patients who develop chronic abnormalities cannot be predicted by the early radiation abnormalities nor are the acute patients more severely affected if affected at all. Associated factors seem to play an important but poorly understood role in the genesis of chronic radiation enteritis including diseases which of themselves affect the intrinsic vascularity of the bowel.

Diagnosis

The diagnosis of radiation enteritis needs to be considered in all patients with gastrointestinal symptoms who have had previous abdominal radiation. Unfortunately, other diseases such as recurrent malignancy, anastomotic obstruction, or diverticulitis can still occur in patients who have been irradiated previously and these frequently confuse diagnostic efforts. It is true, obviously, that only patients who have received an adequate radiation dose (at least 4000 rads), delivered to the abdomen are at risk. However, a history of acute radiation enteritis only affirms that a significant radiation exposure has occurred; it in no way identifies those patients at greatest risk of developing chronic radiation enteritis.

Sigmoidoscopy and barium studies, while the cornerstone of the gastrointestinal armamentarium, may not be diagnostic in patients suffering from radiation enteritis. In these patients, colonoscopy may prove invaluable.[12] Care must be exercised to prevent inadvertent perforation of involved intestine. In particular, excess tension or torque may result in hemorrhage from a friable area of mesentery.

Biopsies should be taken judiciously because of the recognized risk of intestinal perforation at the biopsy site in irradiated bowel. The smaller biopsy accomplished through the colonoscope should have much less risk than larger sigmoidoscopic biopsies.

Histologic examination of biopsies may show fibrosis and endarteritis or the abnormal fibroblasts which are characteristic. The primary significance of tissue evaluation, however, is to exclude a second or recurrent neoplasm. The diagnosis of radiation enteritis depends on a complex of clinical, laboratory, X-ray, and histological findings. It is difficult to be secure on the basis of any one of these alone.

Treatment

Any consideration of the management of radiation enteritis must acknowledge the concept that this disease occurs only after therapeutic radiation. And, while the acute enteritis usually requires no specific treatment, chronic radiation enteritis has no specific treatment and in this sense may be considered an incurable disease. These considerations should engender a healthy respect for the risks of radiation therapy. Unnecessary radiation should be avoided since this dread complication is more easily avoided than treated.

Specific treatment of chronic enteritis must focus on two separate circumstances: treatment of the symptomatic patient and precautions to be taken in the previously irradiated patient who requires abdominal surgery.

Symptomatic patients usually complain of crampy abdominal pain and diarrhea.[13] Pain may be due to fibrotic obstruction or hyperperistalsis. While ischemia is a prominent component of this abnormality, surgically correctable, large vessel ischemia is not a major consideration. Treatment of abdominal pain should be expectant and symptomatic unless physical findings or X-rays demonstrate findings of an acute surgical problem, e.g. peritonitis, free intraabdominal air, etc.[14] Agents which discoordinate intestinal motility, such as opiates, may decrease crampy abdominal pain, but more important, seem to improve intestinal absorption by prolonging contact time. Narcotic addiction should be avoided when possible, but must be considered in the context of an otherwise incurable and very symptomatic disease.

Diarrhea may be multifactorial in nature. Loss of absorptive surface, bacterial overgrowth, and intermittent obstruction may all contribute and should be investigated by standard techniques. Bile salt malabsorption with stimulation of the colon may be a realistic consideration in the presence of ileal involvement and may be amenable to treatment. Oral cholestyramine (one 4g packet four times daily) effectively binds bile salts and offers significant relief from symptoms in some patients. Bacterial overgrowth, identified by quantitative colony counts greater than 10^8 organisms per ml of small bowel contents, can be treated by the intermittent administration of oral antibiotics, particularly directed at anaerobic organisms. The identification of B_{12} malabsorption correctable by oral antibiotics (tetracycline or erythromycin) strengthens the clinical diagnosis, especially when elevated folate levels, from absorption of bacteria-produced folate, can be demonstrated.

Much attention has been directed to the use of steroids for chronic radiation proctitis. Data are controversial and, in general, systemic steroids should be avoided because of the increased catabolic effect and impaired wound healing which result. In patients with rectal involvement, however, particularly when chronic bleeding is the major clinical problem, a trial of steroid enemas, taken at bedtime and retained for as long as possible, seems reasonable and should be continued for at least a month. Objective sigmoidoscopic improvement and subjective relief of symptoms should encourage continued usage, preferably for intermittent courses of therapy separated by rest periods.

Systemic steroids plus azulfidine have been recommended in small, uncontrolled trials.[15] Confirmatory evidence is lacking and wholehearted acceptance should be discouraged. In a very symptomatic and otherwise unmanageable patient, however, a trial for a prescribed period may be justifiable. Newer medications[16] and combinations will certainly be tried and may be of benefit in selected patients.

Surgery in the previously irradiated abdomen challenges the ingenuity and the confidence of even the best technical surgeon. In this arena, intestinal ischemia seems to represent the major limiting factor and often is refractory to any therapeutic intervention. Intestinal anastomoses frequently fail because of inadequate blood supply, resulting in recurrent abscesses, fistulae, and ultimately death. These fistulae are notoriously refractory to nonoperative healing, even with maximal nutritional support. Again, avoidance of surgery unless clearly indicated seems to be a healthy attitude.

Frequently, however, operation cannot be avoided. When this is the case, several points should be kept in mind.[17,18] Only irradiated tissue is liable to radiation damage. Abdominal incisions should be placed outside of radiated areas whenever possible. The smallest operation compatible with successful resolution of the problem should be attempted.[19] Intestinal anastomoses should be avoided whenever possible because of the high failure rate. When necessary, at least one segment of the anastomosis should be healthy, uninvolved intestine. It is preferable to do anastomoses between two normal segments of bowel. Since rectosigmoid involvement is almost universal, end sigmoid colostomy is frequently necessary.[20] While low anastomoses in the pelvis can be accomplished technically, a high failure rate can be expected.[21] A failed low rectal anastomosis involving irradiated bowel usually results in pelvic abscess and/or fistula and requires proximal colonic diversion by colostomy. A well placed colostomy is much easier to care for than a poorly placed fistula and as an initial procedure is frequently preferable to the risk of anastomosis.

While diffuse adhesions are commonly found, extensive enterolysis is not only unsuccessful in many cases, but also may be detrimental. Collateral blood supply, once interrupted, may prove to be the difference between integrity of a segment of bowel and disaster. A specific, limited plan should be designed before embarking on an adventure into obstructed, radiated bowel. Localized segments of involvement should be bypassed or resected *in toto*. Overzealous intestinal resection, however, will only aggravate the malabsorption and diarrhea which already frequently exist.

When surgery is being considered for treatment of obstructive symptoms, preoperative barium studies are essential. In particular, the rectosigmoid area needs to be examined carefully. Areas of narrowing, while not totally obstructing, can cause functional obstruction which may be otherwise unrecognized and be left untreated by an approach to the small intestine only.

Rectovaginal fistulae represent a common yet difficult surgical problem, particularly after combined internal and external radiation for pelvic malignancy. A high failure rate must be anticipated from the outset. In the high risk patient, a totally diverting colostomy is frequently preferable both to the surgeon and to the properly informed patient. In the younger patient, or in patients for whom colostomy is unacceptable, a direct surgical approach may be unavoidable. Attempts at repair per vagina are usually unsuccessful because of the difficulty in separating the resultant rectal and vaginal closures by distance or normal interposed tissue. While this is usually a safe approach and may be indicated as an initial effort at repair, a very high failure rate should be expected.

A trans-sacral approach to the fistula, while providing improved exposure over the vaginal approach and avoiding the need to traverse the abdominal cavity, is still limited by the inability to anatomically separate the resultant suture lines. In addition, the posterior skin closure, notoriously difficult to heal in normal tissue, is further jeopardized by the radiation changes in the skin and soft tissues of the posterior pelvis. This approach should be avoided in the treatment of radiation induced problems.

The currently recommended procedure for repair of rectovaginal fistulas following radiation involves a transabdominal approach combined with synchronous vaginal closure. This allows the interposition of the omentum between the rectum and vagina providing a mechanical barrier to recurrent fistulization and also brings healthy, vascularized tissue into the area. This approach frequently requires extensive adhesiolysis of the small intestine, however, and may result in devascularization of previously marginal areas of bowel with subsequent intestinal fistulae or intraabdominal abscesses.

If the combined abdominovaginal approach is chosen, the tenets of surgery in the irradiated abdomen must be heeded. Operations should be as simple as possible with minimal dissection, and anastomosis should preferably introduce a healthy, well vascularized segment of intestine. An interesting approach to this situation involves division of the proximal colon, above the level of radiation exposure.[22] The distal sigmoid colon is folded over and anastomosed to the defect in the anterior rectal wall. This brings healthy tissue with its normal blood supply into the area and seems to lessen the risk of anastomotic failure. The result is a circle or loop of colon in the pelvis. Proximal diversion by end colostomy is followed after an appropriate interval by taking down the colostomy and performing an anastomosis in an end-to-side fashion to the presenting portion of the previously constructed loop. Alternatively, this anastomosis can be constructed at the initial procedure with proximal diversion by a loop transverse colostomy. While our experience with either technique is limited, it would seem that total colonic diversion is preferable in this situation and, in addition, in case of failure of the pelvic anastomosis or a change of heart by the patient, an end sigmoid colostomy provides a better permanent stoma.

Operative Adjuncts

When surgery is unavoidable in the patient with previous pelvic radiation and resultant enterocolonic complications, attempts must be made to optimize risks in the pre-, intra-, and postoperative period. Optimum nutrition is a necessary prerequisite and, if deficiencies are identified by standard assessment criteria (weight loss; depressed serum albumin or transferrin levels; decreased triceps skin fold thickness, creatinine height index, or total peripheral lymphocyte count) elective surgery should be postponed until vigorous replacement therapy results in normalization. This should be accomplished enterally, when possible, by oral supplements or nasogastric tube feeding, but this may not be possible if gastrointestinal symptoms have been a major or limiting factor. If not possible, a week to ten days of preoperative parenteral nutrition should be provided using currently acceptable techniques. In either case, nutritional deficits should be corrected before surgery is undertaken. The increased complication rate seen after surgery in malnourished patients only compounds the previously described failure rate of surgery in the presence of irradiated bowel.

Careful attention to concomitant cardiac, pulmonary, renal, and hematologic abnormalities preoperatively may minimize postoperative risks. These are particularly likely in patients who have also received multidrug chemotherapy. Specific efforts should be taken to identify abnormalities by appropriate radiologic and biochemical tests. Therapy should be initiated to optimize pulmonary function by physical therapy, nutritional replenishment, and cessation of smoking; cardiac function by pharmacologic intervention; and hematologic parameters by the availability of necessary blood components to correct deficiencies of the formed elements of the blood or clotting factors.

Patients may be identified in whom surgery, while seemingly essential, is precluded by an excessive operative risk. Long-term parenteral nutrition[23,24] has been used effectively in this setting and may postpone or totally circumvent surgical intervention. Inadvertent operative injury to the intestine and colon is common and should be anticipated, even if intestinal procedures are not planned. A formal mechanical bowel prep with supplemental enteral antibiotics to decrease aerobic and anaerobic flora (e.g. aminoglycoside plus erythromycin or metronidozole) will not only be helpful in colonic surgery but may also yield benefits when bacterial overgrowth complicates small intestinal abnormalities. Prophylactic systemic antibiotics, while currently the subject of controversy among surgeons, seem particularly appropriate in this high risk situation. An agent should be chosen which is nontoxic and covers the expected organisms. Currently, the advanced generation cephalosporins seem to be the most appropriate although the recent availability of parenteral metronidazole may have a place in anaerobic coverage.

Careful preoperative consideration of the placement of surgical incisions to avoid creating nonviable abdominal wall segments yet allow adequate, generous exposure is essential. Anticipation of possible colostomy and identification of the most appropriate site by the surgeon or enterostomal therapist before surgery will identify potential stomal difficulties and facilitate subsequent patient adjustment should colostomy be necessary. Skin areas subjected to prior radiation should be identified and avoided if possible. Intraoperative adjuncts would ideally identify well vascularized segments and allow complication-free anastomosis and minimize the amount of resected bowel. It is hoped that prospective studies using the Doppler ultrasound devices and intravenous fluorescein will determine whether these techniques will be helpful.

Radiated microcirculation is an enemy to good hemostasis, resulting in broad oozing surfaces which cannot be controlled by suture or clamps. Electrocautery and topical agents such as thrombin, regenerated cellulose, and microfibrillar collagen should be used to provide complete hemostasis and avoid postoperative intraabdominal or pelvic collections of blood. The time spent in securing hemostasis should be rewarded by fewer postoperative intraabdominal complications.

An appropriate route for maintenance of nutrition should be established before completion of the procedure. Small jejunostomy feeding catheters should be used when this can be done safely. However, if enteral feeding is hazardous because of anastomoses, multiple denuded areas, or concern about viability, intravenous nutrition should be continued postoperatively.

Safe, conservative techniques should be employed whenever possible. The previously irradiated abdomen is no place for surgical creativity or shortcuts. Attention to intraoperative detail and anticipation of possible postoperative complications is essential.

Summary

Chronic radiation enteritis can be expected to be a significant clinical problem in 5–20% of patients receiving pelvic radiation. Surgical intervention in this setting is hazardous and fraught with postoperative complications. The problem is serious enough that adjuvant radiation therapy should be avoided unless specifically indicated. Efforts to protect the intestine when radiation is deemed essential may minimize late radiation sequelae and may merit selective application.[25] No radiation means no radiation enteritis.

In the patient who has incapacitating symptoms or complications of radiation enteritis, surgery may not be avoidable. Recognition of the vascular effects of radiation damage, i.e. obliterative endarteritis, is essential if postoperative complications are to be avoided. Careful preparation of the patient and attention to detail can minimize these risks.

While fibrosis and endarteritis are the primary lesions of chronic radiation damage, it is the ischemia resulting from the vascular injury which is most important to the abdominal surgeon. Intestinal resections and anastomoses should be avoided when possible and should incorporate healthy segments of bowel when unavoidable. An awareness of potential radiation damage and a healthy respect for irradiated tissues improve the likelihood of a successful outcome.

References

1. Morley GW, Seski JC: Radical pelvic surgery versus radiation therapy for stage I carcinoma of the cervix (exclusive of microinvasion). *Am J Obstet Gynecol* 126:785, 1976.
2. Jimenez JA, Beldarrain L, Montalvo J, Roca C: Complications from irradiation of carcinoma of the uterine cervix. *Acta Radiologica Oncology* 19:13, 1980.
3. Bosch A, Frias Z: Complications after radiation therapy for cervical carcinoma. *Acta Radiologica Therapy Physics Biology* 16:53, 1977.
4. Ozarda AT, Shahbazian A. The complications of full-pelvic irradiation with particular emphasis to external beam therapy. *Radiologia Clin* 46:221, 1977.
5. Duggan FJ, Sanford EJ, Rohner TJ: Radiation enteritis following radiotherapy for prostatic carcinoma. *Br J Urology* 47:441, 1975.
6. Donaldson SS, Jundt S, Rigour C, et al: Radiation enteritis in children. A retrospective review, clinicopathologic correlation, and dietary management. *Cancer* 35:1167, 1975.
7. Dirksen PK, Matolo NM, Trelford JD: Complications following operation in the previously irradiated abdominopelvic cavity. *The Amer Surgeon* Pg 234, April 1977.

8. Kinsella TJ, Bloomer WD: Tolerance of the intestine to radiation therapy. *Surg Gynecol Obstet* 151:273, 1980.
9. Burbige EJ, Tarder GL, Belber JP: Malabsorption following radiation therapy. *Am J Gastroenterology* 67:589, 1977.
10. Greenwald R, Barkin JS, et al: Cancer of the colon as a late sequel of pelvic irradiation. *Am J Gastroenterology* 69:196, 1978.
11. Stein RS: Radiation-recall enteritis after actinomycin-D and adriamycin therapy. *Southern Med J* 71:960, 1978.
12. Reichelderfer M, Morrissey JF: Colonoscopy in radiation colitis. *Gastrointest Endoscopy* 26:41, 1980.
13. Cunningham IGE: The management of radiation proctitis. *Aust N Z J Surg* 50:172, 1980.
14. Smith JS, Milford HE: Management of colitis caused by irradiation. *Surg Gynecol Obstet* 142:569, 1976.
15. Goldstein F, Khoury J, Thornton JJ: Treatment of chronic radiation enteritis and colitis with salicylazosulfapyridine and systemic corticosteroids. *Am J Gastroent* 65:201, 1976.
16. Edsmyr F, Huber W, Menander KB: Orgotein efficacy in ameliorating side effects due to radiation therapy. *Curr Therapeutic Res* 19:198, 1976.
17. Stuart M, Failes DG, Killingback MJ, DeLuca C: Irradiation injuries of the large intestine. *Dis Col & Rect* 23:94, 1980.
18. Palmer JA, Bush RS: Radiation injuries to the bowel associated with the treatment of carcinoma of the cervix. *Surgery* 80:458, 1976.
19. Schmitt EG, Symmonds RE: Surgical treatment of radiation induced injuries of the intestine. *Surg Gynecol Obstet* 153:896, 1981.
20. Russell JC, Welch JP: Operative management of radiation injuries of the intestinal tract. *Am J Surg* 137:433, 1979.
21. Anseline PF, Lavery IC, Fazio VW, et al: Radiation injury of the rectum—Evaluation of surgical treatment. *Ann Surg* 194:716, 1981.
22. Bricker EM, Johnston WD: Repair of postirradiation rectovaginal fistula and stricture. *Surg Gynecol Obstet* 148:499, 1979.
23. Lavery IC, Steiger E, Fazio VW: Home parenteral nutrition in management of patients with severe radiation enteritis. *Dis Col & Rect* 23:91, 1980.

24. Miller DG, Ivey M, Young J: Home parenteral nutrition in treatment of severe radiation enteritis. *Ann Int Med* 91:858, 1979.
25. Freund H, Gunderson L, Krause R, Fischer JE: Prevention of radiation enteritis after abdominoperineal resection and radiotherapy. *Surg Gynecol Obstet* 149:206, 1979.

18

Acute Mesenteric Vascular Insufficiency in the Absence of Occlusive Vascular Disease

John M. Stang, M.D.

Introduction and Definition of the Syndrome

Of all vascular disorders of the gastrointestinal tract, the most poorly understood is probably nonocclusive mesenteric vascular insufficiency. This clinical syndrome, known by many other names including the eponym Wilson-Qualheim Syndrome, may be defined as intestinal or colonic ischemia due to functional vascular insufficiency when fixed obstructive lesions cannot be demonstrated and when vasospasm is the presumed mechanism. In effect, this syndrome is Prinzmetal's variant angina of the bowel.

Most of the work in this highly specialized area has been done by one group of investigators, Dr. Scott J. Boley and his colleagues at the Montefiore Hospital and Medical Center in New York.[1–3] Either very little[4,5] or nothing[6] is found in textbooks of cardiovascular medicine, and equally little in the textbooks of surgery.[7]

Incidence

The annual incidence of mesenteric infarction is approximately one in 100,000, or one in 1,000 hospital admissions.[8] Hemorrhagic necrosis of the mucosa of the intestine in the presence of hypotension was probably recognized in the early 19th Century, but it was not until the reports of Wilson and Qualheim[9] and then Ende[10] that the clinical significance of these lesions was known. Nonocclusive mesenteric ischemia contributing to intestinal infarction was believed to occur in approximately one patient in 10 in 1958, and most reports over the next 10–15 years did not much change this incidence.[11–26] Pierce and Brockenbrough[27] suggested that the incidence of nonocclusive ischemic disease was closer to 50%. Boley et al[1] suggested that vasospasm was an important cause of mesenteric vascular insufficiency and described an "aggressive approach."[28,29] They emphasized a 50% incidence of nonocclusive forms of mesenteric vascular insufficiency amongst all forms of mesenteric ischemia and advocated early angiographic investigation of elderly patients with cardiovascular disease who develop abdominal pain, stressing the importance of identification of mesenteric vasospasm which they treated with local infusions of papaverine.[2,3,28,29] In fact, the incidence of vasospastic nonocclusive mesenteric insufficiency in their own series was 15 of 50 patients studied with this diagnosis in mind (incidence = 30%), or 15 of 35 patients ultimately shown to have mesenteric ischemia (incidence = 43%).[29]

Because most hospitals do not employ this aggressive approach, the overall incidence is difficult to estimate. In other reports, the incidence of nonocclusive ischemia is 10%,[30] or even as low as zero.[31] In a group of 32 patients on mechanical ventilators for primary respiratory therapy who required urgent surgical consultation because of gastrointestinal bleeding, abdominal distension, or signs of peritonitis, two patients were thought to have nonocclusive mesenteric vascular insufficiency,[32] although it is not clear how this diagnosis was substantiated. Of perhaps greater importance is the concept that vasospasm plays a role even in patients with a clear-cut obstructive phenomenon such as superior mesenteric arterial thrombosis or embolism, and that therapy should be directed specifically against this component in combination with specific surgical measures.[2,3,28,29]

Etiology

Mesenteric vascular insufficiency may result from a reduction in blood flow, a redistribution of flow, or a combination of the two.[2]

Specifically, the cause of this syndrome may be viewed as a combination of at least three factors and perhaps a fourth.

- Old age seems a prerequisite, perhaps because of an age-related tortuosity of mesenteric blood vessels[33] or perhaps simply because of the underlying subtle atherosclerotic disease common in elderly patients, upon which vasospasm might be superimposed.
- Virtually all such patients have had cardiovascular disease that may cause reduced cardiac output. The mesenteric circulation normally receives more than 20% of the cardiac output, and reductions bring about mesenteric vasoconstriction in response to the customary adrenergic reflex. The mesenteric circulation does employ an efficient autoregulatory mechanism, but this typically fails at arteriolar pressures less than 60–65 mm Hg.[1] The vasospastic response may occur as a delayed phenomenon, explaining the apparent paradox of delayed mesenteric ischemia after correction of a low-output episode.[3] The effects of established vasoconstriction include local hypoxia and tissue injury followed by extravasation of blood, hypovolemia, and impaired mucosal absorption permitting sepsis and toxemia so that the process becomes self-perpetuating.

- The third factor apparently operative in a majority of these patients is the role of digitalis, a well known vasoconstrictor in the mesenteric circulation.[34] This helps to explain the occurrence of the syndrome in patients with congestive heart failure.
- Frank hypovolemia or hypotensive shock is normally accompanied by a vasoconstrictor response in the mesenteric circulation. Apparently, some patients suffer either persistence of this phenomenon after other factors are corrected, or such an exaggeration of this otherwise physiologic response that mesenteric ischemia becomes a predominant pathologic feature of the illness. Boley himself stresses that angiographic studies should not be performed in patients either receiving vasopressors or patients in frank shock, since vasospasm in these circumstances is impossible to interpret. One would expect a decrease in the incidence of nonocclusive mesenteric ischemia in patients treated with vasoactive agents, as the use of dopamine and dobutamine completely replaces the use of levarterenol. Both of the former agents are known to have relatively more beneficial actions on the splanchnic circulation.[35]

Obviously, additional miscellaneous causes will exist in selected patients, for example, the aortoiliac steal phenomenon[36] and ergotism.[37]

Clinical Presentation

Clearly, establishing the diagnosis begins with heightened suspicion in patients with the etiologic precursors. In these patients, the principal clue is abdominal pain which occurs in 75–98% of patients.[2,3] Pain will vary considerably in severity, character, and location, but Boley stressed that any pain severe enough to prompt a call to a physician warrants consideration of the diagnosis of mesenteric ischemia. Disparity between the severity of pain and the meagerness of abdominal findings is emphasized. In nonocclusive mesenteric ischemia, the acute pain is not accompanied by a defecatory urge, unlike that experienced by patients with embolic occlusion of the superior mesenteric artery.

In the absence of pain, other signs may include unexplained abdominal distention, gastrointestinal bleeding, or diarrhea in patients who have progressed closer to impending bowel necrosis. In these patients, signs of peritonitis may be present. Clearly, the goal is to establish the diagnosis early.

Laboratory diagnosis is not conclusive. The leucocytosis of superior mesenteric arterial embolic occlusion may be much less striking in patients with nonocclusive disease.

Angiographic Diagnosis

The approach advocated by Boley and colleagues is to perform early angiography in all acutely ill patients who fit the foregoing description, and the single significant indication may be unexplained abdominal pain. Alternative diagnoses to mesenteric ischemia were also established by this approach.[29] In 15 patients, alternative diagnoses included colonic neoplasm, colonic ischemia, small bowel obstruction, ruptured aortic aneurysm, splenic and renal arterial emboli, diverticulitis, perforated appendicitis, and diabetes mellitus. In 1974, Boley and colleagues summarized the following four criteria for mesenteric vasospasm.[2,38]

- Narrowing at the origins of multiple branches of the superior mesenteric artery.
- Irregularities in intestinal branches.
- Spasm of arcades.
- Impaired filling of intramural vessels.

When mesenteric vasospasm is demonstrated in the presence of mesenteric ischemia, Boley recommends leaving the superior mesenteric arterial catheter in place for local pharmacotherapy.[3]

Combined Pharmacologic and Surgical Therapy

When the diagnosis of mesenteric ischemia has been established and other causes excluded by various diagnostic measures including angiography, treatment of the patient hinges on the presence or absence of an obstructive lesion and the presence or absence of peritonitis. Boley divided these patients into four subsets, although an infusion of papaverine through the angiography catheter is recommended for all four types of patients.[3]

Papaverine affects both cardiac and smooth muscle and relaxes the smooth muscles especially of larger arteries, particularly if spasm is present. This direct action is independent of muscle innervation. Coronary arteries are dilated as well as the mesenteric circulation, making this a safe drug if systemic effects occur. Its effects on the cerebral circulation are also well known. The hepatic metabolism of this drug and direct administration into the splanchnic circulation considerably diminish possible systemic effects. Its action is thought to occur by inhibition of phosphodiesterase, thereby increasing cylic AMP, the modulator of vascular smooth muscle relaxation.[2] Papaverine infusions using a constant infusion pump are continued for 24-hour periods at doses of 30–60 mg per hour. The drug is usually diluted in saline to a concentration of 1 mg per cc. Heparin is not used. Small 25 mg doses of tolazoline are often used during the angiographic procedure to improve angiographic visualization as well as to predict the response to papaverine.

When used as the primary treatment for nonocclusive mesenteric insufficiency, a 24-hour infusion of papaverine is followed by repeat angiography performed 30 minutes after changing the infusion to normal saline. Based on the response of the vasoconstriction, the infusion is either discontinued or continued for up to as long as five days.

The decision to perform a surgical procedure in conjunction with vasodilator therapy for nonocclusive mesenteric ischemia is totally dependent upon the presence of peritoneal signs and suspicion of bowel necrosis.

Additional therapy in such patients includes nasogastric suction, aggressive volume resuscitation as necessary, local and systemic antibiotics as indicated, and strict avoidance of digitalis preparations. Improvement of cardiac output and treatment of cardiac dysrhythmia, if these are present, are paramount, and may include simultaneous administration of positive inotropic agents (dopamine or dobutamine as previously discussed) along with a papaverine selective infusion.

Few studies other than those of Boley and colleagues deal with papaverine and its effect on the mesenteric circulation[39,40] and some fail to confirm the angiographic findings indicative of vasospasm.[40] Williams and Wilson have attempted to develop radioisotopic techniques for evaluation of submucosal blood flow.[41] Studies examining alternative vasodilators are also limited,[39] and may be expected to examine in the near future the efficacy of new vasodilators such as calcium-blocking agents. One study examines the use of thrombolytic agents in this setting.[42]

Mortality

The mortality of this type of mesenteric ischemia has been reported in the past to be over 90%.[8] The improved results of Boley and colleagues appear to recommend their "aggressive approach."[2,29] Of 15 patients with nonocclusive mesenteric ischemia, five had no peritoneal signs and all survived without operation. Seven of 10 patients with peritoneal signs underwent operation and all seven had gangrenous bowel. In two of these the involvement was too extensive for resection. The other five underwent resection, and two survived. Three with peritoneal signs did not undergo the operation; one died before it could be done, and the other two improved with selective vasodilator therapy. The overall mortality for the group of 15 patients was six of 15 or 40%.

Perspective

Acute nonocclusive mesenteric vascular insufficiency can be described as an emergency illness of elderly patients with heart disease, probably under treatment with digitalis. The exact incidence of this disorder is difficult to ascertain. The special experience of a few investigators is most provocative. Their apparent excellent results should provoke at least a greatly heightened awareness of vasospastic bowel disease in elderly cardiac patients who have abdominal pain.

The optimum treatment for such patients requires more confirmatory studies, investigation of alternative diagnostic techniques to urgent angiography, and exploration of other available vasodilating substances if vasospasm is truly the responsible factor. A recent editorial comment mentions the possible role of prostaglandin E_1.[43]

It is possible that the entity so precisely described by Boley et al. is already decreasing in frequency not only because of the altered use of digitalis in the elderly in recent years, but also because of improved treatment of the primary myocardial low output state by systemic positive inotropic or vasodilator agents.

References

1. Williams LF Jr, Kim J-P: Nonocclusive mesenteric ischemia. In *Vascular Disorders of the Intestine.* Boley SJ, Schwartz SJ, Williams LF Jr, (Eds.) Appleton-Century-Crofts, New York 1971; Ch 33, pp 519–30.

2. Boley SJ, Brandt LJ, Veith FJ: Ischemic disorders of the intestines. *Curr Prob Surg* 15:1, 1978.
3. Boley SJ: Early diagnosis of acute mesenteric ischemia. *Hospital Practice* 16:63, 1981.
4. Isselbacher KJ, Adams RD, Braunwald E, Petersdorf RG, Wilson JD, (Eds.) *Harrison's Principles of Internal Medicine.* Ninth Ed. McGraw-Hill, New York 1980, pp 1416, 1438–9.
5. Braunwald E, (Ed.) *Heart Disease. A Textbook of Cardiovascular Medicine.* WB Saunders, Philadelphia 1980, p 522.
6. Rubenstein E, Federman DD, (Eds.) *Scientific American Medicine.* Scientific American, Inc., New York 1981.
7. Schwartz SI, Shires GT, Spencer FC, Storer EH (Eds.) *Principles of Surgery.* Third Ed. McGraw-Hill, New York 1979, p 1439.
8. Ottinger LW, Austen WG: A study of 136 patients with mesenteric infarction. *Surg Gynecol Obstet* 124:251, 1967.
9. Wilson R, Qualheim RE: A form of acute hemorrhagic enterocolitis affecting chronically ill individuals. *Gastroenterology* 27:431, 1954.
10. Ende N: Infarction of the bowel in cardiac failure. *N Engl J Med* 258:879, 1958.
11. Katz AM: Hemorrhagic duodenitis in myocardial infarction. *Ann Intern Med* 51:212, 1959.
12. Ming S, Levitan R: Acute hemorrhagic necrosis of the gastrointestinal tract. *N Engl J Med* 263:59, 1960.
13. Berger RL, Byrne JJ: Intestinal gangrene associated with heart disease. *Surg Gynecol Obstet* 112:529, 1961.
14. Gooding RA, Couch RD: Mesenteric ischemia without vascular occlusion. *Arch Surg* 85:186, 1962.
15. Bachrach WH, Thorner MC: Hemorrhagic enteropathy complicating myocardial infarction. *Am J Cardiol* 11:89, 1963.
16. Boley SJ, Schwartz S, Lash J, Sternhill V: Reversible vascular occlusion of the colon. *Surg Gynecol Obstet* 116:53, 1963.
17. Drucker WR, Davis JH, Holden WD, Reagan JR: Hemorrhagic necrosis of the intestine. *Arch Surg* 89:42, 1964.
18. Heer FW, Silen W, French SW: Intestinal gangrene without apparent vascular occlusion. *Am J Surg* 110:231, 1965.
19. Kligerman MJ, Vidone RA: Intestinal infarction in the absence of occlusive mesenteric vascular disease. *Am J Cardiol* 16:562, 1965.

20. Ming S-C: Hemorrhagic necrosis of the gastrointestinal tract and its relation to cardiovascular status. *Circulation* 32:332, 1965.
21. Musa BU: Intestinal infarction without mesenteric vascular occlusion. *Ann Intern Med* 63:783, 1965.
22. Fogarty TJ, Fletcher WS: Genesis of nonocclusive mesenteric ischemia. *Am J Surg* 111:130, 1966.
23. Bhagwat AG, Hawk WA: Hemorrhagic necrotizing enteropathy. *Am J Gastroenterol* 45:163, 1966.
24. Williams LF Jr, Anastasia LF, Hasiotis CA, et al: Nonocclusive mesenteric infarction. *Am J Surg* 114:376, 1967.
25. Sorensen FH, Vetner M: Hemorrhagic mucosal necrosis of the gastrointestinal tract without vascular occlusion. *Acta Chir Scand* 135:439, 1969.
26. Renton CJC: Nonocclusion intestinal infarction. *Clin Gastroenterol* 1:655, 1972.
27. Pierce GE, Brockenbrough EC: The spectrum of mesenteric infarction. *Am J Surg* 119:233, 1970.
28. Boley SJ, Sprayregan S, Vieth FJ, Siegelman S: An aggressive roentgenological and surgical approach to acute mesenteric ischemia. In *Surgery Annual.* Nyhus LM (Ed.) Appleton-Century Crofts, New York 1973, pp 355–78.
29. Boley SJ, Sprayregan S, Siegelman SS, Vieth FJ: Initial results from an aggressive roentgenological and surgical approach to acute mesenteric ischemia. *Surgery* 82:848, 1977.
30. Hertzer NR, Beven EG, Humphries AW: Acute intestinal ischemia. *Am Surg* 44:744, 1978.
31. Singh RP, Lee STJ: Acute mesenteric vascular occlusion: A review of 40 cases. *Int Surg* 65:231, 1980.
32. Aranha GV, Goldberg NB: Surgical problems in patients on ventilators. *Crit Care Med* 9:478, 1981.
33. Binns JC, Isaacson P: Age-related changes in the colonic blood supply: their relevance to ischemic colitis. *Gut* 19:384, 1978.
34. Shanbour LL, Jacobson ED: Digitalis and mesenteric circulation. *Am J Dig Dis* 17:826, 1972. (Editorial)
35. Leier CV, Heban PT, Huss P, Bush CA, Lewis RP: Comparative systemic and regional hemodynamic effects of dopamine and dobutamine in patients with cardiomyopathic heart failure. *Circulation* 58:466, 1978.

36. Williams LF Jr, Kim RM, Tompkins W, Byrne JJ: Aortoiliac steal a cause of intestinal ischemia. *N Engl J Med* 278:777, 1968.
37. Greene FL, Ariyan S, Stansel HC Jr: Mesenteric and peripheral vascular ischemia secondary to ergotism. *Surgery* 81: 176, 1977.
38. Siegelman SS, Sprayregan S, Boley SJ: Angiographic diagnosis of mesenteric arterial vasoconstriction. *Radiology* 112: 533, 1974.
39. Williams RA, Wilson SE: Effect of intraarterial vasodilators on blood flow in ischemic dog colon. *Arch Surg* 115:602, 1980.
40. Bookstein JJ, Goldberger L, Niwayama G, Nader MJ, Brahme FJ, Jones TA: Angiographic aspects of experimental nonocclusive intestinal ischemic injury. *AJR* 128:923, 1977.
41. Williams RA, Wilson SE: Radioxenon washout for evaluation of vasodilator therapy in mesenteric ischemia. *Am J Gastroenterol* 73:408, 1980.
42. Gurll N, Zinner MJ, Turtine L, Reynolds DG: Vasodilation, fibrinolysis, and thrombolysis with intraarterial infusion of urokinases in the canine superior mesenteric artery. *Gastroenterology* 75:423, 1978.
43. Bynum TE, Jacobson ED: Nonocclusive intestinal ischemia. *Arch Intern Med* 139:281, 1979. (Editorial)

19

Systemic Vasculitis

Michael J. Luzar, M.D.

Intestinal ischemia is one of the life-threatening manifestations of systemic vasculitis. Inflammation in the blood vessel wall with narrowing and obstruction of the vessel lumen leads to ischemia in the area supplied. The incidence of involvement of the gastrointestinal tract varies among the forms of vasculitis. There are multiple classifications of this heterogeneous group of diseases; however, by classifying systemic vasculitides according to their relative importance in producing intestinal ischemia, three groups can be fairly well differentiated:

I. Common occurrence:
   - Polyarteritis nodosa
   - Hypersensitivity angiitis, especially Henoch-Schönlein purpura

II. Less common occurrence:
   - Allergic granulomatous angiitis of Churg and Strauss
   - Wegener's granulomatosis
   - Temporal (giant cell) arteritis

Vasculitis occurring in connective tissue diseases, such as systemic lupus erythematosus, rheumatoid arthritis, and dermatomyositis. (Discussed in Chapter on Connective Tissue Diseases.)
Miscellaneous vasculitides:
Mucocutaneous lymph node syndrome or Kawasaki's disease
Behçet's disease
Cogan's syndrome
Relapsing polychondritis with vasculitis

III. Rare occurrence:
Takayasu's arteritis
Lymphomatoid granulomatosis

The various vasculitides will be described, with special emphasis on those most prominent in producing intestinal ischemia.

Polyarteritis Nodosa

Intestinal vasculitis is a major cause of morbidity and mortality in polyarteritis nodosa (PAN), with the first report of necrotizing arteritis as a distinct entity appearing in 1866.[1]

Pathology

Lesions consist of focal and segmental areas of inflammation involving polymorphonuclear cells and mononuclear cells in medium sized and small vessels. There appears to be a predilection for branching points of vessels, and the entire thickness of the vessel wall is usually involved. Giant cells and granulomas are not seen. Lesions in different areas will reflect different stages of development. Fibrinoid necrosis is common, and the architecture of the vessel wall is severely disrupted. Fibrous scarring and proliferation of endothelial cells lead to vessel occlusion. There may be areas of aneurysmal dilatation at sites of severe lesions.

Autopsy studies have shown that any organ can be involved, but most commonly affected are the heart, kidney, gastrointestinal tract, and peripheral nerves. Less common sites are skeletal muscle, central nervous system, coronary arteries, genitourinary system, and skin. Pulmonary involvement is rare.

Clinical Manifestations

PAN is an uncommon disease, with an incidence of 0.2 per 100,000. The male-to-female ratio is about 1.5:1, and although any age can be affected, the disease is most common in the 40–60 year age range.

Since involvement can be so diffuse, the disease has a wide variety of clinical manifestations. Constitutional symptoms including fever, fatigue, anorexia, and weight loss are common. Arthralgias, and less commonly, arthritis, are not unusual. Skin lesions include nodular lesions along blood vessels, livedo reticularis (Figure 1), ulcerations, and digital ischemia. Involvement of the vasonervorum can lead to nerve infarction and sudden onset of foot drop or wrist drop. Cranial nerve involvement can occur. Other evidence of central nervous system involvement may be seizures, paresis, or paralysis. Coronary arteritis can cause chest pain, congestive heart failure, arrhythmias, or conduction problems. Renal involvement can lead to severe hypertension and renal insufficiency. Thirty percent of patients have a focal necrotizing glomerulitis contributing to renal failure, in which red blood cells and red blood cell casts may be seen, along with significant proteinuria. Renal insufficiency may be the cause of death in up to two-thirds of patients who die of PAN.

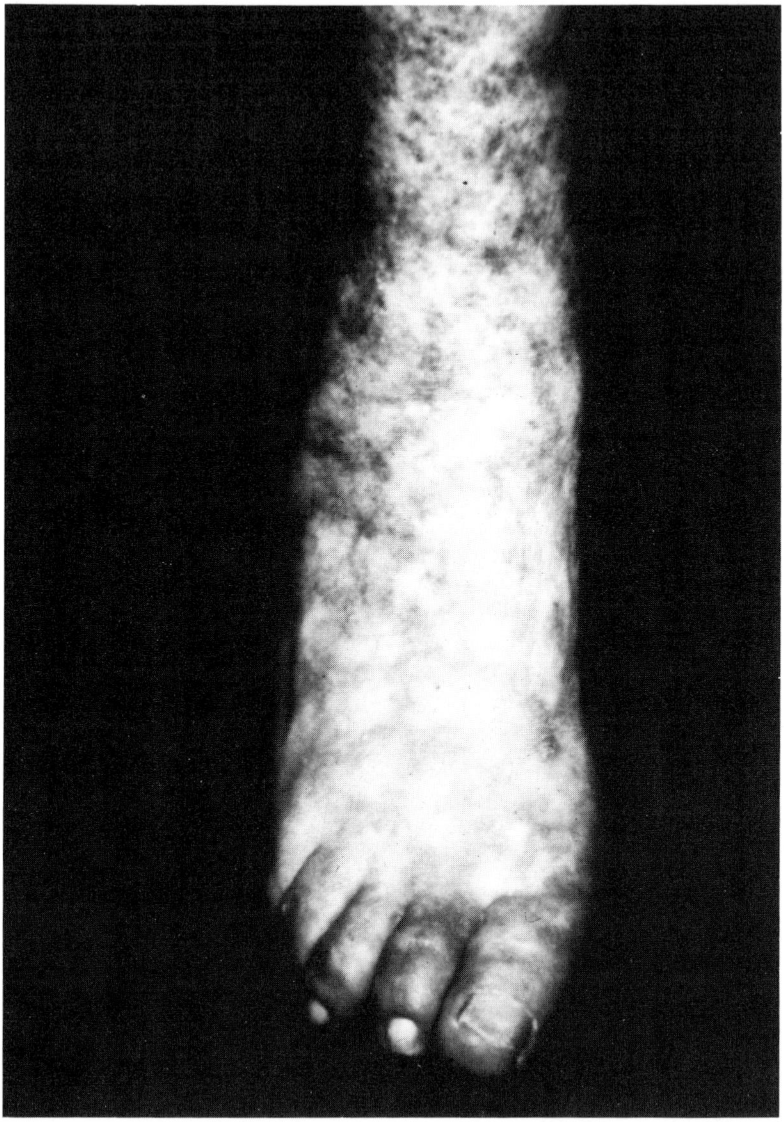

Figure 1. Polyarteritis nodosa. Livedo reticularis of the lower extremity in a patient with PAN.

Gastrointestinal Manifestations

The gastrointestinal tract is one of the most commonly involved areas in PAN.[2] The most common gastrointestinal symptom is abdominal pain. The location of abdominal pain often correlates with specific organ involvement, such as right upper quadrant pain with gallbladder vasculitis[3] or right lower quadrant pain with appendiceal vasculitis.[4] When diffuse abdominal pain is present, mesenteric vasculitis with or without perforation must be suspected.

Gastrointestinal involvement is as important as renal involvement in determining a poor prognosis. In a recent five-year study,[5] 25% of patients had gastrointestinal involvement, and catastrophic complications such as intestinal infarction, perforation, or bleeding occurred in 15%. Seventy-five percent of patients with catastrophic involvement died, and deaths attributable to gastrointestinal vasculitis equalled those attributable to renal insufficiency. In another series,[6] 11 of 17 patients (65%) had abdominal pain or diarrhea, and six of these required laparotomy.

Laboratory Procedures

No specific laboratory abnormality is diagnostic. Common findings include anemia from either chronic illness or blood loss secondary to gastrointestinal involvement, a reactive thrombocytosis from inflammation or bleeding, and leukocytosis. The sedimentation rate is usually elevated. The serum albumin is often low, and the gamma globulins are increased. Serum complement levels are usually elevated, since they act as acute phase reactants. In a minority of patients, the complement levels are decreased, reflecting immune complex activation of the complement cascade. Incidence of positive antinuclear antibodies does not appear to be increased, but low titers of rheumatoid factor are seen more often than in control groups.

The most striking advance in recent years has been the finding of hepatitis B antigen in 10–54% of patients with classic PAN.[7–10] Hepatitis B antigen-antibody complexes are unquestionably related to arteritis in a significant number of patients with PAN, and up to half of the patients who are hepatitis B-positive have abnormal liver function tests.

Diagnosis

Diagnosis rests on either pathologic confirmation by tissue examination or angiographic demonstration of vasculitis. Blind biopsies give a much lower yield than biopsies of clinically involved areas. A sural nerve biopsy will give the highest yield if there is a clinical mononeuritis multiplex or a peripheral neuropathy, a muscle biopsy if there is myopathy. In the proper clinical setting, the finding of a focal necrotizing glomerulitis may be helpful in substantiating the diagnosis.

Abdominal aortography with selective renal, celiac, or mesenteric angiography is very helpful in confirming a suspected diagnosis of PAN. Findings include abnormal variation in the size of vessels, such as beading or fusiform dilatation, complete blockage, or aneurysm formation (Figure 2). Aneurysms are especially frequent at bifurcations of vessels. In a recent series of 17 cases of suspected PAN, 14 were confirmed angiographically, 10 having aneurysms, while four had vasculitis but no aneurysms. Patients with aneurysms had more weight loss, higher blood pressure, and increased incidence of abdominal pain, cardiac involvement, and CNS involvement.[6]

Several conditions may angiographically mimic the multiple aneurysms of PAN, including left atrial myxoma,[11,12] Wegener's,[13] lupus,[14] and allergic granulomatosis of Churg and Strauss.[6] Coronary artery aneurysms have been seen in the mucocutaneous lymph node syndrome.[15] Oral and intravenous drug abusers can develop necrotizing angiitis

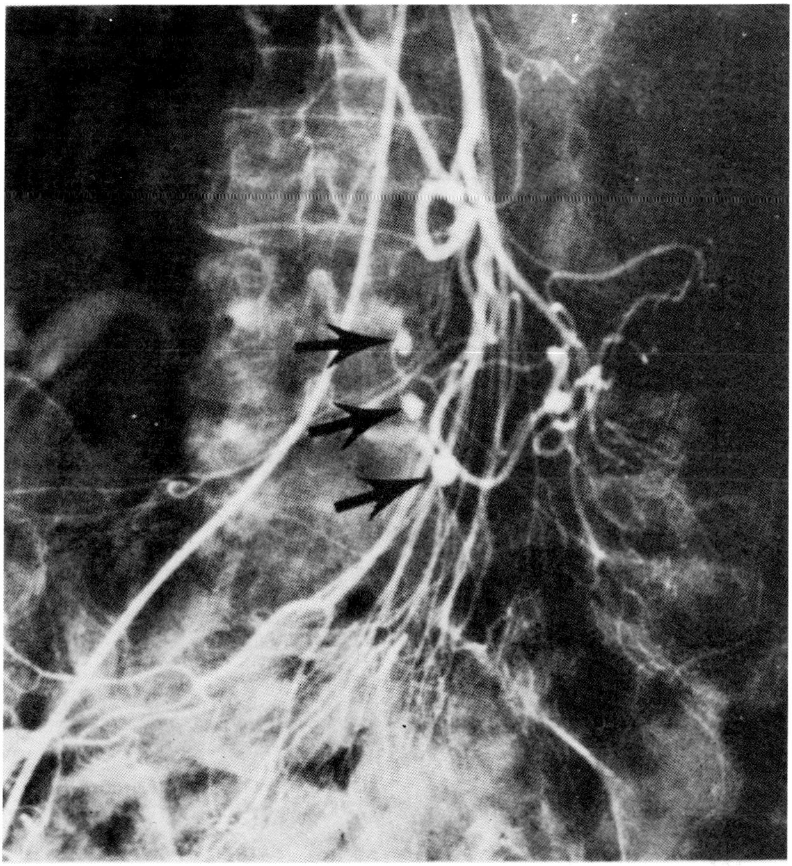

Figure 2. Polyarteritis nodosa. Aneurysms in branches of the superior mesenteric artery in PAN. (With permission from Kelly WN (Ed.) *Textbook of Rheumatology*. WB Saunders Co, Philadelphia 1981.)

indistinguishable from PAN, especially with amphetamine abuse, but it is unclear how many of these patients may also have hepatitis B infection causing a PAN picture. It is well documented that with control of the vasculitis, the aneurysms may resolve.[6,17] Rupture of aneurysms causing intestinal hemorrhage has been documented,[16] as has perirenal and intrahepatic hemorrhage.[6] Angiograms, as do biopsies, give the most precise information when clinical manifestations are present in the areas studied, but they may be positive, even if symptoms are absent.

Treatment

Treatment includes medication to suppress vascular inflammation and supportive measures depending on the areas of vascular damage. Untreated PAN showed a five-year survival of 13%, but with corticosteroid therapy, this increased to approximately 50%.[18] Recent reports suggest that the use of cytotoxic agents in addition to steroids further increases survival.[9,17,19] The usual dose of prednisone is 60 mg per day in divided doses. If oral medication is precluded, methylprednisolone sodium succinate (20 mg I.V. every 8 hours) can be given. Many believe that cytotoxic agents should be used initially along with prednisone, and cyclophosphamide (2–2.5 mg/kg/day) seems to give the most consistent response. However, owing to the multiple problems that accompany cyclophosphamide, such as bone marrow depression, bladder inflammation, increased risk of infection, and occasional occurrence of inappropriate ADH secretion, it should be used only by those familiar with these effects. As the disease comes under control, the prednisone can be gradually changed to a single daily dose and then further tapered over a period of months.

Steroid therapy may necessitate salt restriction, potassium supplements, close observation of blood sugar levels, and antacids to prevent gastritis. Vitamin D and calcium may be needed to retard steroid-induced osteoporosis. Opportunistic infections may occur with steroid or cytotoxic therapy. Symptoms of infection or a perforated viscus may be altered by the anti-inflammatory and immunosuppressive properties of the drugs used to treat PAN.

Additional measures may include medical treatment of hypertension or congestive heart failure, antibiotics for secondary infection of skin ulcers, or surgical intervention for severe visceral hemorrhage or intestinal necrosis.

Hypersensitivity Vasculitis

Not uncommonly, hypersensitivity vasculitis involves the gastrointestinal tract. The two forms most likely to be encountered are cryoglobulinemia and Henoch-Schönlein purpura. Hypersensitivity vasculitis (HV) has diverse causes, but the common factor is the predominate involvement of small vessels with polymorphonuclear infiltration and leukocytoclasis, that is, the presence of nuclear debris from degenerated polymorphonuclear leukocytes. Often, a precipitating antigen can be identified, such as a drug or an infectious agent. Drugs most commonly implicated are penicillin, sulfonamides, and phenylbutazone. Endogenous antigens such as tumor antigens have also been reported to act as sensitizing agents. Studies have shown various immunoglobulins and complement components deposited in the vessel walls of early lesions, strongly suggesting an immune complex-mediated mechanism.

Pathology

There is intense polymorphonuclear leukocytic infiltration of small blood vessels. Nuclear fragments from degenerated leukocytes are seen in perivascular areas. In the acute state, endothelial swelling occurs, often with fibrinoid necrosis of the vessel wall and extravasation of erythrocytes. Later, necrosis of connective tissue about the blood vessels becomes apparent. Different lesions at the same stage of development suggest episodic exposure to the inciting antigen. Immunofluorescent staining often demonstrates IgM, IgG, and C_3 in and around the vessel walls. Less commonly, IgA and fibrinogen are found. The earlier the lesion is biopsied, the greater is the opportunity to show positive immunofluorescence.

Clinical Manifestations

The skin is most frequently involved, exhibiting the classic lesions of palpable purpura.[20–24] Palpability of the lesions is extremely important, since this distinguishes vasculitis from noninflammatory causes of purpura, such as thrombocytopenia. Lesions are usually most prominent over dependent areas such as lower extremities, buttocks, and back, but can occur anywhere. The lesions of gonococcemia, meningococcemia, sepsis from gram-negative bacillae, and subacute bacterial endocarditis can all mimic HV to varying degrees.

Other manifestations[20–24] of HV include fever, weight loss, fatigue, and anorexia. Arthralgias are present in over half the patients, and frank synovitis can occur. Ischemia of the peripheral nerves may lead to a distal sensory or sensory-motor neuropathy. Central nervous system and cranial nerve involvement can occasionally occur. Pulmonary infiltrates, nodules and pleural effusions, pericarditis, and myocarditis have been reported. Renal vasculitis can lead to proteinuria, hematuria, and renal insufficiency. Abdominal pain is common and most often can be attributed to intestinal ischemia and bleeding.

Diagnosis

Diagnosis depends primarily on the clinical presentation, often limited to skin lesions, but at times including a multisystem illness with neurologic, pulmonary, renal, muscle, or gastrointestinal involvement. Skin biopsy will show the typical leukocytoclastic vasculitis. Sural nerve biopsy and nerve conduction studies may be abnormal with peripheral nerve involvement. Electromyograms may show a myopathic process with vasculitis of muscles, and elevated creatine phosphokinase will reflect muscle involvement. A muscle biopsy may be helpful in confirming hypersensitivity vasculitis when evidence of muscle abnormality is present. Barium studies may show evidence of mesenteric vasculitis if gastrointestinal bleeding or abdominal symptoms are present. Chest roentgenograms can be abnormal. Angiography is rarely helpful, since the vessels involved are too small to be visualized adequately.

Hypersensitivity vasculitis is a heterogeneous entity, and gastrointestinal manifestations are likeliest in two forms of the disease.

Cryoglobulinemia

Cryoglobulins are serum proteins, usually immunoglobulins, precipitated by exposure to cold.[25] A distinct clinical syndrome of essential mixed cryoglobulinemia is most common in middle-aged women.[26] The cryoprecipitate usually consists of an IgM immunoglobulin with antibody activity against another immunoglobulin, generally of the IgG class.[27] Recent studies[28] have stressed the finding of hepatitis B antigen or antibody in the serum or cryoprecipitate of over 50% of patients with essential mixed cryoglobulinemia; thus, the label, "essential," may be a misnomer. The classic symptoms include palpable purpura, arthralgias, glomerulonephritis, and extreme fatigue.

Gastrointestinal Manifestations

Intestinal vasculitis has been documented in essential mixed cryoglobulinemia. Episodes of severe abdominal pain occurred in 20% of cases in a large series.[26] At postmortem examination, five of nine patients had evidence of disseminated as well as gastrointestinal vasculitis. In one, diffuse vasculitis of the small and large bowel mucosa was responsible for terminal intestinal hemorrhage.[26] Another report documented intestinal vasculitis mimicking inflammatory bowel disease. The patient's symptoms occurred only in the winter.[29]

Laboratory

Cryoglobulins should be measured in all patients with leukocytoclastic vasculitis. Blood is drawn into a test tube warmed to 37° C without anticoagulant and allowed to clot in an incubator at 37° C. The clot is removed, then the sera spun in a centrifuge at 37° C to remove residual red blood cells. The sera is aspirated, placed immediately at 4° C for 48 to 72 hours, then examined for a cryoprecipitate. Assays for hepatitis B antigen and antibody should be done on the sera and cryoprecipitate due to the recent implication of hepatitis B infection in the pathogenesis of essential mixed cryoglobulinemia. Even if serologic tests for hepatitis B infection are negative in the sera, they may still be positive in the cryoprecipitate.

Other common laboratory abnormalities in cryoglobulinemia include anemia of chronic illness, elevated sedimentation rate, and frequently, low complement levels, since the mixed cryoglobulins act as immune complexes and fix complement. The rheumatoid factor test is often positive in a high titer due to the cryoglobulinemia.

Management

For severe progressive disease, including gastrointestinal vasculitis, steroids and cytotoxic agents should be used. In addition, plasmapheresis has been reported to be beneficial in removing large quantities of circulating cryoglobulins.[25,26] Presently, there are no controlled trials to evaluate therapeutic modalities.

Henoch-Schönlein Purpura

The hypersensitivity vasculitis with the most striking gastrointestinal involvement is Henoch-Schönlein (H-S) purpura. The arthritis and rash were first described by Schönlein in 1837, followed by Henoch's description of the gastrointestinal and renal manifestations in 1874. Anaphylactoid purpura is synonymous with H-S purpura.

Pathogenesis

Immunoglobulins and complement are detected by immunofluorescence in cutaneous vessels and the kidney. IgA is the most abundant and often the only immunoglobulin found in these areas. Serum complement levels are almost always normal. In addition, cases of H-S purpura with congenital absence of C_2 have been reported.[31,32] This and the frequent IgA deposits suggest that the alternate complement pathway is activated, and this has been confirmed in at least one series.[33] Other studies have shown circulating IgA immune complexes.[34,35] However, serum IgA levels, although often elevated, may be normal. The end result of these alterations is a typical leukocytoclastic vasculitis.

Clinical Manifestations

H-S purpura can occur at any age, but is primarily a disease of children with a peak age of onset between 4 and 11 years. There is a slightly greater incidence in males than in females. The most frequent time of onset is the spring, often after an upper respiratory or streptococcal infection. Pathologic changes are those of a typical leukocytoclastic vasculitis. The classic triad of palpable purpura, arthritis, and abdominal pain is present in 60-80% of the cases.

The most common of various rashes that have been described is the classic palpable purpura with a predominantly lower extremity distribution (Figure 3). The rash is usually of short duration, with 43 of 75 patients in one series having a rash less than six weeks.[36] There is no correlation between the severity or the duration of skin involvement and the prevalence or severity of systemic involvement.

Subcutaneous bleeding may occur in the scrotum, eyelids, or back. Edema of the feet and lower legs is common, while edema of the hands, scalp, and periorbital areas may occur. Edema is often due to blood vessel damage, but may be due to the nephrotic syndrome or protein-losing enteropathy.[36]

Arthritis most commonly involves the ankles and knees and is usually transient and nondeforming.[36]

Renal involvement occurs in over 40-50% of cases, is usually mild, but can be severe.[37,38] Renal lesions may vary from mild focal mesangial glomerulitis to diffuse proliferative and necrotizing glomerulonephritis. Immunofluorescence shows predominantly IgA in renal lesions.[39] The prognosis is determined primarily by the extent of renal involvement.[40]

Less common manifestations include pulmonary infiltrates, pleural rubs and effusions, hemoptysis, peripheral neuropathy, and rarely, central nervous system involvement.

Gastrointestinal Manifestations

Any segment of the gastrointestinal tract may be involved, although the jejunum and ileum are most commonly affected. Gastrointestinal vasculitis can cause se-

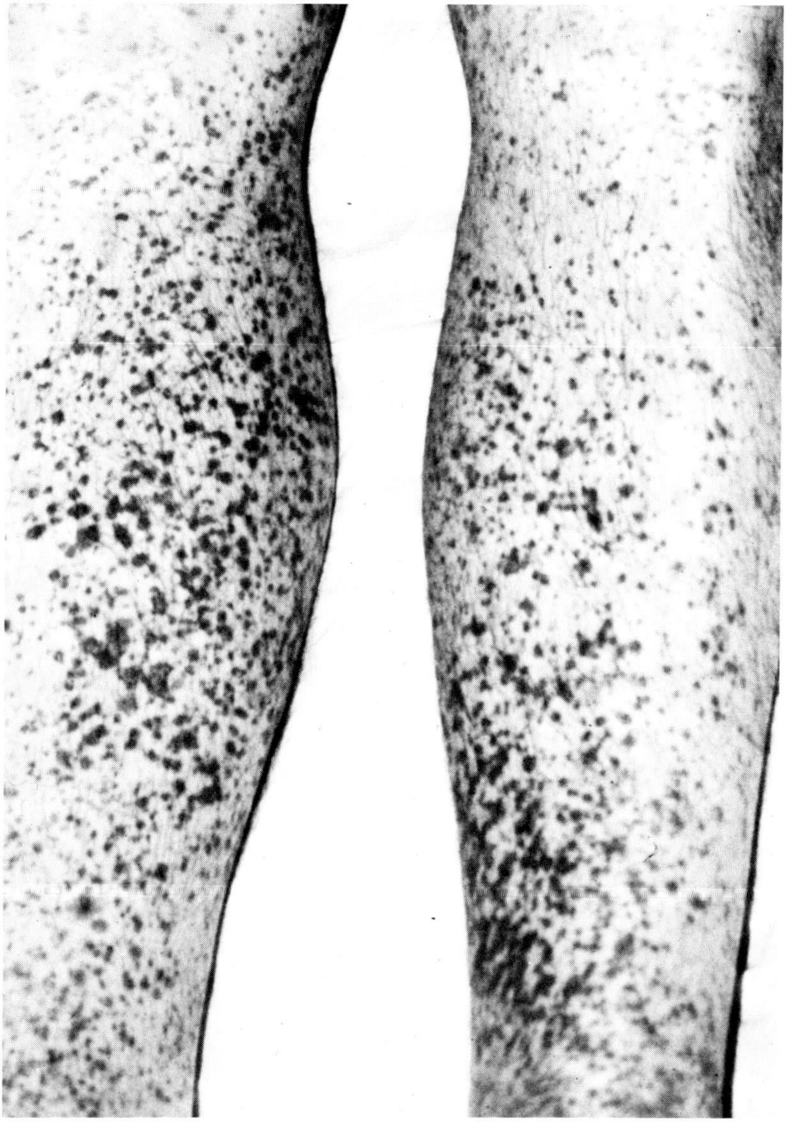

Figure 3. Henoch-Schönlein purpura. Extensive lower extremity purpura in an adult with Henoch-Schönlein purpura. Skin biopsy showed IgA deposits in the vessel walls. Severe intestinal ischemia was present.

vere cramping and abdominal pain. In one series of 139 children, 91 (65%) had either abdominal pain or gastrointestinal hemorrhage.[41] In a series of 77 adults, 34 had colicky abdominal pain as the most common gastrointestinal manifestation. Twenty-three patients had evidence of gastrointestinal blood loss, either occult or obvious.[36] Occasionally bleeding may occur in the absence of abdominal pain.[41]

Intussusception occurs in 2-3% of children and is usually ileocecal or ileoilial. The presence of an abdominal mass is a particularly useful sign in children suspected of having intussusception, and this possibility must always be considered.[41–42] However, a palpable mass may at times be due to bleeding or edema of the bowel wall only.[43] Barium examination of the colon may be helpful in diagnosis.

Other gastrointestinal complications of vasculitis include acute pancreatitis,[44] protein-losing enteropathy,[36] and small bowel perforation.[44a]

Diagnosis

Diagnosis rests on the typical clinical presentation of purpura, arthritis, and gastrointestinal and renal involvement, two or three of which are commonly present. The hemoglobin may be decreased from gastrointestinal blood loss or anemia of chronic illness. The sedimentation rate and platelet count are often elevated due to the ongoing inflammation. Serum IgA levels may be normal or increased. Surprisingly, serum complement levels are almost always normal. Blood urea nitrogen, creatinine, and urinalysis may be abnormal if there is renal involvement. Red blood cell casts are especially helpful in diagnosing active glomerular inflammation. Skin biopsy of a lesion is especially helpful in diagnosing H-S purpura. In contrast to other types of hypersensitivity vasculitis where IgG and IgM are the predominant immunoglobulins, IgA is abundant in lesions of H-S purpura and may be the only immunoglobulin present. Renal biopsy will show various lesions ranging from normal to mild focal mesangial glomerulitis to necrotizing glomerulonephritis. Immunofluorescence of the renal lesions also shows predominant IgA deposition in the glomerulus. Barium studies may show intussusception, mucosal edema, or thumbprinting. Sigmoidoscopy may show bleeding from above or mucosal petechiae.

Management

There have been no controlled trials of the treatment of children or adults with Henoch-Schönlein purpura. It is generally thought that treatment is of benefit for skin, joint, and gastrointestinal manifestations, but of questionable value for renal involvement. Progressive mesenteric vasculitis may respond dramatically to high-dose steroids. Surgical intervention may be needed, especially if nonreducible intussusception or gangrene of the bowel has occurred. Immunosuppressives may be of possible benefit for progressive renal involvement, especially when a trial of steroids in the range of 60 mg a day in an adult fails to produce a response. With the recent finding of circulating IgA complexes in H-S purpura, it is possible that plasmapheresis may be of potential benefit.

Vasculitides in Which Intestinal Ischemia Occurs Less Commonly

Allergic Granulomatosis of Churg and Strauss

Allergic granulomatosis of Churg and Strauss closely resembles periarteritis nodosa (PAN) in the size of blood vessels involved and the major clinical manifestations, except that there is usually a strong history of allergy in patients with this disease. Asthma and allergic rhinitis are common.[45] There is a much higher incidence of pulmonary vasculitis in allergic granulomatosis. Peripheral blood eosinophilia, often to a marked degree, is seen in virtually all cases, while classic PAN has eosinophilia to a modest degree in a small percentage.

The pathologic findings differ from those in PAN in that small, necrotizing granulomas are seen in addition to vasculitis involving medium and small arteries and venules.

Gastrointestinal Manifestations

Owing to the rarity of this disease, data on gastrointestinal involvement are scanty. Allergic granulomas have been reported to involve the stomach, liver, and omentum. In one report, a patient died of perforation of the small bowel with peritonitis and septicemia due to necrotizing granulomatous vasculitis, and an additional patient had granulomas massively involving the ascending colon, mimicking a carcinoma.[45] Gastrointestinal vasculitis has been documented in other reports.[46] Pseudopolyp formation of the colon mimicking chronic ulcerative colitis has also been reported.[45]

Laboratory

Laboratory features are similar to those in PAN, except for striking eosinophilia in virtually all cases and occasionally elevated IgE levels. In the 13 original cases, the absolute eosinophil count ranged from 5000 to 20,000 per cubic millimeter.[47]

Diagnosis

Diagnosis is made by the distinct clinical features, and by biopsy. Besides biopsy of organs mentioned under PAN, lung biopsy is often helpful in allergic granulomatosis due to the significant incidence of pulmonary involvement. Organ biopsy may reveal the distinct eosinophilic granulomas and vasculitis. Angiography may occasionally show aneurysms similar to those seen in PAN[6] and may also show beading or irregularity of vessels suggesting vasculitis, but the role of angiography is less well established than it is in PAN.

Management

High-dose steroid therapy should be used in allergic granulomatous angiitis. There are little data on immunosuppressives. Supportive therapy is similar to that described for PAN.

Wegener's Granulomatosis

Wegener's granulomatosis is a necrotizing granulomatous vasculitis of small vessels, both arteries and veins, which primarily involves the respiratory tract and kidneys. Intestinal involvement has been reported, but is distinctly unusual.

Gastrointestinal Manifestations

Although gastrointestinal vasculitis is not mentioned in many reports, in one series vasculitis involving the small intestines was found at autopsy in one patient and peritonitis attributed to Wegener's in another.[48] A clinicopathologic conference report documented massive splenic necrosis secondary to vasculitis, hepatic vasculitis, and necrotic ulcers of the cecum due to vasculitis.[49] Gastrointestinal vasculitis occurred in three of 16 patients with relatively limited Wegener's, one with angiitis of the gallbladder, and two with small bowel involvement. In one of the patients with small bowel vasculitis, there were nodules in a segment of jejunum, one of which was the cause of gastrointestinal hemorrhage. Pathologically, these nodules consisted of a granulomatous necrotizing angiitis with a dense granulomatous reaction in surrounding tissue.[50]

Laboratory

As in other forms of vasculitis, there is no diagnostic blood test. Complement levels are normal or elevated. Circulating immune complexes are present in some cases, but their role is uncertain.

Diagnosis

Biopsy, usually of nasal mucosa, sinus, lung, or kidney, is needed to confirm the diagnosis. Except for the kidney, the biopsy may show two components, a necrotizing vasculitis and necrotizing granulomas.

Management

Untreated Wegener's is rapidly fatal, with a mean survival of five months, and one-year survival of 18%.[51] Corticosteroids alone are minimally effective in improving survival. Multiple studies have now shown a dramatic increase in survival with the use of cytotoxic agents, with cyclophosphamide the definite agent of choice.[52–55] Chlorambucil and azathioprine have been frequently used, but do not seem to be as effective as cyclophosphamide, and should be reserved for those patients who cannot tolerate cyclophosphamide.

Temporal Arteritis

Gastrointestinal manifestations of temporal arteritis (TA) have been described in occasional patients. Medium or large arteries are involved. Necrosis of the arterial wall occurs with a granulomatous inflammation. Completely normal areas may be interspersed between areas of marked inflammation.[56] The most severely involved vessels are the superficial temporal, ophthalmic, vertebral, and posterior ciliary arteries, and not uncommonly, the carotids, central retinal artery, aortic arch, and its branches.

Clinical Manifestations

Temporal arteritis occurs in elderly people, usually over the age of 50, with a peak occurrence in the 60s and 70s. The female-to-male ratio is 2:1. It is almost always a disease of Caucasians, with only a few cases having been reported in blacks.

The symptoms are varied,[57–59] with fever, weight loss, anorexia, and fatigue occurring in the majority of patients. Psychosis, depression, and dementia have been reported. Headache is often a prominent early manifestation of TA. Scalp tenderness occurs in about half the cases, usually localized to the temporal or occipital arteries. Transient or permanent, partial or complete blindness may occur secondary to ischemia of the optic nerve or tracts. Visual defects are usually permanent. Ischemic jaw claudication occurs in one-third to one-half of patients secondary to facial or maxillary artery involvement.

Polymyalgia rheumatica is present in about half the patients and often is the first clue to the diagnosis. Polymyalgia consists of severe pain and stiffness of the neck, shoulder, and pelvic girdles, more marked in the mornings.

Clinical signs include scalp tenderness and nodules, thickening, irregularity or decreased pulsations of temporal or other superficial arteries. However, the temporal arteries have been completely normal in one-third of patients proved to have arteritis on biopsy. Patients with polymyalgia rheumatica may have decreased motion of hip and shoulder joints and pain on palpation of these areas. Visual field defects will be present if ophthalmic or central retinal artery involvement is present. Scalp and tongue necrosis have been reported.

The aortic arch and its major branches are not uncommonly involved in temporal arteritis. Subclavian, axillary, brachial, and femoral involvement are well documented. Large artery involvement including Raynaud's phenomenon, paresthesias, and intermittent claudication were evident in 34 of 248 patients (14%) in one series.[60] Bruits or decreased pulsations may be detected. Aortic dissection has been implicated as a cause of death.

Gastrointestinal Manifestations

Mesenteric arteritis leading to melena, obstruction, or gangrene has been described.[61–63] Postprandial abdominal pain suggestive of abdominal angina occurred in a patient who was found to have giant cell arteritis of all major aortic branches.[60] In the same report, autopsy of another patient showed pancreatic vasculitis. Cramps and diarrhea controlled by prednisone accompanied symptomatic flares of temporal arteritis in a 75-year-old man.[64]

It is apparent that intestinal vasculitis is an unusual but documented manifestation of temporal arteritis. In addition, aortic dissection resulting from temporal arteritis has the potential to cause mesenteric vascular occlusion.

Laboratory

The most common laboratory abnormality is an elevated sedimentation rate. Anemia of chronic illness is present in the majority of patients. Leukocytosis or thrombocytosis is occasionally seen. Complements are usually elevated, since they act as acute phase reactants. Mild abnormalities of liver function have been documented.[65] Renal function is usually normal, but 10% to 15% of patients may have red blood cells or red blood cell casts on urinalysis, possibly due to mild glomerular ischemia.

Diagnosis

The major diagnostic procedure is temporal artery biopsy. The general consensus is that temporal artery arteriograms are of little benefit in localizing an area for biopsy.[66,67] The importance of obtaining a large segment of artery, at least 2.5 cm or more, as well as multiple sections must be stressed, since skip lesions have been substantiated.[56] In addition, the highest yield is obtained with bilateral biopsies, since 5–10% of lesions are unilateral. Biopsy should be done within one week of initiation of steroid therapy.

Management

The treatment for temporal arteritis is high-dose steroids in the range of 60 mg of prednisone in divided doses initially. Careful adjustment of the steroid dose is mandatory, especially if visual symptoms have been present. Normalization of the sedimentation rate is a good indicator of adequate disease control. Alternate-day steroids, even after initial control with daily steroids, have been shown to be ineffective.[68] Immunosuppressives may be used if steroid side effects are intolerable, and may permit the use of lower doses of steroids.

Miscellaneous Vasculitides

Mucocutaneous Lymph Node Syndrome

This newly described acute illness most often occurs in children under the age of five. The major symptoms are fever, cervical lymphadenopathy, conjunctivitis, erythema of the oral cavity, lips, and palms, strawberry-like swelling of tongue papillae, and desquamation of the skin of the fingertips. Occasionally pericarditis, myocarditis, cardiomegaly, and myocardial infarction occur.

Only 1 to 2% of cases end fatally, but coronary arteritis with myocardial infarction or arrhythmia is the major cause of death. This may occur after other manifestations of the disease have started to resolve. The histologic characteristics of the coronary arteries resembles that in periarteritis nodosa. Diarrhea occurs in 40% of cases.[69,70] Vasculitis, although most common in the coronary arteries, may involve other vessels. Mesenteric vasculitis occurred in six of 29 autopsied cases in one series.[69] In a later series, diarrhea and vomiting were present in 18 of 22 cases that ended fatally. Mesenteric or other gastrointestinal vasculitis was present in ten, hepatic vasculitis in five, and pancreatic vasculitis in eight of the 22 cases at autopsy. Seven of 18 patients with gastrointestinal symptoms failed to have pathologically confirmed vasculitis at autopsy, but 11 of 18 did have vasculitis. In addition, two of four patients without gastrointestinal symptoms had vasculitis at autopsy.[71] However, these series deal with fatal cases. How often diarrhea and vomiting are due to gastrointestinal vasculitis in nonfatal cases is not clear.

Since 98% of patients improve spontaneously, treatment is difficult to evaluate. However, for those who are severely ill, high dose salicylates are generally used. There is an impression that steroids may increase the risk of coronary artery aneurysms.

Behcet's Syndrome

Behcet's syndrome is of unknown etiology and is characterized by recurrent oral and genital ulcerations and iritis. Prevalence is highest in Japan and the Mediterranean countries, although it occurs worldwide. Peak age of onset is in the third decade, and the male:female ratio is approximately 2:1. Familial clustering of cases has been reported occasionally. The pathologic lesion of Behcet's is a vasculitis.[72–74]

In addition to buccal and genital ulcers, other clinical manifestations are varied eye and skin lesions, fever, fatigue, or weight loss. The oral lesions are usually deep and painful, but genital lesions in women may be painless. Eye lesions include episcleritis, keratitis, retinal thrombophlebitis, papilledema, and optic atrophy. Skin pustules may form after mild trauma, such as blood drawing. Superficial thrombophlebitis is common. Deep venous thrombosis of the inferior vena cava or limb veins may also occur. Erythema nodosum may occur early in the course. Other manifestations include peripheral arthritis, spondylitis, and central or peripheral nervous system involvement.

Gastrointestinal Manifestations

Gastrointestinal involvement varies but is included in almost all major reports. One large study from Japan reported manifestations in over 50% of cases.[73] Barium studies, endoscopy, or biopsy were done in 59 patients with Behcet's with gastrointestinal symptoms. Evidence of intestinal ulceration was found in 59% of men and 41% of women. Abdominal pain occurred in 92% of those with intestinal ulcers, while perforation developed in 41% and melena in 25%. The most common area of intestinal ulceration was the ileum and cecum, with the ascending, transverse, descending, sigmoid colon, and rectum involved in decreasing order of frequency. The ileocecal ulcers often perforate. Vasculitis can be found in intestinal vessels of various size including capillaries, arterioles, and venules, and also in areas remote from the ulcers.[74]

Gastrointestinal involvement seems to be much higher in Japan than in other areas. In a series of 32 cases in England, only three had evidence of bowel involvement with large or small bowel ulcerations.[75] A report from Israel of 41 cases of Behcet's revealed no gastrointestinal symptoms.[76] This is one of the few reports of a large series of patients showing no gastrointestinal involvement.

Some believe that Behcet's-like symptoms in the presence of intestinal ulceration may be Crohn's disease or ulcerative colitis with marked extraintestinal manifestations.[76] However, many physicians experienced in the intestinal manifestations of Behcet's consider the radiographic, anatomic, and histologic appearance of intestinal Behcet's to be distinct from that of Crohn's or ulcerative colitis.[74]

Laboratory

There is no diagnostic laboratory test. The sedimentation rate is usually elevated. Complement levels are normal or high. Several studies have shown the histocompatibility antigen HLA-B_5 to have increased prevalence in Behcet's.[72]

Management

Treatment is arbitrary. Most physicians agree that steroids are at best palliative and are often completely ineffective.[74,76] However, prednisone in high doses of 60–80 mg/day may reduce or prevent progression of central nervous system disease. There have been occasional reports of dramatic response to indocin or colchicine in patients with severe organ system involvement.[77] Immunosuppressives seem to be more effective than other forms of treatment, with chlorambucil possibly being preferred.[72,74,78] Data on blood transfusions, transfer factor, and fibrinolytic agents are inconclusive.

Cogan's Syndrome

Cogan's syndrome is characterized by nonsyphilitic keratitis, vestibuloauditory dysfunction, aortitis, and systemic vasculitis involving muscular arteries and veins. Aortitis may develop rapidly leading to severe aortic insufficiency in 10% of cases. Other manifestations include fever, splenomegaly, arthralgias, arthritis, and eosinophilia.

Gastrointestinal involvement is not uncommon, occurring in approximately 25% of cases. Symptoms range from persistent unexplained abdominal pain to peptic and colonic ulcerations.[79] How often gastrointestinal ischemia occurs is not clear.

Steroids and immunosuppressives may be of benefit. There are fewer than 80 reported cases.

Relapsing Polychondritis

Relapsing polychondritis is characterized by recurrent episodes of intense inflammation in the cartilaginous portions of the ear, scleritis, nasal chondritis often leading to a saddle nose deformity, and inflammation of the cartilaginous structures of the airways not uncommonly resulting in tracheal collapse and death from respiratory insufficiency. Other manifestations include aortitis, aortic insufficiency and dissection, or rupture of aortic aneurysms. A generalized systemic vasculitis occurs in 10–25% of cases.[80]

Gastrointestinal involvement with this arteritis has occasionally been reported. In one case, death was due to occlusion of the superior mesenteric artery with infarction of the entire small bowel.[81]

Rare Occurrences of Gastrointestinal Ischemia

Takayasu's Arteritis

Takayasu's arteritis is a large vessel vasculitis typically occurring in young females, showing special prevalence in the Oriental and Latin races, and is an exceedingly rare cause of gastrointestinal ischemia. Pathologically it is a giant cell granulomatous inflammation of the aorta and its major branches.

Gastrointestinal Manifestations

Gastrointestinal ischemia is distinctly unusual in Takayasu's disease and was not mentioned in an early review.[82] In a later report of 84 cases, 51 were studied by aortography and mesenteric involvement was shown in five, but none of the 84 patients had a significant problem with intestinal ischemia.[83] A detailed study of 36 cases from Finland revealed mesenteric artery involvement in one (3%). There were no symptoms of intestinal ischemia.[84]

Autopsy studies of eight cases showed no evidence of mesenteric artery involvement,[85] while another study of 54 patients revealed eight deaths from cardiovascular or cerebrovascular accidents, with no mention of mesenteric involvement on a clinical, arteriographic, or pathologic basis.[86]

Another report of 20 patients tabulated angiographic results according to vessels involved, but failed to indicate any mesenteric artery involvement. None of the patients had symptoms of intestinal ischemia.[87] However, gastrointestinal ischemia with hemorrhage and abdominal pain due to mesenteric artery stenosis has been reported.[88]

Lymphomatoid Granulomatosis

Lymphomatoid granulomatosis (LG) is characterized by angiotrophic and angiodestructive involvement of tissues, especially the lung, with small lymphocytes, plasma cells, histiocytes, and atypical lymphoreticular cells.[89] Granulomas are less well defined than in Wegener's. Clinically, it can closely resemble the pulmonary involvement of Wegener's granulomatosis, with multiple nodular infiltrates of various sizes that tend to cavitate. Skin, kidney, and central nervous system involvement are also common. However, the renal involvement is a diffuse or nodular interstitial infiltrate of atypical cells, not a glomerulitis as in Wegener's. In approximately 15% of patients, LG evolves into a lymphoma.

Several clinical features are also helpful in distinguishing LG from Wegener's. Sinus and upper airway involvement is unusual. Anergy is often present, leukopenia can occur prior to therapy, and the sedimentation rate may be normal.[90]

Gastrointestinal symptoms, including nausea, vomiting, diarrhea, and abdominal pain occurred in four of 152 patients.[89] Autopsies in 72 cases showed that 7% had evidence of gastrointestinal involvement. In another series, four of 40 patients had stomach, small intestine, or liver involvement, but intestinal ischemia was not discussed.[91]

Untreated, LG usually leads rapidly to death. Survival may be increased by cytoxan and steroids.[90,92]

References

1. Kussmaul A, Maier R: Uber eine bischer nicht beschreibene eigenthumliche arterienekainkung (Periarteritis nodosa), die mit Murbos Brightii und rapid furtschreitender allgemeiner. Muskellahmung einhergeht. *Dtsch Arch Klin Med* 1:484, 1866.
2. Zeek PM: Periarteritis nodosa: A critical review. *Am J Clin Path* 226:777, 1952.
3. LiVolsi VA, Perzin KH, Porter M: Polyarteritis of the gallbladder presenting as acute cholecystitis. *Gastroenterology* 65:115, 1973.
4. Hall JW, Shao-Choin S, Macklor W: Arteritis of the appendix. *Arch Pathol* 50:240, 1950.
5. Cohen RD, Conn DL, Ilstrup DM: Clinical features, prognosis and response to treatment in polyarteritis. *Mayo Clin Proc* 55:146, 1980.
6. Travers RL, Allison DJ, Drettle RP, Hughes GRV: Polyarteritis nodosa: A clinical and angiographic analysis of 17 cases. *Sem Arth Rheum* 8:184, 1979.
7. Duffy JD, Lidsky MD, Sharp JT, et al: Polyarthritis, polyarteritis, and hepatitis B. *Medicine* 55:19, 1976.
8. Hunder GG, Conn DL: Necrotizing vasculitis. In *Textbook of Rheumatology*. Kelley WN (Ed.) WB Saunders, Philadelphia 1980, pp 1165–1181.
9. Fauci AS: Polyarteritis nodosa group of systemic necrotizing vasculitides. pp 663–664 in Fauci AS (moderator): The spectrum of vasculitis: Clinical, pathologic, immunologic and therapeutic considerations. *Ann Intern Med* 89 (Part 1):660, 1978.
10. Conn DL, McDuffie FC, Holley KE, Schroeter AL: Immunologic mechanisms in systemic vasculitis. *Mayo Clin Proc* 51:511, 1976.
11. Leonhardt ETG, Kullenberg KPG: Bilateral atrial myxomas with multiple arterial aneurysms: A syndrome mimicking polyarteritis nodosa. *Am J Med* 62:792, 1977.
12. Thomas MH: Myxoma masquerading as polyarteritis nodosa. *J Rheumatol* 8:133, 1981.
13. Baker SB: Unusual renal manifestations of Wegener's granulomatosis. *Am J Med* 64:883, 1978.

14. Longsheth PL, Korobkin M, Palubinskas AJ: Renal microaneurysms in a patient with systemic lupus erythematosus. *Radiology* 113:65, 1974.
15. Clanz S, Bittner SJ, Berman MA: Regression of coronary artery aneurysms in infantile polyarteritis nodosa. *N Engl J Med* 294:939, 1976.
16. Cabal E, Holtz S: Polyarteritis as a cause of intestinal hem orrhage. *Gastroenterology* 61:99, 1971.
17. Fauci AS, Doppman JL, Wolff SM: Cyclophosphamide-induced remissions in advanced polyarteritis nodosa. *Am J Med* 64:890, 1978.
18. Frohnert PP, Sheps SG: Long-term follow-up study of periarteritis nodosa. *Am J Med* 43:8, 1967.
19. Melan H, Patterson R: Periarteritis nodosa: A remission achieved with combined prednisone and azathioprine therapy. *Am J Dis Child* 121:424, 1971.
20. Hunder GG, Conn DL: Necrotizing vasculitis. In *Textbook of Rheumatology,* Kelley WN (Ed.) WB Saunders, Philadelphia 1981. pp 1165–1188.
21. Fan PT, Davis JA, Somer T, Kaplan L, Bluestone R: A clinical approach to systemic vasculitis. *Sem Arth Rheum* 9:248, 1980.
22. Fauci AS: Hypersensitivity vasculitis. pp 664–667 In Fauci AS (moderator): The Spectrum of Vasculitis. Clinical, Pathologic, Immunologic and Therapeutic Considerations. *Ann Intern Med* 89 (Part I):660, 1978.
23. Winkleman RK, Ditto WB: Cutaneous and visceral syndromes of necrotizing or "allergic" angiitis: A study of 38 cases. *Medicine* (Baltimore) 43:59, 1964.
24. Soter NA, Austen KF: Cutaneous necrotizing angiitis. In *Immunological Diseases.* Samter M (Ed.) Little Brown & Co, Boston 1978. pp 993–1001.
25. Brouet JC, Clauvel JP, Danon F: Biological and clinical significance of cryoglobulins: A report of 86 cases. *Am J Med* 57:775, 1974.
26. Furevic PD, Kassab JH, Levo Y: Mixed cryoglobulinemia: Clinical aspects and long-term follow up of 40 patients. *Am J Med* 69:287, 1980.
27. Meltzer M, Franklin EC, Elias K: Cryoglobulinemia: A clinical and laboratory study. *Am J Med* 40:837, 1966.

28. Levo Y, Gorovic PD, Kasab HJ, Zucker-Franklin D, Franklin EC: Association between hepatitis B virus and essential mixed cryoglobulinemia. *N Engl J Med* 296:1501, 1977.
29. Reza MJ, Roth BE, Goldburg LS: Intestinal vasculitis in essential mixed cryoglobulinemia. *Ann Intern Med* 81:632, 1974.
30. Levo Y, Gorevic PD, Kassab HJ: Liver involvement in the syndrome of mixed cryoglobulinemia. *Ann Intern Med* 87: 287, 1977.
31. Gelfand EW, Clarkson JE, Minta JD: Selective deficiency of the second component of complement in a patient with anaphylactoid purpura. *Clin Immunol Immunopath* 4:269, 1975.
32. Sussman M, Jones JH, Almrida JD, Luchmann PJ: Deficiency of the second component of complement associated with anaphylactoid purpura and presence of mycoplasma in the serum. *Clin Exp Immunol* 14:531, 1973.
33. Spitzer RE, Urmson JR, Fornelt ML, et al: Alteration of the complement system in children with Henoch-Schonlein purpura. *Clin Immunol Immunopath* 11:52, 1978.
34. Hall RP, Lawley TJ, Heck JA, Katz SI: IgA-containing circulating immune complexes in dermatitis herpetiformis, Henoch-Schonlein purpura, systemic lupus erythematosus and other diseases. *Clin Exp Immunol* 40:431, 1980.
35. Kauffman RH, Herrmann WA, Meyer CJ, et al: Circulating IgA-immune complexes in Henoch-Schonlein purpura. *Am J Med* 69:859, 1980.
36. Cream JJ, Gumpel JM, Peuchy RDG: Schönlein-Henoch purpura in the adult. A study of 77 adults with anaphylactoid or Schönlein-Henoch purpura. *Quart J Med* 39:461, 1970.
37. Allen D, Diamond LK, Howel DA: Anaphylactoid purpura in children (Schönlein-Henoch syndrome): Review with a follow-up of the renal complications. *Am J Dis Child* 99:833, 1960.
38. Koshimies O, Rapula J, Savilahti E, Volsko J: Renal involvement in Schönlein-Henoch purpura. *Acta Paediatr Scand* 63:357, 1974.
39. Sinniah R, Feng PM, Chen BTM: Henoch-Schönlein syndrome: a clinical and morphological study of renal biopsies. *Clin Nephrol* 9:219, 1978.
40. Levy M: Anaphylactoid purpura nephritis in childhood. Natural history and immunopathology. *Adv Nephrol* 6:183, 1976.

41. Foldt RH: The gastrointestinal manifestations of anaphylactoid purpura in children. *Staff Meetings Mayo Clin* 37:465, 1962.
42. Allen DM: Anaphylactoid purpura in children. *AMA J Dis Children* 99:833, 1960.
43. Wolfsohn H: Purpura and intussusception. *Arch Dis Child* 22:242, 1947.
44. Garner JA: Acute pancreatitis as a complication of Henoch-Schönlein purpura. *Arch Dis Child* 52:971, 1977.
44a. Basu R: Perforation of the bowel in Henoch-Schönlein purpura. *Arch Dis Child* 34:342, 1959.
45. Chumbley LC, Harrison EG, DeRemee RA: Allergic granulomatosis and angiitis (Churg-Strauss Syndrome): Report and analysis of 30 cases. *Mayo Clin Proc* 52:477, 1977.
46. Rosenberg TF, Medsger TA, DeCicca FA, Fireman P: Allergic granulomatous angiitis (Churg-Strauss Syndrome). *J Allergy Clin Immunol* 55:56, 1975.
47. Churg J, Strauss L: Allergic granulomatosis, allergic angiitis and periarteritis nodosa. *Am J Pathol* 27:277, 1951.
48. Fauci AS, Wolff SM: Wegener's granulomatosis: Studies in eighteen patients and a review of the literature. *Medicine* 52:535, 1973.
49. CPC: Wegener's granulomatosis. *Am J Med* 48:496, 1970.
50. Carrington CB, Liebow AA: Limited forms of angiitis and granulomatosis of Wegener's type. *Am J Med* 41:497, 1966.
51. Walton EW: Giant-cell granuloma of the respiratory tract (Wegener's granulomatosis). *Br Med J* 2:265, 1958.
52. Wolff SM, Fauci AS, Horn RG, Dale DC: Wegener's granulomatosis. *Ann Intern Med* 81:513, 1974.
53. Israel HL, Patchefsky AS, Saldana MJ: Wegener's granulomatosis, lymphomatoid granulomatosis and benign lymphocytic angiitis and granulomatosis. *Ann Intern Med* 87:691, 1977.
54. Haynes BF: Treatment of granulomatous vasculitis. pp 671–673 in Fauci AS (moderator): The spectrum of vasculitis. Clinical, pathologic, immunologic and therapeutic considerations. *Ann Intern Med* 89:660, 1978.
55. Reza MJ, Dornfeld L, Goldberg LS, Bluestone R, Pearson CM: Wegener's granulomatosis. *Arth Rheum* 18:501, 1975.
56. Klein RG, Campbell AJ, Hunder GG, Darney JA: Skip lesions in temporal arteritis. *Mayo Clin Proc* 51:504, 1976.

57. Hamilton CR, Shelley WM, Tumulty PA: Giant cell arteritis including temporal arteritis and polymyalgia rheumatica. *Medicine* 50:1, 1971.
58. Hunder GG, Allen GL: Giant cell arteritis: A review. *Bull Rheum Dis* 29:980, 1978.
59. Goodman BW: Temporal arteritis. *Am J Med* 67:839, 1979.
60. Klein RR, Hunder GG, Stanson AW, Sheps SG: Large artery involvement in giant cell arteritis. *Ann Intern Med* 83:806, 1975.
61. Hamrin B, Jonsson N, Hallsten S: Polymyalgia arteritica: Further clinical and histopathological studies with a report of six autopsy cases. *Ann Rheum Dis* 27:397, 1968.
62. Meadows SP: Temporal or giant cell arteritis. *Proc Royal Soc Med* 59:329, 1966.
63. Rusell RWR: Giant-cell arteritis: A review of 35 cases. *Quart J Med* 28:471, 1959.
64. Simkin PA, Healy LA: Giant cell arteritis with polymyalgia rheumatica, loss of vision, and abdominal symptoms occurring during a four-year course. *Arthritis Rheum* 12:147, 1969.
65. Knorring JV, Wasastjerna C: Liver involvement in polymyalgia rheumatica. *Scand J Rheum* 5:197, 1976.
66. Sewell JR, Allison DJ, Tarin D, Hughes RV: Combined temporal arteriography and selective biopsy in suspected giant cell arteritis. *Ann Rheum Dis* 39:124, 1980.
67. Layfer LF, Banner BF, Huckman S, Grainer LS, Golden HE: Temporal arteriography. Analysis of 21 cases and review of literature. *Arthritis Rheum* 21:780, 1978.
68. Hunder GG, Sheps SG, Allen GL, Joyce JW: Daily and alternate day corticosteroid regimens in treatment of giant cell arteritis: Comparison in prospective study. *Ann Intern Med* 82:613, 1975.
69. Tanaka LN, Sekimoto K, Naoe S: Kawasaki's disease relationship with infantile periarteritis nodosa. *Arch Pathol Lab Med* 100:81, 1976.
70. Kawasaki T, Kosaki F, Ottawa S, Shigematsu I, Yanagawa H: A new infantile acute febrile mucocutaneous lymph node syndrome (MLNS) prevailing in Japan. *Pediatrics* 54:271, 1974.
71. Landing FH, Larson EJ: Are infantile periarteritis nodosa

with coronary artery involvement and fatal mucocutaneous lymph node syndrome the same? Comparison of 20 patients from North America with patients from Hawaii and Japan. *Pediatrics* 59:651, 1977.
72. Wright VA, Chamberlain MA: Behcet's syndrome. *Bull Rheum Dis* 29:972, 1978.
73. Shmizu T, Ogino T: Clinico-pathological studies on the intestinal lesions in Behcet's disease—with special reference to entero-Behcet's syndrome. *Stomach Intestine* 7:1649, 1972.
74. Shimizu T, Ehrlich GE, Inaba G, Hayashi K: Behcet's disease (Behcet's syndrome). *Sem Arthritis Rheum* 8:223, 1979.
75. Chamberlain MA: Behcet's syndrome in 32 patients in Yorkshire. *Ann Rheum Dis* 36:491, 1977.
76. Chajek T, Fainaru M: Behcet's disease. Report of 41 cases and review of the literature. *Medicine* 54:179, 1975.
77. Raynor A, Askari AD: Behcet's disease and treatment with colchicine. *J Am Acad Dermatol* 2:396, 1980.
78. O'Duffy JD: Comments on Behcet's syndrome. *Bull Rheum Dis* 29:977, 1978.
79. Cheson BD, Bluming AZ, Alroy J: Cogan's syndrome: A systemic vasculitis. *Am J Med* 60:549, 1976.
80. McAdam LP, O'Hanlan MA, Bluestone R, Pearson CM: Relapsing polychondritis. Perspective study of 23 patients and a review of the literature. *Medicine* 55:193, 1976.
81. Herman JH, Dennis MV: Immunopathologic studies in relapsing polychondritis. *J Clin Invest* 52:549, 1973.
82. McKusick VA: A form of vascular disease relatively frequent in the Orient. *Am Heart J* 63:57, 1962.
83. Nakao K, Ikeda M, Kimata S, et al: Takayasu's arteritis. Clinical report of eighty-four cases and immunological study of seven cases. *Circulation* 35:1141, 1967.
84. Paloheimo JA: Obstructive arteritis of Takayasu's type. *Acta Medica Scand Suppl* 468:1, 1967.
85. Vinijchaikul K: Primary arteritis of the aorta and its main branches (Takayasu's arteriopathy). A clinicopathologic autopsy study of eight cases. *Am J Med* 43:15, 1967.
86. Ishikawa K: Natural history and classification of occlusive thromboaortopathy (Takayasu's disease). *Circulation* 57:27, 1978.
87. Fraga A, Mintz G, Valle L, Floros-Izquierdo G: Takayasu's

arteritis: Frequency of systemic manifestations (study of 22 patients) and favorable response to maintenance steroid therapy with adrenocorticosteroids (12 patients). *Arthritis Rheum* 15:617, 1972.
88. Strachan RW: The natural history of Takayasu's arteriopathy. *Quart J Med* 33:57, 1964.
89. Katzenstein AA, Carrington CB, Liebow AA: Lymphomatoid granulomatosis: Clinicopathologic study of 152 cases. *Cancer* 43:360, 1979.
90. Fauci AS: Lymphomatoid granulomatosis. pp 668–669 in Fauci AS (moderator): The spectrum of vasculitis: clinical, pathologic, immunologic and therapeutic considerations. *Ann Intern Med* 89 (Part 1):660, 1978.
91. DeRemee RA, Weiland LH, McDonald TJ: Polymorphic reticulosis, lymphomatoid granulomatosis. *Mayo Clin Proc* 53:634, 1978.
92. Fauci AS, Haynes BF, Costa J, Katz P, Wolff SM: Lymphomatoid granulomatosis. Prospective clinical and therapeutic experience over 10 years. *N Engl J Med* 306:68, 1982.

20

Connective Tissue Diseases

Michael J. Luzar, M.D.

Connective tissue diseases that can cause gastrointestinal ischemia include systemic lupus erythematosus, rheumatoid arthritis, polymyositis (dermatomyositis), scleroderma, and to a lesser degree, Sjögren's syndrome and mixed connective tissue disease. The etiology of connective tissue diseases is unknown, but all may be manifested by intestinal ischemia due to small vessel vasculitis.

Common clinical manifestations of connective tissue disease include inflammation of the joints, serosal surfaces (pericarditis, peritonitis, and pleurisy), internal organs, and small blood vessels. Histologically, involved areas show alteration of connective tissue, especially fibrinoid degeneration. Laboratory evaluation of these diseases has revealed abnormalities in the humoral and cell-mediated immune systems and their interactions, as well as a high incidence of autoantibodies.

Systemic Lupus Erythematosus

Clinical Manifestations

Systemic lupus erythematosus (SLE) is predominantly a disease of women, with a 9:1 female-to-male ratio. The peak age of onset is between 15 and 45 although the disease can occur at any age. The incidence of lupus is higher in blacks than in Caucasians.

Common clinical manifestations include constitutional symptoms such as fatigue, fever, weight loss, and anorexia. Cutaneous lesions are very common, and some type of skin abnormality is present in 80% of SLE patients. A butterfly rash that typically spares the nasal labial folds is present over the bridge of the nose and the cheeks in about half of lupus patients (Figure 1). Photosensitivity is seen in 20–40% of SLE patients. Sun exposure may not only lead to a severe skin rash, but may exacerbate internal organ involvement. Vasculitic lesions of the skin can be an important clue to underlying vasculitis of internal organs in SLE.

Nasal or oral ulcers occur in 25% of patients. Hair loss may be either diffuse or patchy and occurs in the majority of patients. Cardiopulmonary manifestations include pericarditis or pleuritis, myocarditis, interstitial pulmonary fibrosis, lupus pneumonitis, or pleural effusion. Joint involvement results in synovial thickening or tenderness, especially about the wrists, knees, metacarpophalangeal joints, or proximal interphalangeal joints.

Muscle strength may be decreased due to inflammatory myopathy. Peripheral neuropathy or evidence of central nervous system involvement can occur. A significant percentage of SLE patients may have hepatosplenomegaly or lymphadenopathy. Urine should be carefully examined for evidence of active renal disease such as proteinuria, red blood cells, or red blood cell casts. Roughly one-half of SLE patients have clinical evidence of renal involvement sometime during the course of SLE.

Gastrointestinal Manifestations

Gastrointestinal involvement occurs in 20–30% of patients with active SLE, and intestinal ischemia must be

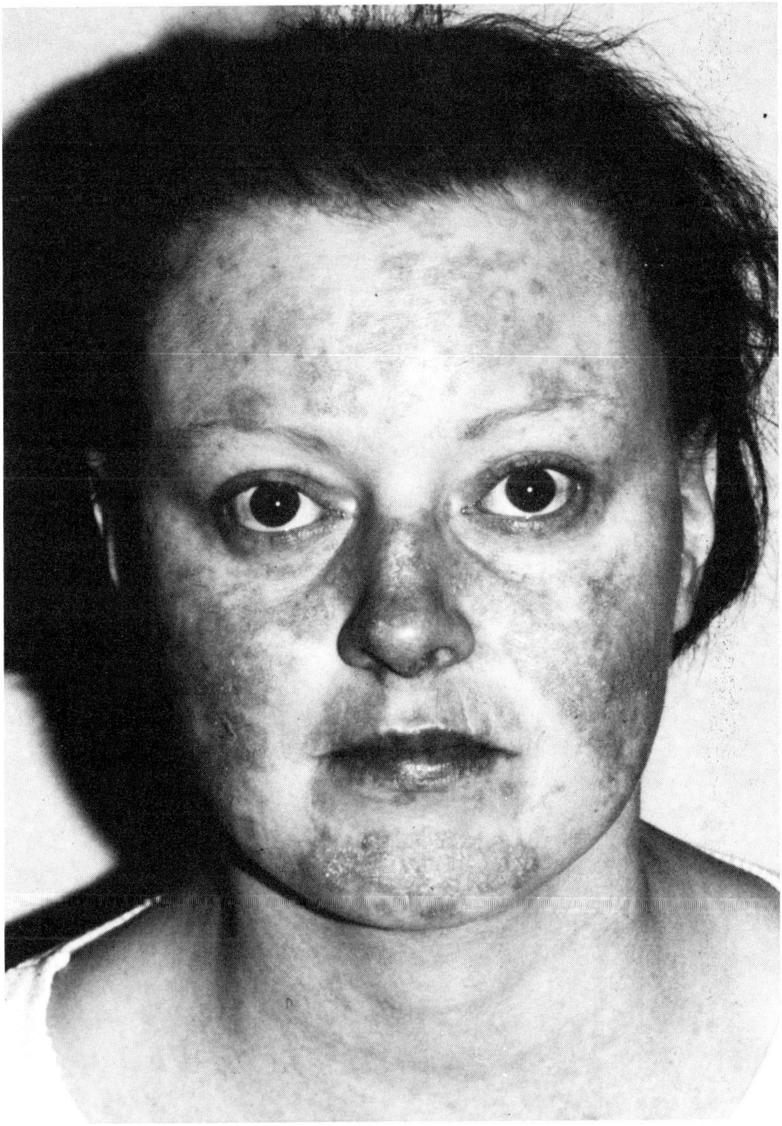

Figure 1. A classic butterfly rash of systemic lupus erythematosus.

considered in any patient with a flare of SLE and abdominal pain.

Intestinal ischemia occurs secondary to vasculitis, producing compromise of the vessel lumen with ischemia in the involved segment of bowel. Superficial mucosal ulcerations are followed by edema and hemorrhage in the wall and finally by necrosis of all or part of the bowel wall, depending on the size of the vessel. The larger the vessel, the more likely will be infarction of the entire thickness of the wall, which can lead to hemorrhage and perforation. Symptoms include crampy abdominal pain, often not well localized, nausea, vomiting, diarrhea, tenderness, distention, rigidity, rebound, and varied changes in bowel sounds. Table I compares the incidence of symptoms in three series of patients with bowel vasculitis secondary to lupus.[1]

In one report,[2] 14 patients with SLE simulated an acute surgical condition of the abdomen; in four the picture was predominantly that of pancreatitis, while ten presented the clinical picture of peritonitis. In five of these 14, surgery or autopsy showed vasculitic involvement of the small arteries in the subserosa and submucosa of the bowel wall. Apparently, none had bowel perforation, although guarding, localized pain, rebound, and to a lesser extent, rigidity were often present. Abdominal symptoms were the initial presenting manifestation of SLE in two of the 14 patients, although evaluation revealed simultaneous renal involvement in both. Thus, all of the patients had additional symptoms or signs of active SLE on thorough evaluation. It was concluded that abdominal involvement in SLE can simulate many different types of abdominal disease. Pollak[2] recommended a 24-to-48-hour trial of steroids before exploratory operation, even if the picture was that of an acute surgical abdomen.

In Rothfield's report,[3] three deaths from intestinal perforation due to vasculitis occurred among 365 lupus patients. Abdominal pain in patients with perforation was usually colicky and well localized in the lower abdomen or

Table I

Symptoms and Physical Findings in Patients with Bowel Vasculitis

	Pollack et al. *n = 10* *Percent*	*Shapero et al.* *n = 20* *Percent*	*Zizac et al.* *n = 8* *Percent*
Nausea	100	65	80
Vomiting	80	60	60
Diarrhea	30	30	60
Distension	90	25	80
Tenderness	100	70	100
Guarding	100	50	20
Rigidity	20		
Rebound	70	55	80
Bowel Sounds			
Normal	50	55	40
Decreased	20	35	20
Absent	20	5	40

(Reprinted with permission from Hoffman BI, Katz WA: The gastrointestinal manifestations of systemic lupus erythematosus. *Seminars Arthritis Rheumatism* 9:239, 1980.)

infraumbilical area. In patients without perforation, the pain was either sharp or colicky and less well localized. Patients without perforation lacked rebound or localized direct tenderness, while those with perforation had these findings. This is in contrast to the other report,[2] in which rebound and localized tenderness did occur without perforation. Episodes of perforation occurred in patients with severe, active SLE in Rothfield's series.[3] The only patients who survived were those who received the earliest surgical intervention, even those with complications such as renal insufficiency. It was also stressed that abdominal pain with signs of peritoneal inflammation in SLE is often due to nonrelated problems, since 15 of the 365 patients had such diagnoses as ruptured ovarian cyst, appendicitis, diverticulitis, and perforated gastric ulcer. It is noteworthy that these patients were in SLE remission at the time they had abdominal pain.

In Zizac's report,[4] five cases of large bowel perforation occurred in 107 patients with SLE. Four of the five died, and perforation of the colon was the most common cause of death in the whole series of patients over a three-year period. At the time of perforation, all five patients had clinical manifestations in other organ systems. Four had vasculitic skin lesions, which stresses the importance of performing a complete examination. Abdominal pain was insidious at onset, intermittent and recurrent for days or weeks before becoming severe and persistent. In four of the five, the pain was initially in the lower quadrant. Abdominal flat plates were normal initially in all five, although three later had free peritoneal air. Four had single perforations, and one had multiple perforations. The average interval from onset to surgical intervention was 30 days, and this stresses the need for keen suspicion by the surgeon. In some of these patients, steroid therapy may have masked the seriousness of the process. The author recommended that lupus patients who have lower abdominal pain with direct or rebound tenderness should undergo exploratory surgery within 24–48 hours if they do not respond to increased steroid dosage.

Intestinal ischemia secondary to mesenteric thrombosis has also been reported in SLE.[5] Often, abdominal pain is generalized, with diffuse tenderness, and no specific diagnosis can be made. Perhaps in these cases, there is peritoneal inflammation, just as other serosal surfaces can become inflamed and cause pleuritis or pericarditis. Peritonitis is well documented in SLE. Autopsy studies have shown evidence of active or past peritonitis in approximately 65% of SLE patients.[6] Ascites, clinically present in up to 10% of patients,[7] may in some cases be secondary to congestive heart failure or nephrotic syndrome.

There are other diverse gastrointestinal manifestations

of SLE. Pancreatitis has been documented,[2,8] and may be due to vasculitis, steroids, or azathioprine. A significant incidence of gastrointestinal hemorrhage may be due to vasculitis, but more commonly is due to drugs such as aspirin or other nonsteroidal anti-inflammatory agents. Coagulopathies, uremia, and stress can all lead to gastrointestinal bleeding. Abnormal esophageal motility and, more rarely, protein-losing enteropathy[9] and malabsorption[10,11] can result from chronic intestinal ischemia. Pneumatosis cystoides intestinalis,[12,13] ileus,[14] and intussusception[15] have also been reported.

Liver enlargement occurs in about 30% of patients. Liver enzyme abnormalities may be due to aspirin.[16,17] Chronic active hepatitis and hepatic vasculitis have also been reported.[18,19]

Besides abdominal symptoms secondary to ischemia, patients may have many of the other manifestations of SLE. The presence of vasculitic skin lesions can be important in increasing the physician's suspicion that the abdominal symptoms may be due to vasculitis. If the diagnosis of lupus has not been made previously, a butterfly rash is an immensely important finding.

Diagnosis

Gastrointestinal roentgenograms are similar to those of patients with intestinal ischemia from other causes. Arteriography has been generally unrewarding, but there are reports of angiographically confirmed mesenteric arteritis[20] demonstrating diffuse irregularities in small mesenteric arteries and localizing the site of bleeding in a patient with arteritis and ileal and colonic ulcers. However, because of the small size of the vessels involved, significant changes on arteriography are uncommon.

If peritoneal fluid is present, it should be aspirated. Lupus peritonitis may produce a sterile effusion. Bowel necrosis secondary to intestinal ischemia may lead to perforation and infectious peritonitis. Paracentesis will help to evaluate the need for surgical intervention, although a walled-off perforation might be missed. Spontaneous bacterial peritonitis has also been reported in systemic lupus.

Laboratory Procedures

The laboratory is helpful in confirming a diagnosis of lupus. Antinuclear antibodies (ANA) are present in almost all patients; probably less than 1–2% will have negative results. There are various patterns of antinuclear antibodies, including speckled, rim, and diffuse, but no pattern is entirely specific for lupus, and it must be remembered that the ANA is positive in a certain percent of normal people and in such diseases as chronic active hepatitis, infections, or other connective tissue diseases.

Nonspecific findings may include thrombocytopenia, leukopenia, anemia, or an elevated sedimentation rate. Thrombocytosis can be seen as a reflection of any chronic inflammatory disorder. Other abnormalities include a positive Coombs test, VDRL, abnormal urine sediment, elevated BUN and creatinine, or abnormalities in prothrombin time or partial thromboplastin time. This is significant in that approximately 15% of SLE patients have a circulating anticoagulant which, depending on the specific type, may or may not lead to bleeding abnormalities during operation. In addition, even if platelet counts are normal, a bleeding time should always be determined on lupus patients prior to operation because they may have abnormalities of platelet function.

More specific tests include complement levels, which are often low in active SLE, and antibodies to double-stranded DNA, which are present in the majority of patients and are very specific for SLE. Cryoglobulins should always be checked, as these can be implicated in vasculitis. In a known Lupus patient, disease activity often, but not always, correlates with a high sedimentation rate and low complement levels.

Management

The mesenteric vasculitis of lupus seems almost always to occur in the setting of active SLE. Acute abdominal symptoms in SLE patients in remission should alert the physician to the more likely possibility of an unrelated abdominal condition, thereby averting the unnecessary delay of a therapeutic trial of steroids. In patients with active SLE, abdominal pain is much more likely to be secondary to lupus, and intestinal ischemia due to lupus vasculitis is a prime consideration. Rebound and localized direct tenderness are extremely worrisome, but do not always imply perforation of ischemic bowel.[4] It is therefore often very difficult to determine whether surgical intervention is needed.

However, patients with SLE and symptoms of an acute abdominal event suggesting a perforated or infarcted bowel treated by early surgical intervention have had much better survival than medically treated patients.[3,4] Although these patients may have an ongoing multisystem disease and not be optimal candidates for operation, the results indicate that an aggressive approach is more successful, once infarction or perforation is suspected on the clinical findings of rebound and localized tenderness. Obviously, at times in retrospect, surgery may not have been needed, but failure to perform surgery when needed is the more serious error.

In early stages of vasculitis, before severe damage occurs to the intestine, medical management may be adequate if it can control and prevent the progression of the inflammatory process. This would consist of high-dose steroids, preferably parenterally to ensure absorption. Many would favor the addition of an immunosuppressive agent, such as cyclophosphamide.

Rheumatoid Arthritis

Rheumatoid arthritis (RA) is the most common of the connective tissue diseases, affecting 2–3% of the population. It is principally a disease of the synovium with an intense lymphocytic synovitis as the primary abnormality. The synovial lining becomes hypertrophied and edematous, with proliferation of blood vessels, fibroblasts, and chronic inflammatory cells. This causes secondary destruction of cartilage, tendons, and periarticular structures. Subcutaneous nodules occur in one-fourth of patients with RA, especially those with more severe disease.

Vascular involvement is not uncommon in rheumatoid arthritis. Small end-artery occlusive lesions lead to ischemic changes of nail beds. A diffuse small vessel vasculitis similar to hypersensitivity vasculitis or a vasculitis resembling periarteritis nodosa is well documented.[21] (See Figures 2 and 3.)

Clinical Manifestations

The male-to-female ratio is 2.5:1, and the peak age of onset is between 20 and 60 years of age. Systemic symptoms such as fever, weight loss, anorexia, and fatigue are very common with active rheumatoid disease. Joint involvement is symmetrical, with synovitis of the small joints of the hands, wrists, knees, elbows, ankles, shoulders, and hips most commonly seen.

Morning stiffness, at times lasting 2–3 hours, is a classic symptom. However, RA is not manifested in the joints alone. Among the many extraarticular manifestations are Felty's syndrome, Sjögren's syndrome, pleuritis, pleural effusions, interstitial lung disease, pulmonary nodules, peri-

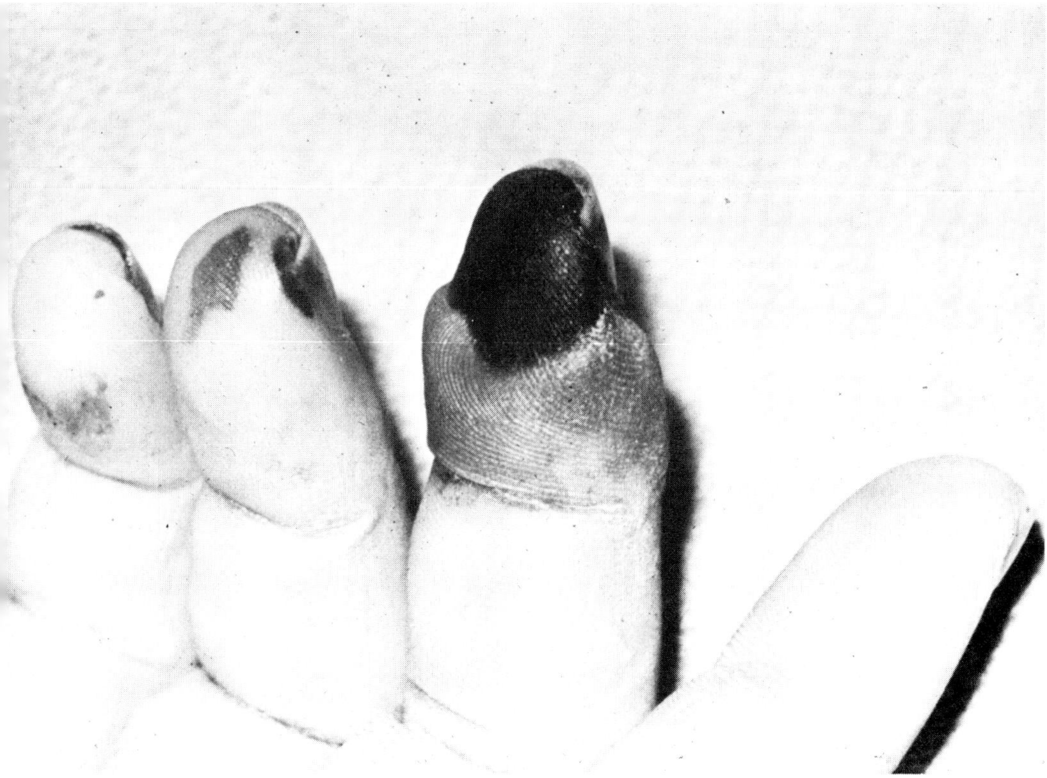

Figure 2. Rheumatoid vasculitis with lesions of several fingers and gangrene of the tip of the middle finger. (From the Clinical Slice Collection on the Rheumatic Diseases, copyright 1972. Used by permission of the Arthritis Foundation.)

carditis, myocarditis, cardiac conduction abnormalities, lymphadenopathy, myopathy, scleritis or scleromalacia, peripheral neuropathies, and entrapment neuropathies.[22]

Diagnosis

Diagnosis of RA rests on the typical joint abnormalities, including synovial hypertrophy, warmth, tenderness, and the appropriate distribution of involvement. In severe

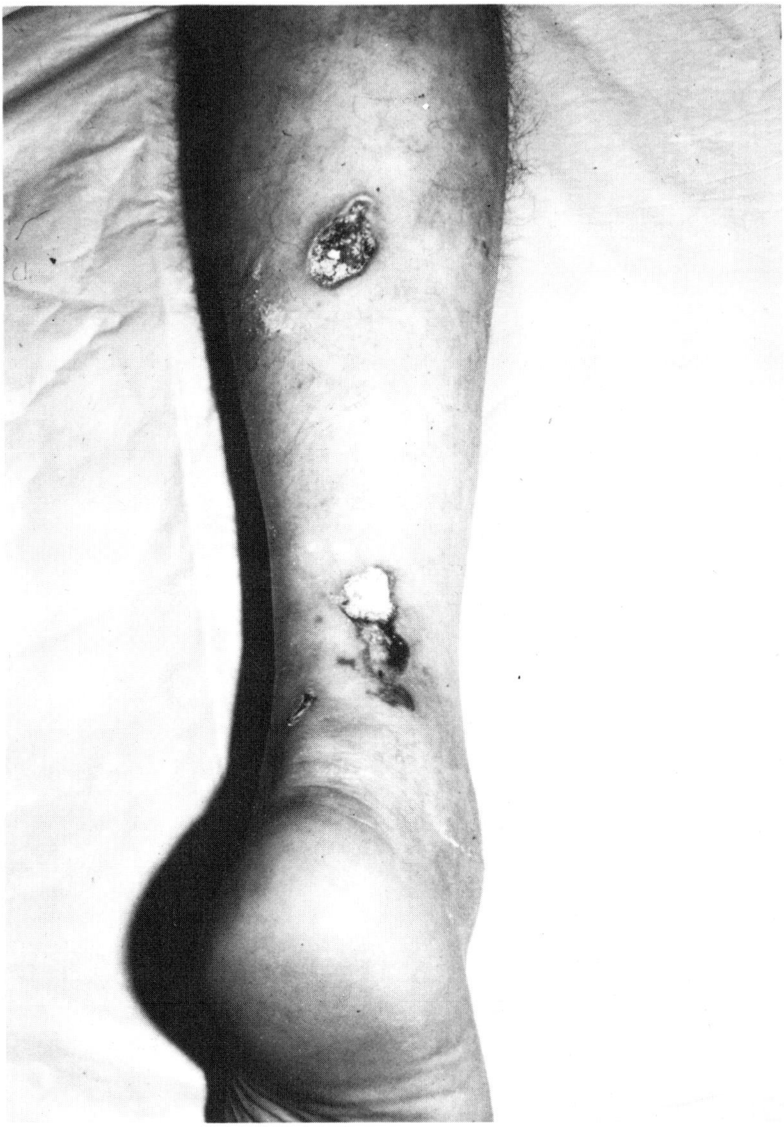

Figure 3. Ulcerative lesions of the leg in a man with rheumatoid vasculitis. He also had mononeuritis multiplex with bilateral foot drop.

cases, ulnar deviation or significant X-ray changes are present. Nodules occur in 25% of cases, and rheumatoid factors in 80%. Presence of the rheumatoid factor is not specific for RA, however, as other diseases such as systemic lupus erythematosus, endocarditis, or essential cryoglobulinemia can be associated with significant rheumatoid factor titers. The history and physical examination can be relied upon to establish the diagnosis.

Gastrointestinal Manifestations

Intestinal ischemia due to vasculitis is a well known complication of RA. Rheumatoid vasculitis is characterized by polyneuropathy, skin infarctions and ulcerations, digital gangrene, and internal organ system changes, especially arteritis of the gastrointestinal tract. Rheumatoid vasculitis occurs in less than 1–2% of all rheumatoid arthritis patients, although in one review,[23] perforation of the gastrointestinal tract occurred in seven of 71 cases with vasculitis. Another recent series of 50 cases of RA vasculitis revealed gastrointestinal involvement in five.[24]

Diagnosis of Gastrointestinal Manifestations

Rheumatoid vasculitis is suspected when skin ulcers, foot or wrist drop, peripheral neuropathy, digital infarcts, or other evidence of vasculitis appears. It may be confirmed by skin, sural nerve, or muscle biopsy. A recent review[24] suggests that rectal biopsy is helpful in diagnosis, although this needs confirmation. Angiography is occasionally helpful in establishing the presence of vasculitis, showing irregularity, narrowing, or blockage of vessels. Contrary to the findings in polyarteritis nodosa, the renal vessels are rarely involved in RA, and aneurysms at the bifurcation of vessels are not seen. Although medium sized arteries can be involved in rheumatoid vasculitis, smaller vessel involvement is more likely. Thus, angiography may not be as helpful as it is in polyarteritis nodosa. Data on angiography in rheumatoid vasculitis are sparse.

Barium studies may show thumbprinting or mucosal abnormalities with intestinal vasculitis. Free air may be present in the peritoneal cavity if bowel perforation has occurred.

The complement levels are usually depressed as a manifestation of immune complex disease with complement consumption. Circulating immune complexes are detected by various methods.[25] Immunofluorescence of skin biopsy specimens from lesions will usually show immunoglobulin deposits in the vessel wall.

Management

Therapy for rheumatoid vasculitis depends on the rapidity of progression of the disease and the areas involved. For bland digital vasculitis without severe organ system involvement, slow acting drugs to control the underlying rheumatoid arthritis, such as gold or D-penicillamine, are appropriate.[26–28] Over 70% of patients respond within 3–6 months. As the rheumatoid synovitis is controlled, the extraarticular manifestations usually regress.

However, in subacute or acute progression of vasculitis, especially when critical areas such as mesenteric vessels or peripheral nerves are involved, more aggressive therapy is appropriate. High daily divided-dose steroid therapy, such as prednisone 15 mg p.o. q.i.d., should be started immediately. Most rheumatologists would favor the addition of an immunosuppressive agent, either azathioprine or cyclophosphamide. In a recent series of five patients, cyclophosphamide proved very effective.[25]

As the disease is controlled, dosage of prednisone and cytoxan can be gradually tapered. If bowel infarction or perforation has occurred, emergency surgical intervention is necessary. Steroids or immunosuppressives may alter the abdominal findings in bowel infarction or perforation and mask the diagnosis, resulting in delayed treatment.

Polymyositis and Dermatomyositis

Polymyositis is an inflammatory myopathy of unknown cause, sometimes associated with vasculitis involving the gastrointestinal tract. When a characteristic skin rash is present, the term dermatomyositis is used.

Clinical Manifestations

The onset of illness is most common between the ages of 30 to 60 years, with a 2:1 female-to-male ratio. The myopathy of polymyositis is typically a painless proximal muscle weakness, usually symmetrical, with subacute or chronic onset over several weeks or months. Rarely, onset may be acute, with severe muscle pain and rapid onset of weakness. Proximal muscles of the hips and shoulders are most commonly involved, but distal muscles can be affected in severe cases. Laryngeal, pharyngeal, and respiratory muscles can also weaken, but it is unusual for ocular muscles to be affected.[29,30]

The term dermatomyositis is used when a typical rash is present. Swelling and a lilac discoloration of the eyelids called a heliotrope rash may be evident, or a dusky, erythematous eruption on the face, forehead, neck, chest, or shoulders can be present. Erythematous flat papules may occur over the metacarpophalangeal and interphalangeal joints, and this is referred to as Gottron's sign. Subcutaneous calcification frequently occurs in children, but is less common in adults. This may lead to flexion contractures about joints. Studies have shown an 8–10% incidence of malignancy in patients with dermatomyositis and polymositis, especially in those over 40 to 45 years of age.[30,31]

Visceral involvement occasionally occurs. Cardiopulmonary manifestations include nonspecific changes in the electrocardiogram, arrhythmias, conduction problems, or cardiomyopathy with heart failure secondary to cardiac muscle inflammation.[30] Interstitial pneumonitis has also been described in less than 1–2% of patients.[32] Approximately 10–20% of patients will have other associated connective tissue diseases, such as lupus.

Gastrointestinal Manifestations

Abdominal pain is more common in childhood disease than in adult onset disease. In six of eight children in one autopsy series, abdominal pain was associated with hematemesis and melena, leading to death.[33] Postmortem examination revealed multiple ulcerations and perforations of the gastrointestinal tract in seven, with intimal proliferation of small blood vessels, thrombosis, and multiple infarctions. These changes involved submucosal, muscularis, and serosal layers. Perforation of one or more viscus occurred in all seven patients with vascular lesions of the gastrointestinal tract.

Subsequent reports confirmed that vasculitis does occur in children, but the incidence appears lower than that in the cited series. Systemic vasculitis also occurs in adult onset disease, and has been reported in four of 142 adults, one of whom died from necrotizing vasculitis of the gastrointestinal tract with intestinal perforation.[30] Others have reported abnormal motility in the esophagus, stomach, or proximal small bowel resembling scleroderma.

Laboratory Findings

Muscle enzymes (CPK, SGOT, SGPT, adolase, and LDH) are elevated in 98% of patients at some time during their illness. The sedimentation rate does not correlate with disease activity. A small percentage of patients will have a positive ANA, rheumatoid factor, or evidence of another connective tissue disease. Cell-mediated cytotoxicity occurs to muscle, but antibody-induced damage does not appear to be a significant factor.

Management

Steroids are the therapy of choice in polymyositis or dermatomyositis, with prednisone given in an initial dosage of 40–60 mg a day. This dose is gradually tapered as the patient responds. Response is determined primarily by an increase in muscle strength. A low maintenance dose is usually needed for a year or more. Immunosuppressives such as azathioprine, cyclophosphamide, or methotrexate are used in patients who fail to respond to steroids within 2–3 months.[29] In rapidly progressive disease, especially when respiratory muscle involvement is significant, steroids and immunosuppressives can be used together initially to ensure an adequate response. In the presence of vasculitis, the use of high-dose prednisone and an immunosuppressive agent is recommended.

Scleroderma

Scleroderma, or progressive systemic sclerosis, is a disorder of skin and certain internal organs, such as the esophagus, intestinal tract, kidney, and cardiopulmonary system. The disease is characterized by inflammation, fibrosis, and degeneration of involved organs and is associated with specific vascular lesions, especially intimal hyperplasia.

Vascular abnormalities are found in all organ systems involved, but clinical intestinal ischemia is extremely rare. Dilatation of the bowel due to sclerodermatous involvement may predispose to volvulus of the colon and intestinal ischemia.[34,35] Small intestinal volvulus has also been reported.[36] Severe vascular disease due to intimal proliferation has been reported as the cause of infarction of the descending colon.[37] However, the major gastrointestinal involvement is related to motility disorders, primarily of the esophagus.

Sjögren's Syndrome

Sjögren's syndrome is a chronic inflammatory disorder of the exocrine glands, especially the lacrimal and salivary glands, with the major manifestations of dry eyes and dry mouth. The spectrum of the disease includes a primary form, a form associated with a connective tissue disease, especially rheumatoid arthritis, and an aggressive form marked by lymphocytic infiltration of vital organs, pseudolymphoma or actual lymphoma.

The pathologic feature is a lymphocytic and plasma cell infiltrate of exocrine glands resulting in glandular atrophy and insufficiency. Extraglandular involvement of internal organs may occur.

Most major reviews do not mention intestinal ischemia. However, vasculitis is a documented, but rare, complication,[38,39] and vascular lesions similar to those of PAN have been reported to involve the small and large intestine in Sjögren's.[40]

Mixed Connective Tissue Disease

Mixed connective tissue disease (MCTD) presents overlapping features of lupus, scleroderma, and polymyositis, with apparently distinct serologic markers.[41–43] Reports of gastrointestinal involvement are rare, although involvement resembling that in lupus or polymyositis has been reported.[44]

References

1. Hoffman BI, Katz WA: The gastrointestinal manifestations of systemic lupus erythematosus: A review of the literature. *Sem Arthritis Rheum* 9:239, 1980.
2. Pollak VE, Grove WJ, Kark RM et al: Systemic lupus simulating acute surgical condition of the abdomen. *N Engl J Med* 259:258, 1958.
3. Rothfield N: Clinical features of systemic lupus erythematosus. In *Textbook of Rheumatology.* Kelly WN, (Ed.). WB Saunders, Philadelphia 1981. pp 1106–1132.
4. Zizic TM, Shulman LE, Stevens MB: Colonic perforations in systemic lupus erythematosus. *Medicine* 54:411, 1975.
5. Carlsen E, Hudson JP: Surgical implications of and splenectomy for collagen disease. *Arch Surg* 74:381, 1957.
6. Ropes MW: *Systemic Lupus Erythematosus.* Harvard Univ Press, Cambridge, 1976. pp 40–41.
7. Dubois EL (Ed): *Lupus Erythematosus: A Review of the Current Status of Discoid and Systemic Lupus Erythematosus and their Variants.* Univ South Calif Press, Los Angeles 1974. p 284.
8. Dubois EL (Ed): *Lupus Erythematosus: A Review of the Current Status of Discoid and Systemic Lupus Erythematosus and their Variants.* Univ South Calif Press, Los Angeles 1974. p 332.
9. Trencham PE, Masl AT: Systemic lupus erythematosus with protein losing enteropathy. *JAMA* 236:287, 1976.
10. Siurala M, Tulkunen H, Toivonen S: Digestive tract in collagen diseases. *Acta Med Scand* 178:13, 1965.
11. Bazinet P, Marin GA: Malabsorption of systemic lupus erythematosus. *Am J Dig Dis* 16:460, 1971.
12. Kleinman P, Moyers MA, Abbott G, et al: Necrotizing enterocolitis with pneumatosis intestinalis in SLE and polyarteritis. *Radiology* 121:595, 1976.
13. Morrison WJ, Siegelman SS: Pneumatosis Intestinalis in association with connective tissue disease. *South Med J* 69:1536, 1976.
14. Brown CH, Shirey EK, Masserick JR: Gastrointestinal manifestations of systemic lupus erythematosus. *Gastroenterology* 31:649, 1956.

15. Herman G: Intussusception secondary to mesenteric arteritis: Complication of systemic lupus erythematosus in a 5-year-old child. *JAMA* 200:74, 1967.
16. Seamon WE, Plotz PM: Effects of aspirin on liver tests in patients with RA or SLE and in normal volunteers. *Arthritis Rheum* 19:155, 1976.
17. Goldenberg DL: Aspirin hepatotoxicity. *Ann Intern Med* 80:733, 1974.
18. Harvey AM, Sholman LE, Tomathy PA, et al: Systemic lupus erythematosus. *Medicine* 33:291, 1954.
19. Dubois EL (Ed): *Lupus Erythematosus: A Review of the Current Status of Discoid and Systemic Lupus Erythematosus and their Variants*. 2nd Ed. Univ South Calif Press, Los Angeles 1974. p 344.
20. Phillips JC, Howland W: Mesenteric arteritis in systemic lupus erythematosus. *JAMA* 206:1569, 1968.
21. Sokoloff L: Pathology of rheumatoid arthritis and allied disorders. In *Arthritis and Allied Conditions*. 9th ed. McCarty DJ Jr (Ed.). Lea & Febiger, Philadelphia 1979. p 429–448.
22. Turner R. Collins R, Nomeir AM: Extraarticular manifestations of rheumatoid arthritis. *Bull Rheum Dis* 29:986, 1978.
23. Schmid FR, Cooper NS, Ziff M, McEwen C: Arteritis in rheumatoid arthritis. *Am J Med* 44:56, 1961.
24. Scott DGI, Bacon PA, Tribe CR: Systemic rheumatoid vasculitis: A clinical and laboratory study of 50 cases. *Medicine* 60:288, 1981.
25. Abel T, Andrews BS, Cunningham PH, Brunner CM, et al: Rheumatoid vasculitis: Effect of cyclophosphamide on the clinical course and levels of circulating immune complexes. *Ann Intern Med* 93:407, 1980.
26. Pearson CM, Dick WC (Eds): Current Management of Rheumatoid Arthritis. *Clin Rheum Dis* 1:215, 1975.
27. Lightfoot RW: Treatment of rheumatoid arthritis. In *Arthritis and Allied Conditions*. 9th Ed. McCarty DJ Jr (Ed.). Lea & Febiger, Philadelphia 1979. p 513–518.
28. Jaffe IA: Rheumatoid arthritis with arteritis. Report of a case treated with penicillamine. *Ann Intern Med* 61:556, 1964.
29. Bohan A, Peter JB: Polymyositis and dermatomyositis. *N Engl J Med* 292:344, 1975.

30. Bohan A, Peter JB, Bowman R, Pearson CM: A computer-assisted analysis of 153 patients with polymyositis and dermatomyositis. *Medicine* 56:255, 1976.
31. Barnes BE: Dermatomyositis and malignancy. A review of the literature. *Ann Intern Med* 84:68, 1976.
32. Duncan PE, Griffin JP, Garcia A, Kaplan SB: Fibrosing alveolitis in polymyositis. *Am J Med* 57:621, 1974.
33. Banker BQ, Victor M: Dermatomyositis (systemic angiopathy) of childhood. *Medicine* 45:261, 1966.
34. Fraback RC, Kadell BN, Nies KM, et al: Sigmoid volvulus in two patients with systemic sclerosis. *J Rheumatol* 5:195, 1978.
35. Budd DC, Nidlinger EL, Sturtz DL, Fouty WJ: Transverse colon volvulus associated with scleroderma. *Am J Surg* 133:370, 1977.
36. Alpert LI, Pichel Warner RR: Systemic sclerosis: Case presenting with tetracycline responsive malabsorption syndrome. *Am J Med* 45:468, 1968.
37. Edwards DH, Lennard-Jones JE: Diffuse systemic sclerosis presenting as infarction of the colon. *Proc Royal Soc Med* 53:877, 1960.
38. Moutsopoulos HM (Moderator): Sjogren's syndrome (Sicca syndrome): Current issues. *Ann Int Med* 92 (Part 1):212, 1980.
39. Shearn MA: *Sjogren's Syndrome.* WB Saunders, Philadelphia 1971. pp 122–124.
40. Cardell BS, Gurling KJ: Observations on the pathology of Sjogren's syndrome. *J Path Bact* 68:137, 1954.
41. Sharp GC, Finn WS, Jan EM: Mixed connective tissue disease. An apparently distinct rheumatic disease syndrome associated with a specific antibody to an extractable nuclear antigen (ENA). *Am J Med* 52:148, 1972.
42. Sharp GC: Mixed connective tissue disease. *Bull Rheumatic Dis* 25:828, 1974.
43. Sharp GC: Mixed connective tissue disease. In *Arthritis and Allied Conditions.* McCarty DJ Jr (Ed.). Lea & Febiger, Philadelphia 1979. pp 737–741.
44. Norman DA, Fleishman NM: Gastrointestinal systemic sclerosis in serologic mixed connective tissue disease. *Arthritis Rheum* 21:811, 1978.

Index